SURGERY - PROCEDURES, COMPLICATIONS, AND RESULTS

LAPAROSCOPY

PROCEDURES, PAIN MANAGEMENT AND POSTOPERATIVE COMPLICATIONS

SURGERY - PROCEDURES, COMPLICATIONS, AND RESULTS

Additional books in this series can be found on Nova's website under the Series tab.

Additional e-books in this series can be found on Nova's website under the e-book tab.

SURGERY - PROCEDURES, COMPLICATIONS, AND RESULTS

LAPAROSCOPY

PROCEDURES, PAIN MANAGEMENT AND POSTOPERATIVE COMPLICATIONS

CHRISTOS IAVAZZO, M.D., PH.D.
EDITOR

New York

For permission to use material from this book please contact us:
Telephone 631-231-7269; Fax 631-231-8175
Web Site: http://www.novapublishers.com

Library of Congress Cataloging-in-Publication Data

ISBN: 978-1-63321-404-0

Library of Congress Control Number: 2014943359

Published by Nova Science Publishers, Inc. † New York

Contents

Preface

This book entitled "Laparoscopy: Procedures, Pain Management and Postoperative Complications" serves to provide a comprehensive, evidence based and updated review of the role of laparoscopy in different surgical specialties. Laparoscopic surgery has changed the way that many surgical conditions are managed. For this reason, techniques, benefits, risks and possible complications, as well as their management are discussed in this book. It starts with the presentation of access techniques for laparoscopic surgery. The role of laparoscopy in spleenectomy and hepatectomy are presented while the applications in colorectal, urological, gynaecological and paediatric operations are also discussed. The book concludes with the presentation of the different complications of laparoscopy and their management.

Written by international experts, this book is a valuable resource for a broad spectrum of clinicians, healthcare professionals and students. This book also includes a good number of tables and images which make it informative and educational. We believe that the information contained in this book will enhance the skills of the surgeon in order to offer excellent preoperative, intraoperative and postoperative care.

Christos Iavazzo, M.D., M.Sc., Ph.D.
Gynaecological Oncology Department,
Christie Hospital, Manchester, United Kingdom
E-mail: christosiavazzo@hotmail.com

In: Laparoscopy
Editor: Christos Iavazzo

ISBN: 978-1-63321-404-0

Chapter 1

Access Techniques for Laparoscopic Surgery

S. M. M. de Castro, M.D., Ph.D.**, *U. K. Coblijn, M.D., W. F. van Tets, M.D., Ph.D. and B. A. van Wagensveld, M.D., Ph.D.

Sint Lucas Andreas Hospital,
Amsterdam, The Netherlands

Abstract

Laparoscopic surgery has revolutionized the field of abdominal surgery. The benefits of this minimal invasive technique include improved visualization of the operative field with magnification, decreased postoperative pain, earlier return to work and normal daily activities, and less postoperative complications such as wound infections, incisional hernia and less adhesion formation compared with open techniques. One major difference with open surgery is the manner of obtaining access to the abdomen. Access techniques can be divided into closed and open introduction. With closed introduction, a device (e.g. Veress needle or a sharp or blunt tipped trocar) is introduced though all layers of the abdominal wall without opening it beforehand. With open introduction, the abdominal cavity is opened under direct sight before the trocar is inserted. The complications that can occur while gaining access to the abdomen are unique for laparoscopic surgery. The most feared complications include bowel injury or major vascular injury. Fortunately these potentially life-threatening complications are uncommon. The techniques for access to the abdominal cavity will be reviewed here.

* Jan Tooropstraat 164, 1061 AE; Number +31 20 510891; E-mail: stevedecastro@me.com.

Introduction

Laparoscopy (Gr *Laparo*-abdomen, *scopie*-to examine) is the art of examining the abdominal cavity and its contents. It requires the insertion of a cannula through the abdominal wall and into the abdominal cavity in order to visualize and examine the abdomen and its contents. Laparoscopy in abdominal surgery is increasing in popularity throughout the world. Laparoscopic surgery was first pioneered in the early 20th century. In 1902 Georg Kelling performed the first laparoscopic procedure in dogs in Germany. In 1910 Hans Christian Jacobaeus reported the first laparoscopic operation in humans in Sweden. He used rigid cystoscopic instruments to perform diagnostic procedures in the abdomen. In 1911 he published an article titled "Über die möglichkeit die zystoskopie bei untersuchung seröser höhlungen anzuwenden" (The possibilities for performing cystoscopy in examinations of serous cavities) in the journal Münchner Medizinischen Wochenschrift. The technique was adopted and refined the following decades but was only performed by a selected number of physicians for diagnostic purposes.

The introduction of the microprocessor and advancements in the camera was a major step forward for laparoscopy. This made it possible to perform more complex procedures. In 1972, Clarke published and recorded a gynaecological laparoscopic procedure. In 1975, Tarasconi, from the Department of obstetrics and gynaecology of the University of Passo Fundo Medical School, Brazil, started his experience with laparoscopic salpingectomy. This was first reported in the Third AAGL Meeting, Hyatt Regency Atlanta, November 1976 and later published in The Journal of Reproductive Medicine in 1981 [1]. In the 1980's the first solid state camera was introduced. It was now possible to magnify the image and project it on a screen.

In 1981, Semm, from the Universitats Frauenklinik, Kiel, Germany, performed the first laparoscopic appendectomy. Following his lecture on laparoscopic appendectomy, the President of the German surgical society wrote to the board of directors of the German gynecological society suggesting suspension of Semm from medical practice. Subsequently, Semm submitted a paper on laparoscopic appendectomy to the American journal of obstetrics and gynecology, which was rejected and considered unacceptable for publication because the technique was considered not ethical. His paper was eventually published in the Journal of Endoscopy. Nowadays, the laparoscopic appendectomy is one of the most performed abdominal laparoscopic procedures.

Complications can occur when gaining access to the abdominal cavity during laparoscopic surgery. The closed technique with the Veress needle or open technique are the two principal techniques used to gain access to the abdominal cavity. Secondary trocar insertion can also result in complications.

Complications can be divided into vascular and visceral injuries. Vascular lesions can occur when epigastric vessels in the anterior abdominal wall are injured or the great vessels in the back of the abdominal cavity are damaged. Visceral lesions can occur in any organ but in particular in the colon, usually when adhered to the anterior abdominal wall.

In a review article in the Netherlands in 1994, 145 perioperative complications were recorded on a total of 25764 laparoscopies (5.7 per 1000) of which 83 (57%) during trocar insertion and the remaining 62 (43%) during the course of the operation [2]. In this study, 0.3

per 1000 injuries were caused by the Veress needle, 1.9 per 1000 by the primary trocar and 0.8 per 1000 by the secondary trocar. These figures are probably underestimated.

Risk Factors for complications associated with trocar introduction include previous abdominal surgery (in particular, the median abdominal incision), peritoneal infections and large intra-abdominal tumours.

To minimize introduction related injuries, several techniques, instruments, and approaches have been introduced during the last century. These include the Veress needle or closed entry [3], the open (Hasson) entry technique [4], direct trocar insertion without prior pneumoperitoneum [5,6], use of shielded disposable trocars [7], optical Veress needle, [8] optical trocars [9] and radially expanding trocars [10] Each of these methods of entry enjoys a certain degree of popularity according to the surgeon's training, experience, and bias, and according to regional and interdisciplinary variability. The present chapter will discuss the most accepted access techniques used in laparoscopic surgery and provide best evidence.

Standard Procedure

Preoperative Measures

It is recommended to have conventional instruments available in the case of an emergency conversion to laparotomy is needed for serious vascular injury. To reduce bladder lesions when inserting trocars suprapubically the patient should be encouraged to urinate or be catheterized (preferably one time) before the procedure. The same hold true for the stomach in case of upper abdominal trocar or Verres needle insertion. In the latter case, a gastric tube could be inserted to deflate the stomach and reduce possible injuries since the stomach can be significantly inflated during induction of general anaesthesia.

The anatomy of the patient deserves attention. Patient weight and abdominal circumference have enormous effect on the position of the umbilicus, in most cases the preferred site for introduction of the first trocar. The umbilical site will be relatively low when performing a laparoscopic appendectomy in a morbidly obese patient. On the other hand, a laparoscopic cholecystectomy in a morbidly obese patient via the umbilicus will result in an enormous distance between gallbladder and camera. The superior anterior iliac spine is a useful landmark when the umbilicus has migrated caudally due to obesity.

Trocar Design

Trocars can be divided into cutting and non-cutting. A cutting trocar has sharp blades at the tip of the obturator. The trocar goes through tissues cutting a small hole around it. Cutting trocars can be made of metal with a pyramidal or conical shape or of plastic with an integrated knife. A non-cutting trocar has a blunt tip and expands the tissue radially, so that the surrounding tissue is damaged less. Another distinction can be made between disposable and reusable trocars.

Disposable trocars have the advantage they need not to be cleaned and in case of bladed trocars always have a sharp knife and contain no magnetic parts. They are, however, considerably more expensive compared to disposable trocars [11,12]. Nowadays, all disposable trocars have a threaded or rough surface around the shaft, in such a way that they are better fixed in the skin. Then there are the shielded cutting trocars. These trocars have a covering shield, which shoots as a screen over the knife after the peritoneum has been passed. The intended benefit is that there is no injury to visceral organs during entry, but this advantage is not yet proven. [13] Reusable trocars are usually made of metal. It is important to realize that during insertion of a disposable trocar less cutting power is needed than with a reusable trocar, because the point is not subject to wear. Figure 1 shows an example of a commonly used trocar.

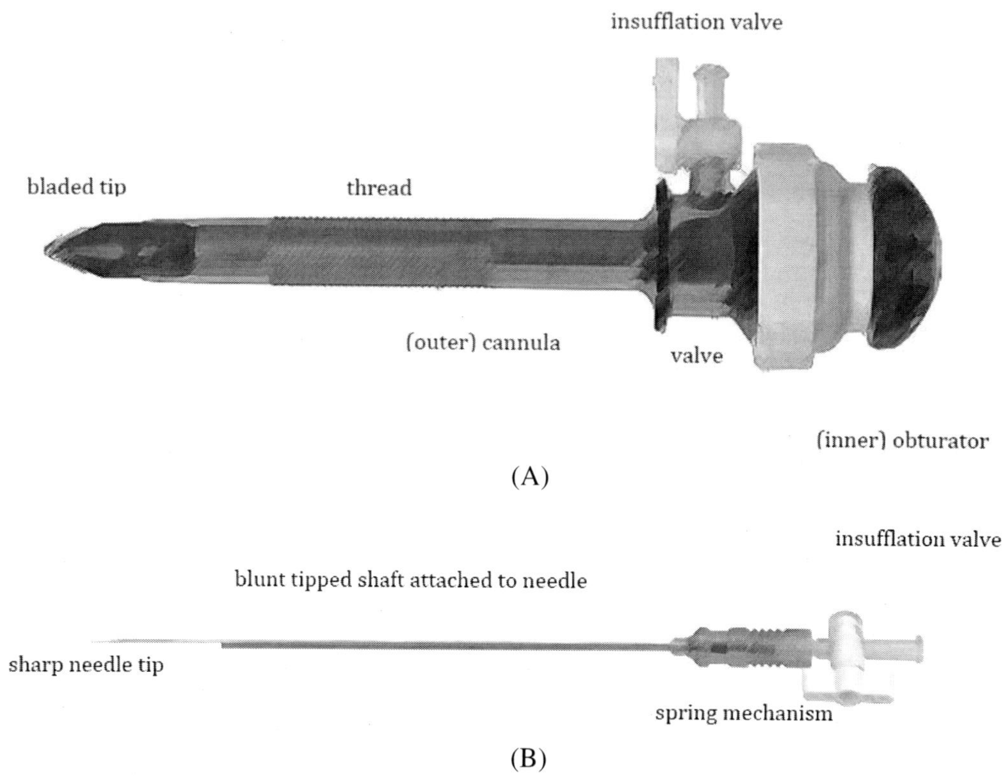

Figure 1. (A) Basic design of a Trocar. (B) Basic design of a Veress Needle.

Closed Entry (Classic) Laparoscopy

The classic or closed entry laparoscopic technique requires cutting of the abdominal skin with a scalpel, insufflation of gas (generally CO^2) into the abdomen and insertion of a penetrating trocar system into the abdomen. Following removal of the obturator from the cannula, an illuminated telescope through the cannula examines the abdominal cavity. The Veress needle is the most popular tool to achieve a pneumoperitoneum. The n spring loaded needle shoots back over the sharp tip once the pressure is gone (e.g. when entering the abdominal cavity) Most gynaecologists practising laparoscopy worldwide use the Veress needle to obtain pneumoperitoneum and subsequently insert the trocar to access the abdomen [14]

Before the insertion of the Veress needle, the needle has to be checked by the surgeon. Does the inner and outer shaft fit well together? Is the opening for the insufflation of gas free of any obstruction? Patency should be tested for insertion by means of insufflation or rinse with saline. Is the spring functioning correctly? Does the sharp stylet shoot back after the pressure is withdrawn?

Firstly a small incision is made in the skin where the Veress needle will be inserted. Two popular sites for Veress needle insertion include Palmer's point and sub umbilical. Palmer's point is located in the left upper abdomen, mid clavicular and 3cm subcostal. [3] When using this site it is advisable to deflate the stomach with a nasogastric tube to prevent injury. When inserting at the umbilical site, the abdominal wall is lifted, preferably by hand, and the Veress needle is inserted perpendicularly between the plane of the operating table and 45 degrees, until the fascia is passed. The needle carrying hand rests on the abdominal wall in order to promote controlled entrance. Fixation of the abdominal wall near the umbilicus is done by lifting the skin around the umbilicus by hand or clamp. This maneuvre creates as much distance as possible between fascia and great vessels. A Cochran review based on 1 RCT with inadequate statistical power concluded that lifting of the abdominal wall did not prevent serious complications. [15] However, there were significantly more failed entrances seen when the abdominal wall was lifted. Theoretically, not fixing the abdominal wall could result in compression of the abdomen during insertion reducing the distance between the abdominal wall and retroperitoneal structures and increasing the risk of injury. While passing the fascia of the anterior rectus sheath and then the parietal peritoneum, the stylet will shoot back as a 'click ' when the intra-abdominal cavity has been reached. The advantage of Palmer's point is that when introducing the Verres needle either ometum or stomach can be potentially lacerated. In contrast when introducing via the umbilicus there is a chance of puncturing the more fragile small bowel.

There are several tests including the double click test, the hanging drop test, the aspiration test, and the initial five pressures at the time of insufflation test to allow one to check whether the end of the Veress needle is located free in the peritoneal cavity, and is not occluded with omentum or inserted into an organ. There is no scientific evidence that these tests are 100% accurate.

In a recent study, the different tests were evaluated and it was concluded that a low initial intra-abdominal pressure (<10 mm Hg) at the start of insufflation, followed by a free flow of CO^2, is probably the most valuable [16]. The trocar is introduced when the pneumoperitoneum has been established. An incision is made under or above the umbilicus depending on the abdominal circumference. The trocar is the introduced perpendicular to the fascia. During introduction the abdominal wall is fixated with one hand. In many modern trocars it is possible to perform this step under direct vision with the camera in the shaft. The abdominal wall can also be splinted using temporary hyperdistension (abdominal pressure of 20-25 mmHg). This makes introduction considerably easier since the abdominal wall is more rigid and doesn't give way. [17]

Open Laparoscopic Entry or Hasson Technique

The Hasson trocar system was initially developed for laparoscopy in patients who have had a previous laparotomy [18,19] Hasson first described this open entry technique in 1971. After seeing benefit of this open access technique many surgeons started performing this technique routinely in all patients. The reported benefits include prevention of gas embolism, reduction of preperitoneal insufflation, and prevention of possibly visceral and major vascular injury. Generally, an open introduction is performed by making a transverse incision in the sub umbilical region using the skin lines. Take care not to make the incision too small or too large. Too small will result in damage to the skin and too large will result in diminished grip and accidental removal of the trocar when removing instruments. The upper skin flap is retracted with surgical tweezers. The lower flap is retracted using a small right angled retractor (e.g. Langenbeck). Subcutaneous tissue is dissected till the linea alba and the rectus sheath is visualized using the umbilical ligament as a guide. The umbilical insertion is located and dissected free from the surrounding tissue. Subsequently the umbilical insertion is grasped with a Kocher or a towel clamp and elevated creating a mountain like elevation of the rectus. The umbilicus is incised transversely or longitudinally at the junction with the rectus (linea alba).

The incision should not penetrate the peritoneum in order to prevent visceral injury due to adhesions with the peritoneum. Preferably, the incision is big enough to be able to dissect down to the peritoneal cavity under direct vision. Alternatively, a closed Mayo scissor or haemostat is gently stabbed into the peritoneum, holding the stays up. The give-way of the peritoneum can be felt as peritoneum is perforated. Moving the closed mayo scissor against the anterior abdominal wall gives a frictionless feel of the smooth peritoneum confirming entry. Adhesions can also be detected this way. If suspected, the surgeon should insert his finger to feel all around inside the abdominal cavity to feel any possible adhesion. Small adhesions can be broken with a gentle sweeping movement of finger. Blunt trocar should be inserted for the first port after visualizing the intra-peritoneal viscera. If the incision is too big a purse string suture should be apply to hold the port in proper position and prevent the loss of pneumoperitoneum. The open technique is favoured by surgeons and considered by some to be indicated in patients with a previous midline laparotomy.

Relative contraindications for umbilical entry (also apply for the Veress needle) include: previous midline incision, morbid obesity, portal hypertension with a possible recanalized umbilical artery (which can occur with advanced cirrhosis of the liver), umbilical abnormalities such as urachal cyst or sinus and to some extend a umbilical hernia.

Direct Trocar Entry

In 1978, Dingfelder published a paper on direct entry into the abdomen with a trocar [5] The suggested advantages of this method were similar to the Hasson method and include reduced rate of failed pneumoperitoneum and preperitoneal insufflation, and a reduced rate of the more serious CO_2 embolism [20]. Laparoscopic entry is initiated with only one blind step (trocar) instead of two (Veress needle insufflation and trocar). The direct entry method is faster than any other method of entry [21] It was the least used laparoscopic access technique in during the nineties but is increasingly being used [22]. The technique begins with an infraumbilical skin incision wide enough to accommodate the diameter of a sharp trocar. The anterior abdominal wall must be adequately elevated by hand, and the trocar is inserted directly into the cavity, aiming towards the pelvic hollow. Alternatively, the abdominal wall is elevated by pulling on two towel clips through the abdominal skin on either side of the umbilicus, and the trocar is inserted at a 90 degree angle.

Disposable Shielded Trocars

Disposable shielded "safety" trocars were introduced in first in 1984. These trocars are designed with a shield, which partially retracts and exposes the sharp tip as it encounters resistance through the abdominal wall. As the shield enters the abdominal cavity, it springs back and covers the sharp blade on the tip of the trocar. These trocars were intended to prevent the sharp tip from injuring intra-abdominal content. However, even when a shielded trocar functions properly and is used according to the specifications, there is a brief moment when the sharp trocar tip is exposed and unprotected as it enters the abdominal cavity. In the presence of pneumoperitoneum with the Veress needle, disposable shielded trocars have been shown to require half the force needed of a reusable trocar. Increased entry force frequently results in loss of operator control and over thrusting of the trocar, which is a potential cause of serious vascular and visceral injuries [23].

Optical Trocar (Endopath Optiview)

The Endopath Optiview optical trocar comprises a hollow transparent obturator and a cannula. The optical trocar can be used directly, without pre-insufflation. The assistant may grasp the abdominal wall with towel clips, while the surgeon inserts the visual trocar [24] Twisting the handle advances the winged trocar tip to dissect successive tissue layers on its way towards the abdomen under direct camera view. Obviously this method is less suited for thin and cachectic patients. Experience with such methods is limited, and large-scale studies are lacking [25].

The retention of the push-through trocar design necessitates considerable axial force to propel the trajectory, with no mechanism to offset overshoot. Hybrid trocars have been designed with a insufflation hole in the tip of the obturator. Upon immediate penetration of the peritoneum under direct visualization, the peritoneal cavity is inflated. In seconds, pneumoperitoneum is established at up to three times the rate of alternative methods with only a 3mm intrusion of the tip into the peritoneal cavity. Figure 2 shows an example of how the optiview is used.

This technique combines some benefits of the Veress needle and optical non-bladed trocar creating a safe entry. These trocars seem promising but it must be kept in mind that there are no studies, which show that these trocars are superior.

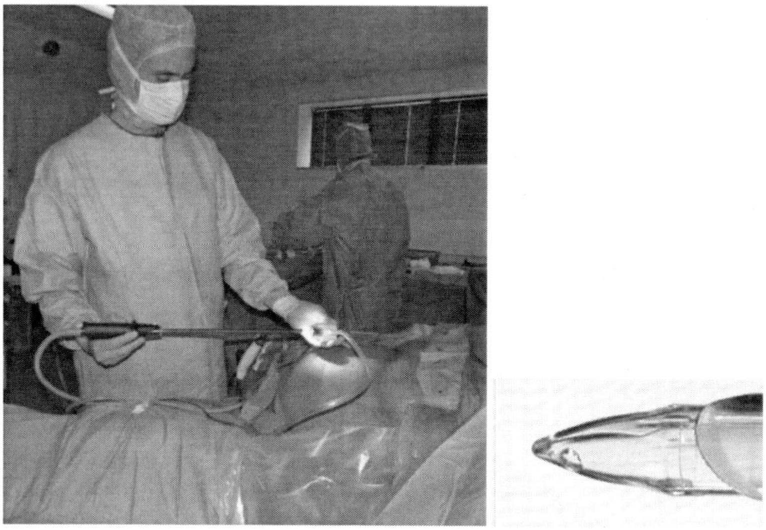

Figure 2a. An obese patient has been draped and is in the French position. The optiview trocar with insufflation is being assembled and the camera is inserted in the cannula. Insert is a close-up of the tip with the insufflation hole just 3mm away from the tip.

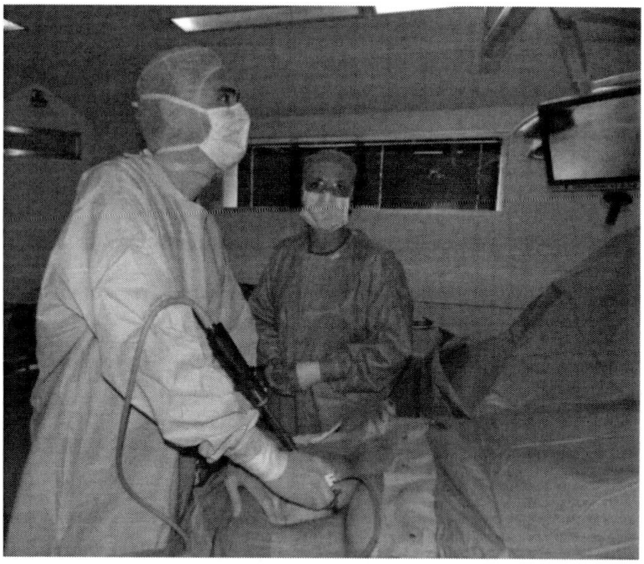

Figure 2b. The skin incision has been made and the trocar is introduced with the insufflation set on maximum flow with a maxium pressure of 16mmHg. The trocar is introdoced in a twisting manner while the surgeom kan focus on the screen. Here the anterior rectal sheet has been perforated showing the muscle layer (far screen).

Visiport Optical Trocars

The Visiport Plus optical trocar consists of an obturator with a blunt clear dome at the distal end that encloses a crescent shaped knife blade. When the trigger is squeezed, the blade extends approximately 1mm and immediately retracts. This action permits a controlled, sharp dissection of the tissue layers. The pistol grip handle includes a trigger and, at the proximal end, an opening accommodating a 10mm laparoscope. The 10 mm 0° laparoscope permits complete visualization as the obturator passes through the abdominal wall. It is advised that, as with other visual trocars, the Visiport optical trocar is to be inserted only after CO2 insufflation.

When insufflation is complete, the Veress needle is withdrawn. The location of introduction is determined and an incision is made in the skin. The Visiport optical trocar is palmed by the surgeon's dominant hand and held perpendicular to the supine patient's CO^2 distended abdomen. Once the exact anatomical position of the trocar tip is verified on the monitor, downward axial pressure is applied while activating the trigger. Then downward pressure is relieved, the trigger released, and the trocar tip position verified on the monitor again.

This entry sequence is repeated until the peritoneal cavity is entered. The trigger is not fired until the exact anatomical position of the trocar tip is known. One major drawback of this system is the steep price. The Visiport optical trocar comes in only one diameter and accommodates only a 10 mm laparoscope.

Radially Expanding Access System

The radially expanding access system was introduced in 1994. It consists of a 1.9 mm Veress surrounded by an expanding polymeric sleeve. The abdomen may first be insufflated using the Veress needle. The needle is removed, and the sleeve acts as a tract through the abdominal wall that can be dilated up to 12 mm by inserting a blunt obturator with a twisting motion. The force required to push this trocar through the abdomen in pigs is 14.2 kg compared with forces of 4 to 6 kg needed for disposable trocars [23] Radially expanding trocars have lost popularity after its introduction and are seldom used nowadays. They do have blunt tips that may provide some protection from injuries but required greater entry force compared with disposable trocars. They are also considered the most time consuming method to obtain access and are more expensive.

Main Trocar Placement

There is a simple preoperative test that can help to identify a safe region for Veress needle insertion in the scarred abdomen. The preoperative detection of anterior abdominal wall adhesions by ultrasonic scanning is a simple and reliable technique and can be considered in selected cases [26].

Secondary Tocar Placement

The secondary trocars should be inserted under direct camera vision. There is no systematic research into how secondary ports are safe. The site of insertion should be based on triangulation. Diaphany through the abdominal wall might be helpful to prevent injury to the blood vessels such as the epigastric vessels. A prospective observational study showed that 64% of the superficial epigastric vessels were identified in this way. With laparoscopic visualization from the peritoneal cavity, up to 82% of the deep and superficial epigastric vessels were visualized. These methods are less effective with the increase of body mass index (BMI) [27]. Extra attention must be paid to the suprapubic trocar with respect to the boundary of the bladder. The visualization of the bladder can be difficult. This is the reason why it is recommended to deflate the bladder prior to surgery. When in doubt, one could temporary fill the bladder retrogradely to assess the boundaries.

Removal of the Trocars

The secondary trocars should be removed under direct vision while the primary can be removed with the camera in the shaft. The main trocar can perforate an adhesive bowel loop which will only be notices when removing the trocar under sight. The same holds true for bleedings which are not seen when the trocar tamponades the bleeding vessel. The bleeding will become apparent only after the trocar is removed under sight. Another reported complication is herniation of bowel or omentum after trocar removal. When removing the trocars, the positive intra-abdominal pressure can force an intestinal loop or omentumslip through the trocarport and a herniation can occur.

Residual CO^2 left inside the abdominal cavity sometime causes considerable discomfort like chest pain and referred shoulder pain. This discomfort is caused by residual CO^2 gas that is trapped in the sub diaphragmatic recesses and then irritates the diaphragm, leading to referred pain in chest and shoulder. This pain is more prominent when patient sits upright. It is advisable to actively desufflate the abdomen with the suction device to prevent postoperative shoulder pain. If the suction device in not used, the last most cranial trocar should be unscrewed to allow all the air to escape while the patient is in the trendelenburg position.

Closing the Fascia After Removal

In the medical literature there were no RCTs, which analysed the occurrence of port herniation in relation to closing the fascia. With the closure of the fascia one does not rule out the occurrence of a herniation. Kadar et al. reported that three of the six hernias which were found, occurred after the fascia was closed [28]

Sound medical and scientific literature, which might show that closing fascia defects can reduce the risk of port site herniation is not available. Another important aspect is the size threshold above which the risk herniation of increases. The majority of reported herniation was found in ports ≥ 10 mm. This is reported in retrospective cohort studies, case series and case reports where no adequate analysis of incidences in specific size is possible [29–32] Only in the retrospective cohort study of Kadar et al., incidences of 0.23 % and 3.1 % are given by fascia defects of 10 and 12 mm, respectively.28 The power of this study is not sufficient for an accurate estimation of incidence and risk calculations.

In general, in the literature it is recommended to close the fascia defects ≥ 10 mm to prevention herniation [28,29]. Examination of the same literature, however, shows that there is no good evidence. Closing a fascia defects may not necessarily be associated with a decrease in the incidence of port site herniation but can also cause complications like nerve constriction, superficial vascular injury and bowel injury. The incidences of these complications are unknown and are expected to be lower than the incidence of port herniation after laparoscopy.

Evidence Surrounding Different Introduction Methods

In a Cochrane review studies comparing closed and open introduction were pooled [33] A wide variety of endpoints including mortality, vascular or visceral damage, gas emboli and trocar infections were included. There was no difference found between closed or open introduction. The Australian college of surgeons also performed a systematic review and pooled 5 non-randomised studies [34]. They found a significant higher risk over visceral injury (RR 2,17; 95%-BI: 1,14–4,10) in the open group while there was a trend towards more vascular injury (RR 0,68; 95%-BI: 0,16-2,84) in the Veress Group. These results should be interpreted with caution. They are probably subject to bias since the open technique was more often performed in patients with previous abdominal surgery. These patients obviously have a higher risk for visceral injury.

At this time, there is not convincing evidence that the open entry technique is superior to or inferior to the other entry techniques currently available. The open entry technique does have a lower incidence of vascular injuries, but this is balanced by a potentially higher incidence of bowel injury. Instead of dissecting down at the umbilicus on suspected bowel adhesions, an alternative site of entry may be more appropriate, such as the left upper quadrant. This could possibly decrease the rate of bowel injury, as these sites are rarely affected by adhesions and have been shown to be safe in small studies when hepatosplenomegaly and stomach distension have been excluded.

Many different alternate trocar systems have been developed since the advent of laparoscopic surgery. The main design goal is to ease introduction and reduce the risks of introduction. The Cochrane review found no RCTs that compare direct vision introduction with Veress needle introduction. There are some observational studies showing no reduction in the risk of vascular and intestinal injuries. In these studies the introduction under vision was significantly faster compared to the Veress needle.

The Cochran review shows that radially expanding access trocars have advantages in terms of reduced trocar opening bleedings and less extraperitoneal insufflation and introduction failures [33,35,36] There are no trials or comparative studies with sufficient power which analyse the safety of the hybrid technology compared with conventional closed or open technique. There does not appear to be an increased or reduced risk of vascular or intestinal injury from retrospective studies [37]. There is no systematic research into how secondary ports can safely be inserted. Prospective observational study showed that with transillumination, 64% of the superficial epigastric vessels was identified and this was 82% when combined with laparoscopic visualization (from the peritoneal cavity) of the deeper epigastric vessels [27]. This method is less effective in patients with a high BMI. The secondary ports are inserted under direct vision in order to prevent visceral and vascular lesions Special attention should go to the suprapubic trocar with respect to the boundary of the bladder. The visualization of the bladder can be difficult. If the boundary of the bladder is not clear, the bladder can be filled retrogradely.

Overall, injury associated with abdominal entry is rare. The difference between the various techniques is minimal in retrospective studies. A randomised controlled trial would need thousands of patients to detect a difference. It is advisable that one should perform the technique he/she is most comfortable with.

Special Condiderations

Adhesions

Adhesions in the umbilical region can occur in up to 50 % of the patients who have had a median laparotomy, and up to 23 % of patients who have a low transverse (Pfannenstiel) incision. Adhesions around the umbilicus were seen in approximately 0.68% of the patients without abdominal surgery in their history. A Veress needle or trocar should never be introduced near a location where adhesions are expected in context to a previous laparotomy. Interestingly, there is no clear evidence concerning preforming a laparoscopy via the umbilicus after previous laparoscopy and many gynaecologists and surgeons simple use the previous access route.

The most preferred alternative entry point in patients who have undergone previous laparotomy is the upper left quadrant of the abdomen. In this area adhesions are rare, except for cases in which surgery in that area has previously been performed or if there is splenomegaly. Most used it the point of Palmer (3 cm subcostal in the midclavicular line).

Pregnancy

The only published guideline on laparoscopy in pregnancy is written by the SAGES (2007), the American Association of Gastrointestinal Surgeons [38] From a gestation of 12 weeks, the volume of the uterus increases rapidly. Due to the increased size of the uterus, there is a higher risk of injury to the uterus or other intra-abdominal organs [39]. The American guideline concludes that, on basis of the opinion of experts, in the second and third trimesters of pregnancy the location of the entrance is adapted to the fundus level and shifts from the umbilicus to subcostal region. The expert panel suggest that if one elevates the abdominal wall at the entrance, both the closed and the open entrance technique should be safe [38].

The Thin Patient

Children and extremely thin patients (anorectic or cachectic patients with a BMI < 18) have the greatest risk of retroperitoneal vascular injury at the entrance. The aorta is less than 2,5 cm away from the skin. For this reason, extra caution should be used when the primary entrance is gained. Preferably, the Hasson technique should be used or insertion at the point of Palmer is recommended.

The Patient with Obesity

Obese patients (BMI > 30kg/m^2), who are undergoing laparotomy, run a significantly larger risk of overall complications. Laparoscopic surgery has proven to have particular advantages in these patients. Depending on the fat and the habitus of the patient, a closed introduction with the Verress needle at the location of the umbilicus, or at Palmer's point can be used. The preferred location for entrance is where the subcutis is expected to be thinnest. When the needle is inserted vertically and reaches the fascia, the average distance from the umbilicus to the peritoneum is 6 cm. So even in extremely obese patients a Veress needle with standard length can be used.

Direct optical trocar entry might seems to be the preferred technique in (morbidly) obese patients. In large series in bariatric surgery there are no reports of introduction related injury. However, there are no randomised or prospective studies.

Conclusion

Obtaining abdominal access can be performed with minimal risk of complications. Gynaecologist generally prefer the Veress needle introduction while laparoscopic surgeons prefer the open technique. There is no evidence that the open entry technique is superior or inferior to the closed techniques. Other variants on the open or closed technique are available and have similar complication rates. The Left upper quadrant (e.g. Palmer's point) laparoscopic entry should be considered in patients with suspected or known periumbilical adhesions. Shielded trocars may be used in an effort to decrease entry injuries but there is no evidence that they result in fewer complications during laparoscopic access. Radially expanding trocars are not recommended because the force required for entry is significantly greater than with disposable trocars. The visual entry cannula system and newer hybrid systems with insufflation capabilities may represent an advantage over traditional trocars, as it allows a clear optical entry, whilst insufflating and dissecting the tissue. This theoretical advantage seems promising but has not been proven yet.

References

[1] Tarasconi JC. Endoscopic salpingectomy. *J Reprod Med.* 1981; 26: 541–545.

[2] Jansen FW, Kapiteyn K, Trimbos-Kemper T, Hermans J, Trimbos JB. Complications of laparoscopy: a prospective multicentre observational study. *Br J Obstet Gynaecol.* 1997; 104: 595–600.

[3] Palmer R. Safety in laparoscopy. *J Reprod Med.* 1974; 13: 1–5.

[4] Hasson H. A modified instrument and method for laparoscopy. *Am J Obs Gynecol.* 1971; 110: 886–887.

[5] Dingfelder JR. Direct laparoscope trocar insertion without prior pneumoperitoneum. *J Reprod Med*. 1978; 21: 45–47.

[6] Byron JW, Fujiyoshi CA, Miyazawa K. Evaluation of the direct trocar insertion technique at laparoscopy. *Obstet Gynecol*. 1989; 74: 423–425.

[7] Nezhat FR, Silfen SL, Evans D, Nezhat C. Comparison of direct insertion of disposable and standard reusable laparoscopic trocars and previous pneumoperitoneum with Veress needle. Obstet. Gynecol. 1991 p. 148–150.

[8] Riek S, Bachmann KH, Gaiselmann T, Hoernstein F, Marzusch K. A new insufflation needle with a special optical system for use in laparoscopic procedures. *Obstet Gynecol*. 1994; 84: 476–478.

[9] Kaali SG. Introduction of the opti-trocar. *Am Assoc Gynecol Laparosc*. 1993; 1: 50–53.

[10] Turner DJ. A new, radially expanding access system for laparoscopic procedures versus conventional cannulas. *J Am Assoc Gynecol Laparosc*. 1996; 3: 609–615.

[11] Adler S, Scherrer M, Rückauer KD, Daschner FD. Comparison of economic and environmental impacts between disposable and reusable instruments used for laparoscopic cholecystectomy. *Surg Endosc*. 2005; 19: 268–272.

[12] Paolucci V, Schaeff B, Gutt C, Morawe G, Encke A. Disposable versus reusable instruments in laparoscopic surgery--a controlled study. Zentralbl. Chir. 1995 p. 47–52.

[13] Bhoyrul S, Vierra MA, Nezhat CR, Krummel TM, Way LW. Trocar injuries in laparoscopic surgery. *J Am Coll Surg*. 2001; 192: 677–683.

[14] Corson SL, Chandler JG, Way LW. Survey of laparoscopic entry injuries provoking litigation. *J Am Assoc Gynecol Laparosc*. 2001; 8: 341–347.

[15] Briel JW, Plaisier PW, Meijer WS, Lange JF. Is it necessary to lift the abdominal wall when preparing a pneumoperitoneum? A randomized study. Surg. Endosc. 2000 p. 862–864.

[16] Teoh B, Sen R, Abbott J. An evaluation of four tests used to ascertain Veres needle placement at closed laparoscopy. *J Minim Invasive Gynecol*. 2005; 12: 153–158.

[17] Tsaltas J, Pearce S, Lawrence A, Meads A, Mezzatesta J, Nicolson S. Safer laparoscopic trocar entry: it's all about pressure. *Aust N Z J Obstet Gynaecol*. 2004; 44: 349–350.

[18] Hasson HM, Rotman C, Rana N, Kumari NA. Open laparoscopy: 29-year experience. *Obstet Gynecol*. 2000; 96: 763–766.

[19] Huber DH. Open laparoscopy. Commentary. *Biomed Bull*. 1984; 5: 5.

[20] Catarci M, Carlini M, Gentileschi P, Santoro E. Major and minor injuries during the creation of pneumoperitoneum. A multicenter study on 12,919 cases. *Surg Endosc*. 2001; 15: 566–569.

[21] Byron JW, Markenson G, Miyazawa K. A randomized comparison of Verres needle and direct trocar insertion for laparoscopy. Surg. Gynecol. Obstet. 1993 p. 259–262.

[22] Molloy D, Kaloo PD, Cooper M, Nguyen T V. Laparoscopic entry: a literature review and analysis of techniques and complications of primary port entry. *Aust N Z J Obstet Gynaecol*. 2002; 42: 246–254.

[23] Tarnay CM, Glass KB, Munro MG. Entry force and intra-abdominal pressure associated with six laparoscopic trocar-cannula systems: A randomized comparison. *Obstet Gynecol*. 1999; 94: 83–88.

[24] McKernan JB, Finley CR. Experience with optical trocar in performing laparoscopic procedures. *Surg Laparosc Endosc Percutan Tech*. 2002; 12: 96–99.

[25] Angelini L, Lirici MM, Papaspyropoulos V, Sossi FL. Combination of subcutaneous abdominal wall retraction and optical trocar to minimize pneumoperitoneum-related effects and needle and trocar injuries in laparoscopic surgery. *Surg Endosc*. 1997; 11: 1006–1009.

[26] Kolecki R V, Golub RM, Sigel B, Machi J, Kitamura H, Hosokawa T, *et al.* Accuracy of viscera slide detection of abdominal wall adhesions by ultrasound. Surg. Endosc. 1994 p. 871–874.

[27] Hurd WW, Amesse LS, Gruber JS, Horowitz GM, Cha GM, Hurteau JA. Visualization of the epigastric vessels and bladder before laparoscopic trocar placement. *Fertil Steril*. 2003; 80: 209–212.

[28] Kadar N, Reich H, Liu CY, Manko GF, Gimpelson R. Incisional hernias after major laparoscopic gynecologic procedures. *Am J Obstet Gynecol*. 1993; 168: 1493–1495.

[29] Tonouchi H, Ohmori Y, Kobayashi M, Kusunoki M. Trocar site hernia. *Arch Surg*. 2004; 139: 1248–1256.

[30] Montz FJ, Holschneider CH, Munro MG. Incisional hernia following laparoscopy: a survey of the American Association of Gynecologic Laparoscopists. *Obstet Gynecol*. 1994; 84: 881–884.

[31] Azurin DJ, Go LS, Arroyo LR, Kirkland ML. Trocar site herniation following laparoscopic cholecystectomy and the significance of an incidental preexisting umbilical hernia. *Am Surg*. 1995; 61: 718–720.

[32] Nezhat C, Nezhat F, Seidman DS. Incisional hernias after operative laparoscopy. *J Laparoendosc Adv Surg Tech A*. 1997; 7: 111–115.

[33] Ahmad G, O'Flynn H, Duffy J, Phillips K, Watson A. Laparoscopic entry techniques. *Cochrane Database Syst Rev*. 2012;

[34] Merlin TL, Hiller JE, Maddern GJ, Jamieson GG, Brown AR, Kolbe A. Systematic review of the safety and effectiveness of methods used to establish pneumoperitoneum in laparoscopic surgery. *Br J Surg* [Internet]. 2003; 90: 668–679.

[35] Bhoyrul S, Payne J, Steffes B, Swanstrom L, Way L. A randomized prospective study of radially expanding trocars in laparoscopic surgery. *J Gastrointest Surg*. 2000; 4: 392–397.

[36] Feste J, Bojahr B, Turner DJ. Randomized trial comparing a radially expandable needle system with cutting trocars. *JSLS*. 2000; 4: 184.

[37] Sharp HT, Dodson MK, Draper ML, Watts DA, Doucette RC, Hurd WW. Complications associated with optical-access laparoscopic trocars. *Obstet Gynecol*. 2002; 99: 553–555.

[38] Soper NJ. SAGES' guidelines for diagnosis, treatment, and use of laparoscopy for surgical problems during pregnancy. Surg. Endosc. 2011. p. 3477–3478.

[39] Halpern NB. Laparoscopic cholecystectomy in pregnancy: a review of published experiences and clinical considerations. *Semin Laparosc Surg*. 1998; 5: 129–134.

In: Laparoscopy
Editor: Christos Iavazzo
ISBN: 978-1-63321-404-0

Chapter 2

Modified Laparoscopic and Open Splenectomy and Azygoportal Disconnection for Portal Hypertension

Dou-Sheng Bai, M.D., Jian-Jun Qian, M.D., Ping Chen, M.D., Jie Yao, M.D., Xiao-Dong Wang, M.Sc., Sheng-Jie Jin, M.Sc. and Guo-Qing Jiang*, M.Sc.

Department of Hepatobiliary Surgery,
Clinical Medical College of Yangzhou University, Yangzhou, China

Abstract

Background: Laparoscopic splenectomy and azygoportal disconnection (LSD) using many different surgical techniques has become increasingly popular for treatment of cirrhotic patients with bleeding portal hypertension and secondary hypersplenism. We have developed an even less invasive technique, modified laparoscopic splenectomy and azygoportal disconnection (MLSD), and identified clinical outcomes of modified laparoscopic and open splenectomy and azygoportal disconnection (OSD) in patients with portal hypertension.

Methods: Between January 2010 and May 2013, 115 cirrhotic patients with portal hypertensive bleeding and secondary hypersplenism had underwent MLSD (n=44) or OSD (n=71) . Their Clinical outcomes including demographic, intraoperative, and postoperative variables were evaluated retrospectively.

Results: All patients experienced successful MLSD. None suffered conversion to open surgery or had significant perioperative complications. For MLSD, operation time was significantly longer than OSD ($P < 0.0001$), but estimated intraoperative blood loss

* Corresponding author: Guo-Qing Jiang, MSc, Department of Hepatobiliary Surgery, Clinical Medical College of Yangzhou University, 98 West Nantong Rd, Yangzhou 225000, China. E-mail: jgqing2003@hotmail.com; Tel: 86-514-87373272; Fax: 86-514-87990188.

† Drs. Dou-Sheng Bai, Jian-Jun Qian, and Ping Chen contributed equally to this work.

($P<0.0001$); volume of intraoperative blood transfusion ($P<0.05$); visual analog scale pain score on the first postoperative day ($P<0.0001$); times to first oral intake ($P<0.0001$), passage of flatus ($P<0.001$), and off-bed activity ($P<0.0001$); postoperative hospital stay ($P<0.0001$); postoperative days of temperature >38.0°C ($P<0.0001$) and white blood cell counts on postoperative days 1 ($P<0.0001$) and 7 ($P<0.05$) were significantly reduced in the MLSD group. The lower percentage of patients experiencing postoperative complications was found significantly in the MLSD group than in the OSD group (15.91% [7/44] vs 36.62%[26/71], ($P<0.05$).

Conclusions: The less invasive MLSD group involving the use of an electromechanical morcellator provides expedient recovery and minimal postoperative pain and scarring. It is a feasible, effective, and safe surgical procedure for liver cirrhosis patients with portal hypertensive bleeding and hypersplenism.

Keywords: Liver cirrhosis, Portal hypertension, Devascularization, Laparoscopy, Morcellator

Introduction

In Asia, patients with liver cirrhosis, portal hypertensive bleeding and secondary hypersplenism has been widely accepted the surgical treatment of OSD. However, the liver function of those patients is usually very poor, and OSD, which involves a large surgical incision, is associated with high morbidity rates.

Jiang et al. [1] reported patients after OSD had higher the overall complication rate than after laparoscopic splenectomy and azygoportal disconnection (LSD) (42.31% [11/26] vs 19.23% [5/26], $P < 0.05$).

Safe, minimally invasive alternatives are therefore necessary. However, the laparoscopic technique is much more challenging when performed in patients with cirrhosis, portal hypertension, and splenomegaly. These were many techniques for LSD including the use of cumbersome intracorporeal bags to draw massively enlarged spleens, creation of enlarged incisions to morcellate and draw splenic issues, and hand-assisted laparoscopy [1-11]. Indeed, the less invasive laparoscopic techniques have been shown to be safe and feasible in patients with portal hypertension.

We herein report modified laparoscopic splenectomy and azygoportal disconnection (MLSD) with a new technique that greatly reduces impairments. An electromechanical morcellator was used to remove massively enlarged spleens from the abdominal cavity through the existing incision.

To the best of our knowledge, this is the first report of the use of an electromechanical morcellator to extract the entire massive splenic tissue in LSD. Nevertheless, the safety of laparoscopic splenectomy for patients with portal hypertensive bleeding and hypersplenism secondary to liver cirrhosis is still unclear [12-14]. We therefore investigated whether our MLSD is more effective and safer than OSD for patients with portal hypertension.

Materials and Methods

Patients

Between January 2010 and May 2013, the clinical records of 115 patients diagnosed with liver cirrhosis, portal hypertensive bleeding, and secondary hypersplenism were retrospectively analyzed in our department; among them, 44 accepted MLSD and 71 underwent OSD. During the preoperative discussion, all patients were informed that MLSD is a minimally invasive procedure but was in the experimental stage compared with typical OSD. The selection of procedure was based on the patient's decision. All operations were performed by the same surgical team. This study was approved by the Ethics Committee of Clinical Medical College of Yangzhou University. All patients provided written informed consent. Pre- and intraoperative patient data retrospectively collected included age, gender, etiology of cirrhosis, Child-Pugh classification, the model for end-stage liver disease score, longitudinal diameter of the spleen, preoperative hemoglobin concentration, operation time, estimated intraoperative blood loss, and volume of intraoperative blood transfused. Postoperative data included visual analog scale pain score on the first day after surgery; times to first oral intake, initial passage of flatus, and off-bed activity; number of days with temperature >38°C; postoperative hospital stay; perioperative complications; and white blood cell counts on days 1 and 7.

Using direct interview, Visual analog scale pain score was evaluated by a questionnaire that rated pain intensity on a scale of 0-10 [15-17], with 0 representing no pain and 10 representing very severe pain.

Modified Laparoscopic Procedures

Laparoscopic Splenectomy

Under general anesthesia, patients were placed in the supine position with legs parted. Thirteen mmHg pressure was skept in the abdomen insufflated with carbon dioxide. A five-port method was chosen for MLSD (Figure 1). A 10 mm port (port A) was placed through the umbilicus for a 10 mm, 30-degree angled laparoscope. Under direct visualization, a 5 mm port (port B) was placed in the right midclavicular line just below the costal margin; a 10 mm port (port C) was placed in the right midclavicular line halfway between the costal margin and the umbilicus; a 12 mm port (port D) was placed in the left midclavicular line halfway between the costal margin and the umbilicus; and a second 10 mm port (port E) was placed in the left anterior axillary line below the border of the spleen. Port C and E were the main ports used for the LigaSure vessel-sealing device (Covidien, Boulder, USA), and port D was the main port used for the linear laparoscopic vascular stapler (EndoGIA) and the electromechanical morcellator (TSCS, Hangzhou, China).

The most important manipulation in this stage is blocking up the splenic artery. This can reduce the rate of conversion to an open surgical procedure and should thus be performed as early as possible at the beginning of MLSD. To expose the splenic artery, the reverse Trendelenburg position was chosen, with the surgeon on the right side of the patient. The procedure began by opening the gastrocolic ligament to enter the lesser sac. After dividing the splenogastric ligament (excluding the short gastric vessels for the time being), the paries posterior gastricus was lifted using a single 5 mm laparoscopic goldfinger retractor (YIDA, Hangzhou, China) avoiding gastricus impairment by gripping forceps and the splenic artery was carefully dissociated above the tail of the pancreas (Figure 2) and tightly clipped with a hem-o-lock.

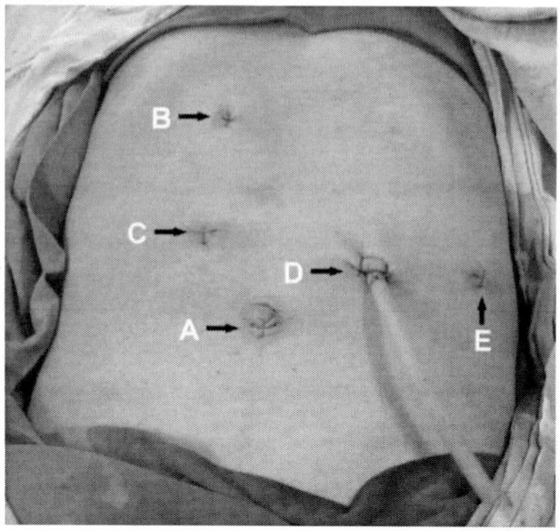

Figure 1. Trocar positions for modified laparoscopic splenectomy and azygoportal disconnection.

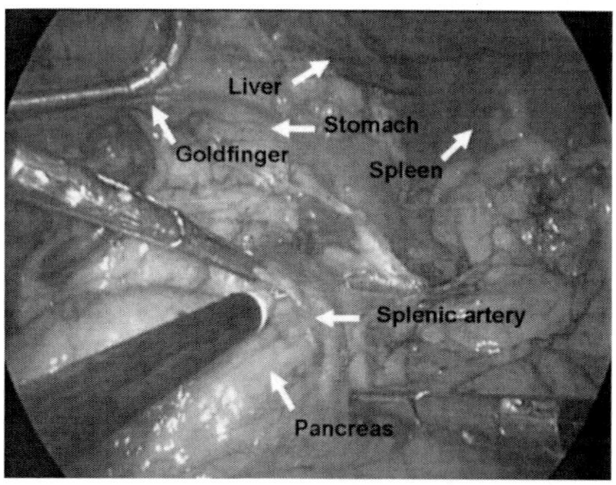

Figure 2. Exposure of splenic artery by a single 5-mm laparoscopic goldfinger retractor.

The lower pole of the spleen was lifted by the bar of a tube-type forceps, and the flexura lienalis coli was pushed by a 5 mm laparoscopic goldfinger retractor, resulting in good exposure of the splenocolic ligament, which was divided using an electric hook. The posterior view of the splenic wall was best obtained by gradually sliding the above-mentioned instruments from the lower to the upper pole of the spleen.

The retroperitoneum between the left diaphragm and the posterior margin of the spleen, the splenorenal ligament, and the splenophrenic ligament were then dissected with the LigaSure vessel-sealing device. The proximal stomach was elevated in the upper right direction using a 5 mm laparoscopic goldfinger retractor, resulting in better exposure of the short gastric vessels for easier dissection (Figure 3). Following laparoscopic mobilization, the spleen and splenic artery and vein were transected en bloc using a linear laparoscopic vascular stapler through port D. Splenectomy was performed by carefully dissecting the splenic hilum to protect the tail of the pancreas. The dissected spleen was then placed in the left subphrenic space.

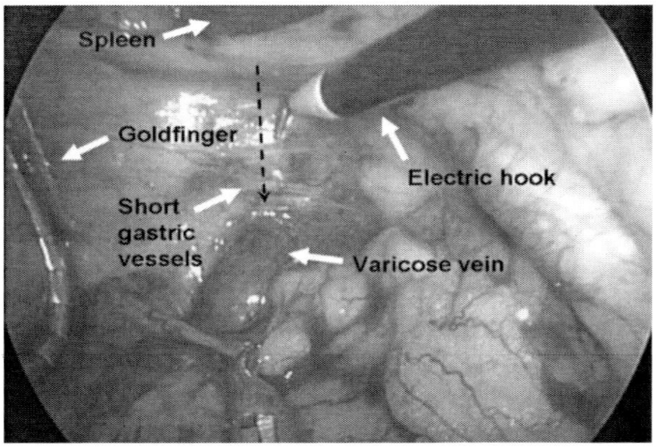

Figure 3. Exposure and division of short gastric vessels. Peritoneum viscerale of the short gastric vessels was divided along the dotted line.

Laparoscopic Azygoportal Disconnection

The patient was placed in the reverse Trendelenburg position, with the LigaSure vessel-sealing device used through trocar C. The dissociated length of the distal esophagus was ≥8 cm. In the authors' view, the optimal flow of laparoscopic azygoportal disconnection performed was from back to front, from below to above, and from left to right. Thus, the order of disconnection of the paraesophageal venous collaterals should carried out in the following order: (1) the posterior surface of stomach, including the posterior gastric veins; (2) the left lateral surface of the distal esophagus; (3) the left inferior phrenic veins; (4) the posterior surface of the distal esophagus; (5) the gastric coronary vein; (6) the anterior surface of the distal esophagus; (7) the gastrohepatic ligament; and (8) the right lateral surface of the distal esophagus (Figure 4). The advantages of this procedure are that it is ordered, convenient, and fast.

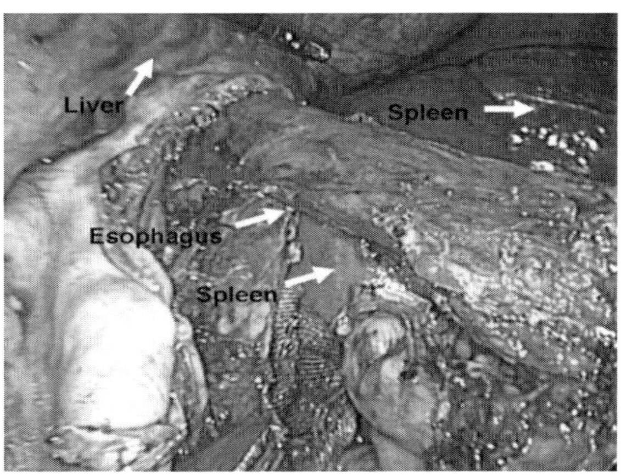

Figure 4. Dissociation of the distal esophagus between the two diaphragmatic crura.

Laparoscopic Spleen Extraction

Patients were maintained in the reverse Trendelenburg position. An electromechanical morcellator, consisting of a motor-driven cutting tube, was inserted directly into the abdominal cavity through port E, and a large claw forceps that can grasp spleen tissues was inserted through the tube (Figure 5). As the electromechanical morcellator potarys spleen tissue from the lower pole in the direction of the upper pole, the retractor should push the upper pole in the direction of the pelvic cavity. During this procedure, the large claw forceps grasped the spleen through the motor-driven cutting tube, pulling it back while pressing the splenic tissue against the cutting edge of the rotating tube; the rotation was triggered by a hand switch. A cylindrical tissue sample (Figure 6) was removed from the tube by applying a measured pulling force.

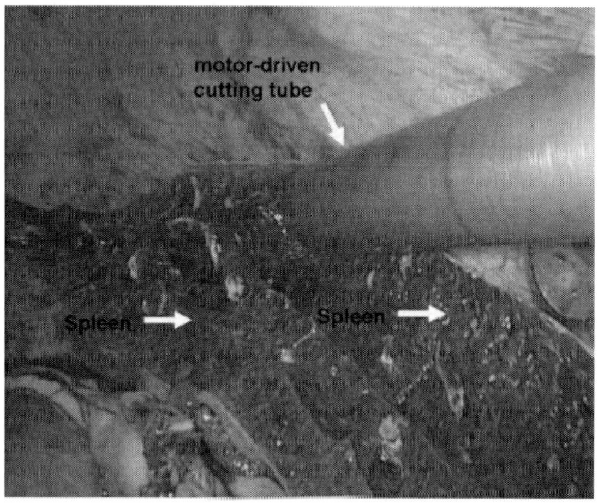

Figure 5. Extraction of spleen by rolling electromechanical morcellator.

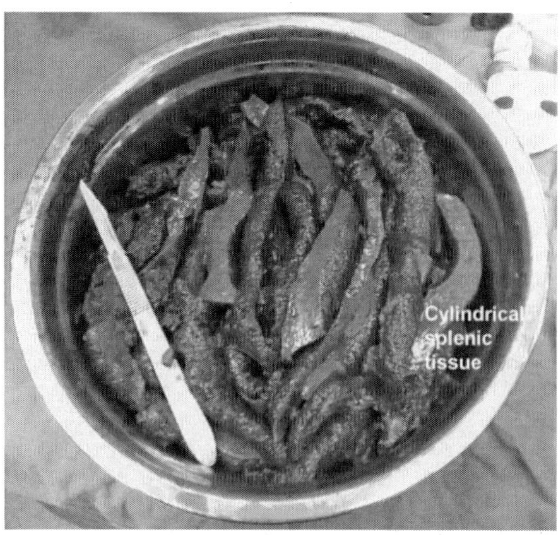

Figure 6. Cylindrical the splenic tissue.

This procedure was repeated until the entire spleen was removed by the electromechanical morcellator. The entrance of the tube should be in view during the entire procedure to prevent damage to the surrounding organs. The entire upper quadrant was irrigated from right to left and from above to below with sterile saline, and the operation area was carefully inspected for bleeding.

Open Procedures

OSD was performed through either a left subcostal incision or a midline laparotomy using traditional methods. Splenectomy was performed before azygoportal disconnection.

Statistical Analysis

Data are presented as the mean ± standard deviation, median/range, or percentages (%). Group means were compared using Student's t test or the Mann-Whitney U test, as appropriate. Percentages were compared using chi-square tests. P values < 0.050 were considered statistically significant. All statistical analyses were performed using SPSS 13.0 software (SPSS, Chicago, IL, USA).

Results

From January 2010 and May 2013, MLSD was performed on 44 patients (27 males, 17 females) with cirrhosis, portal hypertensive bleeding, and secondary hypersplenism and was successful in all patients. No conversion to open operation happened. These patients ranged in age from 37 to 75 years with a mean age of 54.98±10.41 years, had been admitted owing to repeated variceal bleeding. Total 29 patients' Liver cirrhosis stage was Child-Pugh A and 15 was Child-Pugh B. Liver damage was caused by chronic hepatitis B in 23 patients, by chronic hepatitis C in 3, by schistosomes in 6, by alcoholic cirrhosis in 3, and by autoimmune liver cirrhosis in 9. All 44 patients had splenomegaly, with ultrasound, computed tomography or magnetic resonance showing that spleen diameters ranged from 13.5 to 25.0 cm.

The results of MLSD were compared with those of 71 patients (41 males, 30 females) who underwent OSD during the same time period. These patients ranged in age from 31 to 73 years with a mean age of 52.46±10.33 years, and were also admitted owing to repeated variceal bleeding. Total 39 patients' liver cirrhosis stage was Child-Pugh A and 32 was Child-Pugh B. Liver damage was caused by chronic hepatitis B in 46 patients, by chronic hepatitis C in 5, by schistosomes in 9, by alcoholic cirrhosis in 4, and by autoimmune cirrhosis in 7. Spleen diameters ranged from 12.5 to 26.3 cm.

Baseline demographic and clinical characteristics of the modified and OSD groups are shown in Table 1. No significant differences existed between group, including in age, gender, etiology of cirrhosis, Child-Pugh classification, the model for end-stage liver disease score, longitudinal diameter of the spleen, or preoperative hemoglobin concentration. All patients were discharged in good condition.

The perioperative details of the two groups are shown in Table 2. Contrast to those undergoing OSD, median operation time was significantly longer in patients undergoing MLSD ($P < 0.0001$). The volume of intraoperative blood transfused ($P < 0.05$), and median intraoperative blood loss ($P < 0.0001$), however, were much lower in the MLSD group. Visual analog scale pain score on the first day after surgery was significantly lower in the MLSD group ($P<0.0001$). Similarly, mean times to first oral intake ($P < 0.0001$), initial passage of flatus ($P < 0.001$), initial off-bed activity ($P < 0.0001$) and median hospital stay ($P < 0.0001$) were significantly shorter after MLSD. The overall postoperative complication rate was lower in patients who underwent MLSD than in those who underwent OSD (15.91% vs. 36.62%, $P < 0.05$). In the MLSD group, none of the patients experienced incisional complications, although one experienced four had asymptomatic portal vein thrombosis and a pancreatic fistula. Of the patients undergoing OSD, one had a pancreatic fistula, seven had asymptomatic portal vein thrombosis, nine had incisional complications (1 incisional hernia, 5 Superficial surgical site infections [SSI], and 3 Deep SSI), three had pneumonia, two had Organ Space SSI, and three required emergency laparotomy for bleeding after OSD. In contrast, no emergency laparotomy for bleeding emerged in the MLSD group.

Table 1. Baseline demographic and clinical characteristics of the MLSD and OSD groups

Variable	MLSD (n=44)	OSD (n=71)	*P* value
Gender, m/f, n	27/17	41/30	*P*=0.701
Age, mean ± SD, years	54.98±10.41	52.46±10.33	*P*=0.209
Etiology, n			
HBV cirrhosis	23	46	*P*=0.183
HCV cirrhosis	3	5	*P*=0.963
Schistosome cirrhosis	6	9	*P*=0.882
Alcoholic cirrhosis	3	4	*P*=0.796
Autoimmunity liver cirrhosis	9	7	*P*=0.111
Child-Pugh classification, A/B, n	29/15	39/32	*P*=0.244
MELD, mean ± SD	3.32±2.27	3.49±2.57	*P*=0.712
Longitudinal diameter of spleen, mean ± SD, mm	179.45±27.88	185.44±33.24	*P*=0.321
Hemoglobin concentration, mean ± SD, g/dl	104.16±26.95	95.34±28.14	*P*=1.000

Abbreviations: *MLSD*, modified laparoscopic splenectomy and azygoportal disconnection; *OSD*, open splenectomy and azygoportal disconnection; *HBV*, hepatitis b virus; *HCV*, hepatitis C virus; *MELD*, the model for end-stage liver disease score; *IQR*, interquartile range.

Compared with OSD group, the mean number of postoperative days with temperature >38.0°C was significantly shorter in MLSD group (4.09±3.16 vs. 6.89±3.55 days, $P < 0.0001$). Seven patients in the MLSD and two in the OSD group did not suffered fever postoperatively, making the rate significantly higher in the MLSD than in the OSD group (15.91% vs. 2.82%, $P<0.05$). Although median white blood cell count in the two groups was similar at admission ($P>0.05$), median white blood cell counts on postoperative days (11.45 [range, 5.2-17.4]×10^9/L vs. 16.9 [range, 6.1-33.90]×10^9/L, $P < 0.0001$) and 7 (8.4 [range, 5-

23.1]×10^9/L vs. 9.5 [range, 4.9-38]×10^9/L, $P < 0.05$) were significantly lower in the MLSD group than in the OSD group.

The percentage of patients with normal WBC counts on postoperative days 1 (34.09% vs. 4.22%, $P<0.0001$) and 7 (81.82% vs. 54.93%, $P<0.01$) were all significantly higher after MLSD lower after OSD.

Table 2 Intraoperative and postoperative characteristics of the MLSD and OSD groups

Variable	MLSD (n=44)	OSD (n=71)	*P* value
Operation time, median (range), min	210 (140-390)	180 (110-300)	*P*<0.0001
Estimated blood loss, median (range), ml	150 (50-800)	300 (50-1200)	*P*<0.0001
Blood transfused, median (range), ml	0 (0-400)	0 (0-700)	*P*=0.024
VAS pain score on the first day, mean ± SD	2.50±0.85	5.06±1.08	*P*<0.0001
Time to first oral intake, mean ± SD, days	1.52±0.63	2.76±0.62	*P*<0.0001
Time to first flatus, mean ± SD, days	2.36±0.97	3.18±1.00	*P*=0.0004
Time to off-bed activity, mean ± SD, days	2.59±0.69	5.96±0.93	*P*<0.0001
Postoperative hospital stay, median (range), days	10 (7-18)	15(7-28)	*P*<0.0001
Perioperative complications, n	7	26	*P*=0.017
Incisional complications	0	9	*P*=0.035
Incisional hernia	0	1	
Superficial SSI	0	5	
Deep SSI	0	3	
Pneumonia	0	3	*P*=0.436
Organ Space SSI	0	2	*P*=0.697
Emergency operation for bleeding	0	3	*P*=0.436
Pancreatic fistula	2	1	*P*=0.672
Asymptomatic portal vein thrombosis	5	8	*P*=1.000

Abbreviations: *MLSD*, modified laparoscopic splenectomy and azygo*port*al disconnection; *OSD*, open splenectomy and azygoportal disconnection; *IQR*, interquartile range; *VAS*, visual analog scale; SSI, surgical site infections.

Discussion

With the recent significant progress in laparoscopic skills and advances in technical instruments, endoscopic surgery involving improved and advantageous techniques is performed in almost all fields of conventional abdominal surgery. However, the laparoscopic technique is much more challenging when performed in patients with cirrhosis, portal hypertension, and splenomegaly. Patients who undergo conventional spleen extraction by LSD have complained of pain associated with the enlarged or hand-assisted incision to remove the spleen, thus obviating the advantages of laparoscopic surgery.

In contrast, MLSD with postoperative abdominal pain being rare owed to laparoscopic spleen extraction without enlarging any incision. In addition to entailing less postoperative pain than OSD, the extremely minimally invasive MLSD method is accompanied by more rapid recovery and lower incisional complication rates, owing to the extremely small incisions required. Of the 44 patients in our MLSD group, there were no incisional complications. Compared with the OSD group, the incision complication rate was significantly lower in the MLSD group (0% vs. 12.68%, $P<0.05$).

Because of the lower rate of abdominal pain in patients, MLSD may be associated with other benefits. For example, the absence of pain may have improved patients' appetite and gastrointestinal function, shorten postoperative times to oral intake and first flatus, respectively. Furthermore, reduced pain may also have promoted the recovery of pulmonary function, shortening the time to first off bed activity, and may also decrease the incidence of pulmonary complications.

In addition, the better visual field during MLSD than OSD may allow better inspection for bleeding, reducing the incidence of postoperative bleeding.

Although gastric fundus perforation as a complication has been reported after LSD [6, 10], none of the patients in our MLSD group suffered it. To our knowledge, thermal damage to the gastric wall caused by the LigaSure vessel-sealing device or devices that divide short gastric vessels is the main factors leading to gastric perforation. To avoid perforation, three steps were necessary before cutting the short gastric vessels. First, in order to increase splenic activity, most of the ligaments surrounding the spleen must be divided. Second, a 5 mm retractor the proximal stomach was lift toward the upper right by a 5 mm retractor, while the upper pole of the spleen was pushed toward the lower left by the bar of a tube-type forceps. Final, in order to spread out the length of the short gastric vessels to a certain extent, the visceral peritoneum of the short gastric vessels should be divided in advance (Fig. 3). Thus, full exposure of the short gastric vessels with sufficient length to avoid thermal damage to the gastric wall was gained.

Compared with OSD, MLSD is also significantly associated with shorter the number of days that patients had a postoperative temperature >38.0°C. Moreover, although pre-admission white blood cell count was similar in the two groups, white blood cell counts on postoperative days 1 ($P < 0.0001$) and 7 ($P < 0.05$) were significantly lower after MLSD than after OSD. These findings were consistent with each other, since high white blood cell count is related to high temperature. In contrast, between patients undergoing LSD and OSD, another study [6] reported there was no significant difference in day 7 white blood cell count (7.7 [range, 4.2-13.9] vs. 7.4 [range, 3.4-29.4], $P = 0.7673$). Thus, our findings suggest that MLSD maybe generate less inflammatory reactions compared with LSD and OSD.

Selective devascularization with ligation division of the esophagus, cardia, and proximal stomach without splenectomy has demonstrated similar results to those obtained with splenectomy [18]. Surgical disconnection does not change portal flow, thereby decreasing hepatocellular damage and encephalopathy [19]. Patients with splenectomy suffered from portal vein flow alteration frequently. This may damage liver function [20].

The risk of spontaneous bleeding is significantly increased by severe thrombocytopenia due to hypersplenism. It can postpone diagnostic or therapeutic procedures for cirrhotic patients, such as liver biopsy, interferon therapy, and hepatocellular carcinoma resection. Furthermore, bacterial infections may induced by leukocytopenia due to hypersplenism. In the present study, laparoscopic splenectomy was performed on all patients with platelet count of $\leq 50\times10^9$/L, and most of them suffered leukocytopenia. If patients with esophageal varices did not have severe thrombocytopenia and leukocytopenia due to hypersplenism, esophageal devascularization with splenic preservation may benefit patients.

The results of the present study presented indicate that MLSD is technically feasible and safe, and is preferable to OSD. MLSD was associated with minimal postoperative pain and scarring and faster postoperative recovery than OSD. It may become the gold standard for splenectomy and azygoportal disconnection.

Disclosure

Drs. D.-S. Bai, J.-J. Qian, P. Chen, J. Yao, X.-D. Wang, S.-J. Jin, and G.-Q. Jiang have no conflicts of interest or financial ties to disclose.

References

[1] Jiang XZ, Zhao SY, Luo H, Huang B, Wang CS, Chen L, Tao YJ (2009) Laparoscopic and open splenectomy and azygoportal disconnection for portal hypertension. *World J Gastroenterol* 15:3421-3425.

[2] Helmy A, Abdelkader Salama I, Schwaitzberg SD (2003) Laparoscopic esophagogastric devascularization in bleeding varices. *Surg Endosc* 17:1614–1619

[3] Wang Y, Ji Y, Zhu Y, Xie Z, Zhan X (2012) Laparoscopic splenectomy and azygoportal disconnection with intraoperative splenic blood salvage. *Surg Endosc* 26: 2195-2201.

[4] Yamamoto J, Nagai M, Smith B, Tamaki S, Kubota T, Sasaki K, Ohmori T, Maeda K (2006) Hand-assisted laparoscopic splenectomy and devascularization of the upper stomach in the management of gastric varices. *World J Surg* 30:1520–1525.

[5] Wang YD, Ye H, Ye ZY, Zhu YW, Xie ZJ, Zhu JH, Liu JM, Zhao T (2008) Laparoscopic splenectomy and azygoportal disconnection for bleeding varices with hypersplenism. *J Laparoendosc Adv Surg Tech A* 18:37–41.

[6] Zheng X, Liu Q, Yao Y (2013) Laparoscopic Splenectomy and Esophagogastric Devascularization Is a Safe, Effective, Minimally Invasive Alternative for the Treatment of Portal Hypertension With Refractory Variceal Bleeding. *Surg Innov* 20:32-9.

[7] Hashizume M, Tanoue K, Akahoshi T, Morita M, Ohta M, Tomikawa M, Sugimachi K (1999) Laparoscopic splenectomy: the latest modern technique. *Hepatogastroenterology* 46:820-824.

[8] Hong DF, Zheng XY, Peng SY, Gao M, Wu JG, Cao Q (2007) Laparoscopic splenectomy and pericardial devascularization for treatment of portal hypertension due to liver cirrhosis. *Zhonghua Yi Xue Za Zhi* 87:820-822.

[9] Wang Y, Zhan X, Zhu Y, Xie Z, Zhu J, Ye Z (2010) Laparoscopic splenectomy in portal hypertension: a single-surgeon 13-year experience. *Surg Endosc* 24:1164–1169.

[10] Xin Z, Qingguang L, Yingmin Y (2009) Total laparoscopic versus open splenectomy and esophagogastric devascularization in the management of portal hypertension: a comparative study. *Dig Surg* 26:499-505.

[11] Li SL, Li YC, Xu WL, Shi BJ (2009) Laparoscopic splenectomy and periesophagogastric devascularization with endoligature for portal hypertension in children. J Laparoendosc *Adv Surg Tech A* 19:545–550.

[12] Zhu JH, Wang YD, Ye ZY, Zhao T, Zhu YW, Xie ZJ, Liu JM (2009) Laparoscopic versus open splenectomy for hypersplenism secondary to liver cirrhosis. *Surg Laparosc Endosc Percutan Tech* 19:258–262.

[13] Habermalz B, Sauerland S, Decker G, Delaitre B, Gigot JF, Leandros E, Lechner K, Rhodes M, Silecchia G, Szold A, Tar-garona E, Torelli P, Neugebauer E (2008) Laparoscopic splenectomy: the clinical practice guidelines of the EuropeanAssociation for Endoscopic Surgery (EAES). *Surg Endosc* 22:821–848.

[14] Trelles N, Gagner M, Pomp A, Parikh M (2008) Laparoscopic splenectomy for massive splenomegaly: technical aspects of initial ligation of splenic artery and extraction without hand-assisted technique (case report). *J Laparoendosc Adv Surg Tech A* 18:391–395.

[15] Chapman CR, Casey KL, Dubner R, Foley KM, Gracely RH, Reading AE (1985) Pain measurement: an overview. *Pain* 22:1-31.

[16] Hoffmann NE, Bischof JC (2002) The cryobiology of cryosurgical injury. *Urology* 60:40-49.

[17] Gage AA, Baust J (1998) Mechanisms of tissue injury in cryosurgery. *Cryobiology* 37:171-186.

[18] Pin-Wen L, Ygn-Sheuy S (1992) Effects of splenectomy andsplenic artery ligation on the portal pressure in portal hypertensive rats. *J Surg Res* 53: 621–624.

[19] Chaib SA, Lessa BS, Cecconello I, Felix WN, Chaib E (1983) A new procedure for the treatment of bleeding esophageal varices by transgastric azygoportal disconnection. *Int Surg* 68: 353–356.

[20] Orozco H, Mercado MA, Martinez R, Tielve M, Chan C, Vasquez M, Zenteno-GuichardG, Pantoja JP (1998) Is splenectomy nec-essary in devascularization procedures for treatment of bleeding portal hypertension? *Arch Surg* 133: 36–38.

In: Laparoscopy
Editor: Christos Iavazzo
ISBN: 978-1-63321-404-0

Chapter 3

Single Incision Laparoscopic Splenectomy

Ioannis D. Gkegkes,[1] M.D. and Christos Iavazzo,[2] M.D., Ph.D.
[1]First Department of Surgery, General Hospital of Attica "KAT", Athens, Greece
[2]Gynaecological Oncology Department, Christie Hospital, Manchester, United Kingdom

Abstract

Recent advances in the surgical technique have favoured the development of minimally invasive procedures. Currently, the laparoendoscopic single-site surgery has accomplished conventional operations through a single incision with the utilization of common laparoscopic instruments. The application of single incision laparoscopic technique on the resection of spleen appears to be the natural evolution of the laparoendoscopic surgery. Even though, nowadays, this "scarless" technique seems to have good clinical outcomes, further technical improvement is required to establish the single-incision laparoscopic splenectomy as a common practice procedure.

The evolution of minimally invasive techniques has presently made feasible a great variety of major open surgery to "scarless surgery". Twenty years after the first laparoscopic splenectomy was performed, laparoendoscopic resection of spleen became a commonly utilized technique, safe and valuable in the hands of well-trained surgeons. [1] Currently, the development of laparoendoscopic single site surgery (LESS), which represents a novelty in the field of surgical technique, was became reality thanks to the overcome of technical issues, such as the absence of specifically designed single port systems, the lack of articulating instruments, the instrumental crowding and decreased visualization have restrained the broad use of the single-port surgical technique. [2] The introduction of single-port technique in the realization of splenectomy represent a important advance in minimally invasive surgery.

Shorter hospital stay, reduced morbidity, less postoperative pain and complications a well as better cosmetic outcome are the already known benefits of single-port surgery. Regarding the single-incision laparoscopic splenectomy (SILS), the clinical evidence is not sufficient in order to state with clearness the real potentialities of this new technique. [3] The selection of the single-port system used is correlated not only to the technical properties of each device but also to patient's body type. Moreover, one of the most frequent causes for conversion to laparotomy is the uncontrolled bleeding. According to the till now published studies, the rate of conversion are relatively low, similar to the published rates of conversion for a variety of laparoscopic operations. [3,4] Also, the rates of complications (intra-operative and post-operative) and of patients' deaths related to the single-port technique were comparable to the low incidence of the conventional laparoscopy. [4,5] Among the published evidences, there are 2 studies where SILS was applied in the management of splenic trauma. [6,7] Regarding the blunt trauma of the spleen, there are many risk factors that make obligatory the open surgical treatment (Injury Severity Score [≥20], high grade of splenic injury [grade III or more], presence of hemoperitoneum in ≥2 recesses, low Glasgow Coma Scale score). An open surgical management is the preferred approach in order to have a better overall view of the abdominal cavity and to control possible damages. Both traditional laparoscopic approach and SILS are not advisable for the treatment of splenic injury superior to grade I (haematoma subcapsular, <10% surface area / Laceration capsular tear, <1cm parenchymal depth). [8]

Single-port technique also presents some limitations. The utilization of the umbilicus or the periumbilical area as an entry point restricts the number of patients who may be suitable candidates for SILS due to the patients' elevated BMI. The use of either flexible endoscopes or proximally curved coaxial instruments with double bending may increase the intra-abdominal visualization of the surgical field, by passing the effect of instrument crowding. [9] Also, the installation of surgical ports with a large outer cap can increase the distance between instruments, increasing the triangulation and at the same time decreasing the effect of instrument crowding. A further limitation of the technique is that the handling of the laparoscopic instruments can possibly create CO_2 leakage from the entry point of the port system, interrupting the required stability of pneumoperitoneum in order to complete the entire operation. [3]

Surgical Technique

The patient is placed in reverse Trendelenburg position with the legs open. The surgeon is positioned between the patient's legs and the monitor is on the patient's left side. A periumbilical vertical incision (up to 40 mm) is made while the abdominal fascia is exposed and an absorbable suture is applied to it. Through the incision is positioned a multichannel single site device with the use of a Mayo-Guyon clamp. Pneumoperitoneum is established with the insufflation of carbon dioxide through the specific cannula, located on the multichannel single site device, at a constant pressure of 10 to 12 mm Hg in order to prevent gas embolism. Firstly, a high-definition camera is inserted while 2 or more laparoscopic instruments can be safely and easily inserted into the abdominal cavity under vision. Consequently, the body of the patient is adjusted into a semilateral or lateral position with the intention to expose the spleen. The splenocolic ligament and the splenogastric ligament were dissected using the LigaSure vessel sealing system (Covidien Valleylab, Boulder, CO, USA), rendering the splenic hilum visible. The splenic artery is clamped and dissected with the use of an endoscopic stapler. Subsequently, with the utilization of an intestinal retractor on the lower pole of the spleen, the rest of the splenic ligaments (such as the splenophrenic, splenorenal, and splenocolic ligaments) can be dissected with the use of harmonic shears. When the spleen is entirely free of its attachments, the resected specimen can be extracted, in a plastic bag, from the abdominal cavity through the umbilical hole after removal of the single-port device. In cases in which the splenic specimen has large dimensions, it can be morcellated with Pean forceps, under laparoscopic visualization. Careful hemostasis is achieved and a single drain may be placed at the splenic fossa. The peritoneal cavity is inspected and examined for any active hemorrhage. Both the fascia and the skin are closed separately.

The improvement of the existing port technology may establish SILS as a standard procedure in the near future. Even though the published data regarding the learning curve for the SILS are not sufficient, it is suggested that inexperienced surgeons should gain firstly sufficient dexterity on advanced multiport laparoscopy in order to be able to proceed to single incision technique. Therefore, at the beginning, it is advisable to avoid the performance either partial spleen resection or splenectomy.

References

[1] Rhodes M, Rudd M, O'Rourke N, et al. Laparoscopic splenectomy and lymph node biopsy for hematologic disorders. *Ann Surg.* 1995;222:43–46.

[2] Iavazzo C, Gkegkes ID. Single-site port robotic-assisted hysterectomy: a systematic review. *Arch Gynecol Obstet.* 2014 Apr;289(4):725–31.

[3] Gkegkes ID, Mourtarakos S, Iavazzo C. Single-incision laparoscopic splenectomy: a systematic review. *JSLS* 2014.[Article in press]

[4] Habermalz B, Sauerland S, Decker G, et al. Laparoscopic splenectomy: the clinical practice guidelines of the European Association for Endoscopic Surgery (EAES). *Surg Endosc.* 2008; 22:821–48.

[5] Telem D, Chin EH, Colon M, et al. Minimally invasive surgery for splenic malignancies. *Minerva Chir.* 2008;63:529–40.

[6] Hong TH, Lee SK, You YK, et al. Single-port laparoscopic partial splenectomy: a case report. *Surg Laparosc Endosc Percutan Tech.* 2010;20:e164–e166.

[7] You YK, Lee SK, Hong TH, et al. Single-port laparoscopic splenectomy: the first three cases. *Asian J Endosc Surg.* 2010;3: 33–35.

[8] Moore EE, Cogbill TH, Jurkovich GJ, Shackford SR, Malangoni MA, Champion HR. Organ injury scaling: spleen and liver (1994 revision*).* *J Trauma.* 1995 Mar;38(3):323–24.

[9] Jung YW, Kim SW, Kim YT. Recent advances of robotic surgery and single port laparoscopy in gynecologic oncology. *J Gynecol Oncol.* 2009;20:137–44.

In: Laparoscopy
Editor: Christos Iavazzo

ISBN: 978-1-63321-404-0

Chapter 4

Laparoscopic Liver Surgery

J. M. Ramia*[*,1], R. De la Plaza[1], F. Adel[1], M. Goergen[2], J. Garcia-Parreño[1] and J. S. Azagra[†2]

[1]Unidad de Cirugía Hepatobiliopancreática, Servicio de Cirugía General y Aparato Digestivo, Hospital Universitario de Guadalajara, Guadalajara. Spain

[2]Unité des Maladies de l'Appareil Digestif et Endocrine (UMADE), Centre Hospitalier de Luxembourg, Luxembourg

Abstract

Consolidation of laparoscopic liver surgery (LLS) has been slow due to its technique complexity, so liver has been one of the last abdominal organs treated by Minimal Invasive Surgery. First, only small resections of benign tumors located in easier segments were performed. Nowadays, every liver surgical technique made by open laparotomy, has been done by laparoscopic approach. LLS has several advantages to open approach: less blood loss, less postoperative pain, less analgesics, quicker oral intake, less hospital stay, less postoperative adherences and better cosmesis.

We have performed a literature review talking about: types of LLS, its surgical tips and tricks and results published in each disease treated by LLS (liver metastasis, hepatocellular carcinoma).

We could conclude that LLS is safe and feasible without increasing morbidity or mortality, and oncological results are comparable to those obtain by open approach. Minor hepatectomies in favourable segments (II al VI) are now the gold standard. Major hepatectomies or LLS in right posterior sector are not performed in many centers because they are technically demanding.

* CORRESPONDENCE: J.M. Ramia, C/General Moscardó 26, 5-1, Madrid 28020. (Spain), e-mail: jose_ramia@hotmail.com, Tlf: 0034-616292056

† Unité des Maladies de l'Appareil Digestif et Endocrine (UMADE), Centre Hospitalier de Luxembourg, 4 rue Barblé, L-1210, Luxembourg, Tel : +352 44 11 63 80, Fax : +352 44 11 62 74, Azagra.JS@chl.lu

Laparoscopic Liver Surgery

Laparoscopic liver surgery (LLR) is one of the last minimally invasive surgery techniques to have become consolidated. This is probably due to the fear of bleeding, the long learning curve, the need for adequate equipment for parenchymal section, the difficulty of access to certain segments, and the fear of gas embolism [1-13].

Initially, only small resections were performed in benign and small tumors localized in "favorable" segments (II to VI) [2,3,5,7,14-21]. Today, all liver surgery techniques involving laparotomy, for benign or malignant lesions localized in any segment, can be carried out via a laparoscopic approach, although major hepatectomies are not often performed [2,3,5,6,14,16-20,22-30].

Once an approach for small peripheral liver lesions attempted by only a few surgeons, LLR has now become the gold standard for certain procedures. Its use has increased exponentially in recent years [3,12,13,26,27]. Nguyen's et al. literature review published in 2009 included 2804 LLR [12], but today the number of LLR cases performed is far higher, and a search in PubMed (November 2013) for the term "laparoscopic liver surgery" yielded 5485 citations. At some specialized liver surgery units, between 25% and 80% of hepatectomies are performed via laparoscopic approach [2,6,12,31].

LLR presents a number of advantages over laparotomy surgery: lower blood loss, less postoperative pain and analgesic consumption, earlier oral intake, shorter hospital stay, fewer postoperative adhesions and better cosmetic results [1,2,6-10,12-15,21,25,26,28,30-34]. More importantly, the results obtained with LLR show that is safe, feasible and efficient when used in patients with either benign or malignant lesions [9,11,12,20]. But it should be borne in mind that the feasibility of LLR and the excellent results should never change the surgical indications, especially in benign tumors [6,12,27].

Classical contraindications for LLR are non-tolerance of pneumoperitoneum, adhesions from previous surgeries that impede laparoscopic vision, lesions very close to major vessels (portal vein or inferior vena cava) or the hepatic hilum; very large tumors, central or bilateral, the need for biliary or vascular liver resections and reconstructions, and tumors that require extensive periportal lymphadenectomy [4,6,12,16,19,26]. Probably today only intolerance of pneumoperitoneum and severe adhesions are real contraindications for LLR; the contraindications of tumor size and proximity to large vessels are debatable [16,19].

Conversion to open surgery should never be considered as a failure of LLR. Conversion rates vary widely according to the published series (0-55%), although the average is around 5% [1-4,6,12]. The most common cause is bleeding; others are proximity to large vessels, macroscopically positive or questionable margins, and lack of progress in surgery [2,4,6,12].

Morbidity associated with LLR ranges from 10 to 15%, and is highest in patients with hepatocellular carcinoma (HCC). Its mortality rate is below 1% [1,2,12]. Though there may be a selection publishing bias, it seems that morbidity and mortality in LLR are lower than in laparotomic surgery [2,4,6,12,13]. Some authors claim that the morbidity rate is related to the LLR technique (major hepatectomy vs minor) and lesion site, but others do not confirm these results [25,34]. The hepatectomy-related morbidity and mortality published in LLR (biliary fistulas and postoperative bleeding) are lower than or similar to those previously published in open surgery [1,2,21]. But the rate of decompensation in cirrhotic patients, cardiopulmonary complications, intra-abdominal abscesses, wound-related complications and rate of incisional hernia in LLR are lower than in open surgery [2,5,6].Economic studies show that LLR does not increase the total cost because the greater expense of the intraoperative devices is offset by the shorter hospital stay and lower complication rate [6,12,13,17,21]. Cannon et al. reported that LLR implies an average saving of $11,000 per patient, though the saving in cancer patients was less ($6000) and in right hepatectomy patients LLR cost $1300 more than open surgery [13].

No randomized controlled trials (RCT) have compared LLR and the laparotomy approach [7]. Croome et al. and Simillis et al. conducted two meta-analyses comparing the two approaches and concluded that LLR is better than open surgery in terms of intra-operative blood loss, postoperative pain and hospital stay, and obtains similar oncological outcomes such as survival and affected margins [1,2,5,12,16,19,35]. With regard to blood loss, it is believed that the role of the pneumoperitoneum and careful dissection made possible by the magnification provided by the laparoscope favors a reduction in bleeding [2]. Surgical time was initially higher in the LLR techniques than the open approach due to the initial learning curve, but now surgical times are very similar or may even be shorter in LLR [1,5,12]. The need for clamping and hilar clamping time is comparable in the two approaches [1].

Types of LLR

Three techniques have been used to perform LLR: pure laparoscopy, hand-assisted laparoscopy, and hybrid [4,12,15,21,24,28,36]. Other technical options are robotic surgery and single incision laparoscopic surgery (SILS).

Pure Laparoscopy

The pure laparoscopic technique involves intra-abdominal mobilization and parenchymal liver transection and subsequent removal of the laparoscopic specimen by extension of a trocar incision or usually a suprapubic accessory incision [4,24]. Initially used to wedge resections or minor hepatectomy, it is currently used for liver surgery of all kinds [4]. According to Nguyen's et al.' worldwide review, it is the most frequently performed technique, accounting for 75% of cases: in a Korean multicenter study it was applied in as many as 89% [3,6,12].

Hand Assisted Laparoscopic Surgery (HALS)

Hand-assisted laparoscopic surgery is used to perform hepatectomy by means of a hand-port and removal of the specimen through the hand-port incision [4,24]. It is more popular in the U.S. than in Europe [27]. Its main advantages are easier surgical field exposure, retention of tactile sensation, use of the hand to control bleeding and, in theory, a higher quality of cancer surgery. Its main disadvantages are the need for a larger incision than pure LLR, hand fatigue due to the use of the hand-port, and air leakage around the trocar [2,17,4-6,13,17,30,36]. In Nguyen et al's 2009 review [12], only 17% of cases published involved use of the hand-port, and even fewer (11%) in the Korean multicenter study by Park et al. [3]. Probably these figures will have fallen today, as HALS was used more when experience with LLR was limited. Initially, this technique was recommended for major hepatectomy and localized lesions in posterior segments, but today these situations are mostly approached using the pure technique [6]. HALs has also been used when there is no progression in pure laparoscopy in order to avoid conversion to laparotomy [1,6,12].

Hybrid

In this technical option, the liver is mobilized laparoscopically but liver transection is performed outside the abdomen after removing the liver via a mini-incision [17,24]. In the review by Nguyen et al. (12,36) the hybrid approach was used in only 2% of cases of LLR. This approach involves certain technical variations: the use of a medium or subcostal incision line, the use of a hand-port or a pure laparoscopic approach [4,36]. It has been used in living donor transplantation or in LLR programs as an initial approach for reducing the learning curve time [6].

Robotics

The first robotic LLR was performed by Giulanotti in 2003 [29]. In 2013 Reggiani et al. published a systematic review of the literature including 235 robotic LLR [9]. Theoretically, robotic surgery should perform better than conventional laparoscopic technique because it improves accuracy and vision, and is not affected by fatigue and tremor [9,15,29,30]. Robotic surgery appears to be particularly useful during hilar and hepatocaval dissection and for vascular or biliary reconstructions (29]. Clinical characteristics of patients undergoing robotic LLR and the results obtained are similar to those associated with the non-robotic approach: the tumors are less than 5 cm, 66% of the lesions are malignant, the conversion rate is 6-8%, 13% of patients present complications, and survival in cancer patients is similar [9]. in the robotic approach is the rate of major hepatectomy is higher, probably due to the better vision and control provided by the robot, and because the surgeons who routinely perform robotic surgery are very experienced [4,9,29,30]. In a study comparing laparoscopic vs robotic left lateral sectionectomy no significant increase in operative time or postoperative stay was observed [9]. Economic studies show that robotic surgery is more expensive than the LLR, but the learning curve may be shorter and the quality of the biliary or vascular reconstructions is substantially higher [6,9,17].

SILS

The SILS technique is another option for minor resections [4,21,37-43]. The main problems for liver surgery SILS are the learning curve, the loss of instrument triangulation, problems of vision because the camera and instruments are parallel, high cost and the risk of incisional hernias (14.19). An extensive bibliographical search revealed very few instances of

SILS used for liver surgery, mainly laparoscopic fenestration of simple cysts and small liver resections. The lesions were always located in favourable segments [14,19]. In any case, the surgeon's feeling is that liver SILS surgery is complex, technically demanding and not always feasible. In addition, additional ports may be required [18,19]. In a report of a small series of seven patients undergoing robotic surgery and SILS published in 2013 [30], the authors concluded that this combination facilitates LLR.

Technical Points in LLR

Anesthesia

Central venous pressure (CVP) should be maintained between 2-4 mm Hg during liver transection in order to minimize bleeding. The accurate measurement of CVP requires catheterization of a central line, which makes fast-track programs difficult. That is why should be avoided in minor resections [10,13]. The risk of gas embolism in LLR has been shown to be as low as 0.3% when working at pressures below 12 mm Hg.

Position

Several positions are standardly used in LLR but the two most frequent [13] are supine and left lateral decubitus. Surgeons may be on the left side of the patient or in the French position (surgeon between the legs). The best position depends on the location of the tumor. The supine position is useful for lesions in the left liver and anterior segments of the right liver, and lateral decubitus for posterior segments [13,21].

Trocars

There are many possible ways of placing trocars for LLR. The classical LLR technique uses five trocars (two 12 mm and one 10 mm, or three 12 mm, and two 5 mm). One 12 mm trocar is placed in the supra-umbilical region and the other two in the half-clavicular line, and the 5 mm trocars are placed in the epigastrium or the left hypochondrium and right hypochondrium. The surgeons who use a 5mm camera may replace the 12 mm umbilical trocar with a 5 mm one [45].

For lesions in the right liver (right hepatectomy and right posterolateral sector) three 12 mm trocars (supraumbilical, right midclavicular line and right flank) and two 5 mm trocars are often used, located in the epigastrium and more lateralized in the right flank [28]. Some authors use a sixth trocar to perform the Pringle maneuver [46]. (Fig.1) There are few reports of the use of three trocars [13,37,44]: in selected patients, those with peripheral lesions smaller than 5 cm can be performed with only three trocars instead of the classical five.

Intraoperative Ultrasound

The advent of laparoscopic intraoperative ultrasound has been vital for LLR because it allows intraoperative study of the liver parenchyma. It identifies lesions not visualized using imaging methods, determines the precise location of the great vessels and makes it possible to use the extra-Glissonian approach [6,26]. (Fig.2)

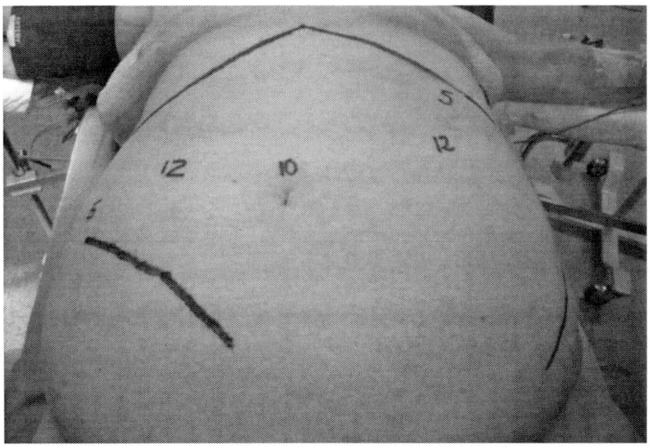

Figure 1. Position of trocars for laparoscopic liver resection.

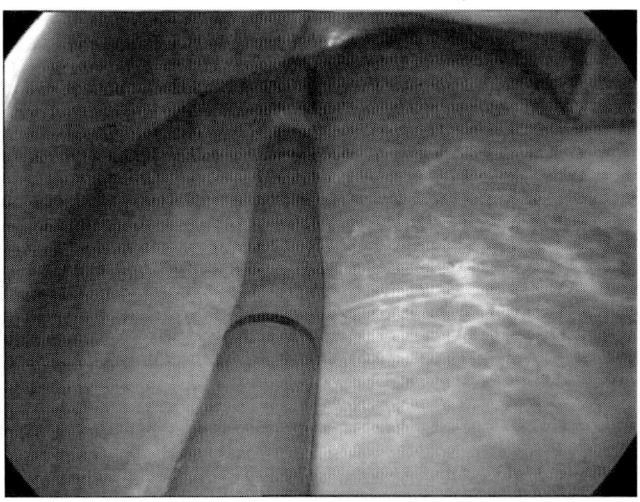

Figure 2. Laparoscopic Intraoperative ultrasound.

Pringle Maneuver

In the early days of LLR, hilar clamping was firmly recommended to decrease blood loss using an intracorporeal tourniquet technique, as described by Cherqui [37-44,46]. Rotellar et al. have recently described a new method for extracorporeal tourniquet triad clamping which is easy, cheap, and effective [12,46]. The series published show that in a variable percentage of patients (12.5% to 89%), LLR was performed without the Pringle maneuver [5,12,46]. Our policy is that in liver resections for small peripheral tumors, or in segmentectomies in favorable segments, it is not strictly necessary to perform hilar clamping, although it is advisable to prepare for any contingency [4,5].

Liver Parenchymal Transection

Liver parenchymal transection is a key point in liver surgery, because most of the bleeding events occur at this stage [12,46]. Currently, there are many possibilities for liver transection and none of the systems used have been shown to be superior in randomized control trials [4,13,21]. The choice of method depends on the surgeon's personal experience and preferences [13]. Transection can be performed with ultrasonic scalpel, sealants, mono or bipolar scalpel, clips and staplers (Figure 3) [4,5]. Staplers can be used to dissect the parenchyma or just to cut the great vessels; usually vascular loads of 25 mm [5,6] are used. (Figure 4)

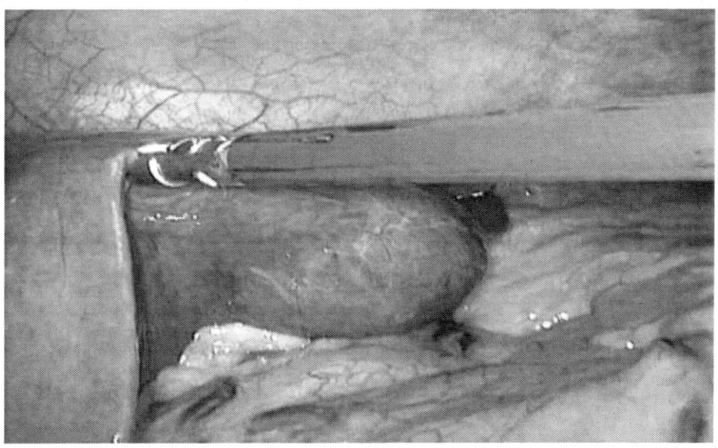

Figure 3. Parenchyma resection with Ligasure (R).

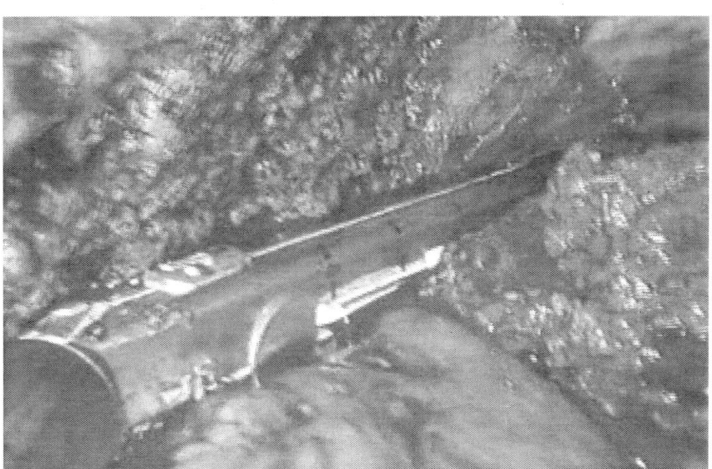

Figure 4. Parenchyma resection with staplers.

Removal of the Surgical Specimen

The surgical specimen is introduced into a bag and extracted by extending one of the 12 mm trocars, usually the umbilical trocar, or by performing a new incision usually made in the suprapubic area. Surgeons who use HALS extract the specimen through the hand-port.

LLR Surgical Techniques

Minor Hepatectomies and Wedge Resections

Approximately 70% of the cases published until 2009 were atypical resections (45%) or minor hepatectomies (25%) [12]. The first non-anatomic liver resection was performed by Gagner et al. [8]. In this type of resection, especially those located in favorable segments, there is a clear international consensus regarding the benefit of LLR over laparotomy. Indeed, LLR is considered the gold standard [4,5,14].

Left Lateral Sectionectomy

In 1996, Azagra et al. published the first report of laparoscopic left lateral sectionectomy (LLS) [3,12,47]. Twenty per cent of the LLR published until 2009 were LLS [12]. LLS is safe and feasible, and many authors now regard it as the approach of choice for lesions in the left lateral sector [14,18,19,48-50]. The popularity of the laparoscopic approach in this segment is due to its good accessibility [12,18,49,50]. Comparative studies of open and laparoscopic procedures are inconclusive; although the open procedure is faster, postoperative pain, hospital stay, and complication rates all appear to be lower with laparoscopic LLS [31,49,50,51].

Major Hepatectomy (Figure 5 and 6)

The first major hepatectomy using laparoscopy was performed in 1997 [52]. This technique requires extensive experience in laparoscopic and liver surgery and is not widely used [4,12,14,32,33]. Fear of intraoperative bleeding and its technical complexity (involving large vessel dissection and extensive parenchymal transection) have halted its expansion [12,27,33]. Initially only a very small number of surgeons applied this surgical procedure and its use has grown very slowly [12,33].

In 2009, in the review by Nguyen et al. only 17% of LLR were major hepatectomies [12]. In 2013, a multicenter study of ten European services with high experience in LLR included 495 major hepatectomies, which accounted for 22% of all LLR performed at these units. Seventy per cent were right hepatectomies, 80% were performed for malignant lesions and the conversion rate was 10% [27]. The number of extended right and left hepatectomies performed was very small; the multicenter study by Tzanis et al. included only 34 (7% of all major hepatectomies) [12,27]. The rate of major laparoscopic hepatectomies at units performing LLR ranges between 4 and 40% [27].

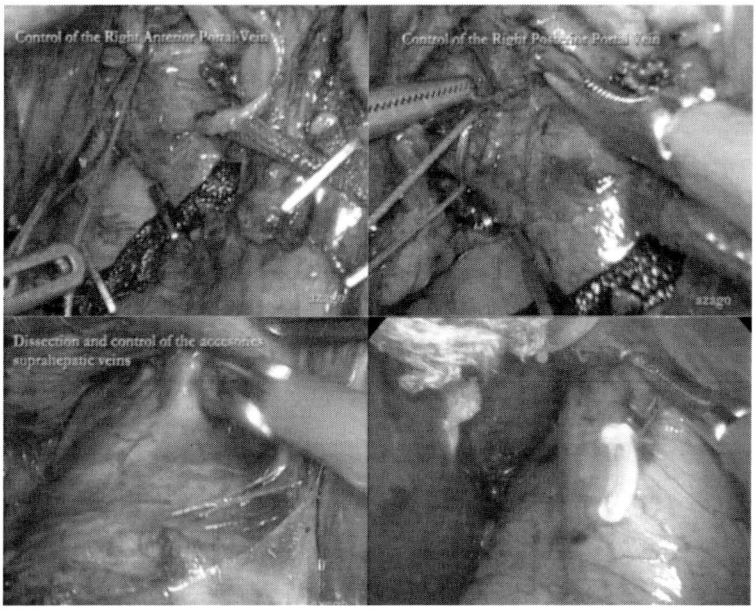

Figure 5. Vascular control: right posterior and anterior portal vein, accessory veins to inferior cava vein.

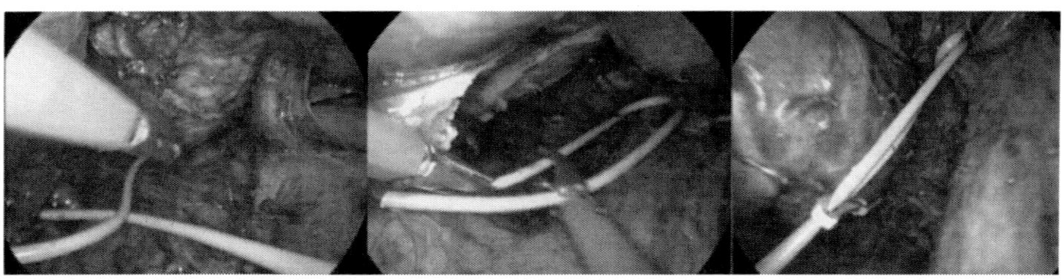

Figure 6. Control or right hepatic vein.

The published results of major hepatectomy for LLR show that when performed by surgeons with extensive experience it is a safe and efficient technique (24). Surgeons should select the best candidates: tumors far away from the transecting line or great vascular structures or large tumors. Some authors suggest that laparoscopy an extra-Glissonian approach facilitates major laparoscopic hepatectomy [11,14,45]. The hanging maneuver can be helpful for major hepatectomy (Figure 7).

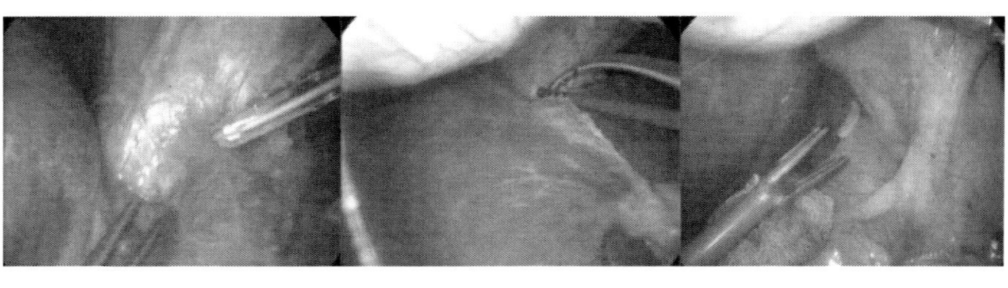

Figure 7. Hanging maneuver by laparoscopy.

Obviously, major laparoscopic hepatectomy always involves major bleeding, longer operative time and hospital stay than minor laparoscopic hepatectomy [12,24,32,33]. The mortality published in major laparoscopic hepatectomy is no greater than 1% [6].

Few studies have compared major hepatectomy using laparoscopic and open approaches. The review by Lin et al. reported lower blood loss and shorter portal clamping time, less morbidity and fewer severe complications, and shorter stay in the LLR group. The slight increase in operative time is likely to disappear as more experience is accumulated [14,24].

Combined Liver and Colorectal Surgery

Multiple series have shown that combined and sequential surgery in patients with synchronous LM obtains similar results. Additionally, in patients undergoing two-stage (TS) liver resection, if combined surgery is not performed three operations are required [5]. In 2010, Karoui et al. published a series of 33 patients with two-stage surgery combined with colorectal surgery, with good results (21% morbidity and 0% mortality) [5,8,9]. Combined laparoscopic colorectal tumor surgery and LM surgery presents certain advantages (easier access to both intra-abdominal regions, preservation of the abdominal wall, postoperative recovery room, and staging) without increasing morbidity or hospital stay, but it is not widely used [8-10].

Two Stage Laparoscopic Liver Resection

There are very few reports of two-stage (TS) laparoscopic liver resection. Machado et al. and Jain et al. reported totally laparoscopic two-stage liver resection almost simultaneously in 2010 (11,53). Later, in 2012, Robles et al. published two more totally laparoscopic two-stage hepatectomies [54]. The longest reported experience is a series of eight IS partial/total TS laparoscopic liver resection, five cases with laparoscopy in the first stage and laparotomy in the second, one conversion to laparotomy, and only two totally laparoscopic cases [55].

The first step of a TS can usually be performed by laparoscopic approach, because it is often a minor wedge resection in left lobe associating colon surgery and/or right portal vein ligation [11,55-7]. Laparoscopic ligation of the right portal vein, though feasible and successful, has been performed in very few patients [56]. The advantages of the laparoscopic first stage are: the reduction of intra-abdominal adhesions, appropriate oncological staging, less pain and shorter hospital stay, faster recovery and maintenance of the integrity of the abdominal wall [55,58]. The second part of TS (major hepatectomy) can be performed by laparoscopy or laparotomy, but as we noted above, the performance of major hepatectomy requires high technical skill [3,6].

Radiofrequency Ablation

Radiofrequency ablation (RFA) for treating LM or HCC can be performed by percutaneous, laparoscopy, or laparotomy approaches [17,59]. The percutaneous route is normally used. When laparotomy is used, the RFA is usually combined with some kind of hepatectomy. Laparoscopic RFA is usually performed in complex lesions located near large vessels or deep in the liver parenchyma which require major hepatectomy in patients who are unfit for surgery [60]. RFA has obtained acceptable oncological outcomes and may be an alternative in high-risk patients for performing hepatectomy (Child B) [17,59,61]. The advantage of laparoscopic RFA over the percutaneous approach is the theoretical lower rate of recurrence [61].

ALPPS

Associated Liver Portal vein ligation and Partition for Staged hepatectomy (ALPPS) has recently been described by experienced teams in short series of selected patients. It obtains good results in terms of liver hypertrophy and low rates of post-operative liver failure [22,62,63]. It comprises right portal vein ligation and in-situ liver splitting during the first surgical stage to obtain adequate left lobe hypertrophy and complete right hepatectomy with a very short delay (10 days) [62,63]. Therefore, the laparoscopic approach is promising because it may decrease the physiological response to two major surgeries, reducing levels of pain and blood requirement. From the technical perspective, laparoscopic ALPPS is extremely demanding, and very few surgeons have performed it; however, the experience demonstrates once again that, in expert hands, all forms of liver surgery can be performed via laparoscopy [22,23].

Diseases Treated by LLR

1. Benign Lesions

Gagner et al. performed the first LLR for a benign lesion in 1992 [21]. Today, around 40% of lesions treated with LLR are benign [3]. All types of benign liver cyst (simple cyst, polycystic, cystadenomas, and so on), solid lesions (hemangioma, focal nodular hyperplasia, liver cell adenoma, angiomyolipoma, and pseudotumors) and miscellaneous (hepatolithiasis, liver abscesses) have been treated by LLR [4,13,16]. We stress that he criteria for resection of benign liver lesions should not be expanded due to the existence of LLR: the surgical indications are symptomatic lesions, diagnostic doubt or complications [4,13,16]. Because of their unusual features, we now make some comments on liver cystic lesions and liver hydatid disease.

Liver Cysts

Although in 2008 the consensus conference of Louisville stated that fenestration of cysts should not be considered as LLR, we will briefly comment on this topic [64]. Before the emergence of LLR, open fenestration was used to treat symptomatic simple cysts. Now, except in extreme cases, this technique has been replaced by a laparoscopic approach [65].

In 2011 Qiu et al. conducted a systematic literature review comparing open and laparoscopic approaches for treating simple cysts including 657 patients [65]. In spite of the methodological weaknesses of some of the articles reviewed, Qiu et al. concluded that the laparoscopic approach has a shorter operating time, shorter hospital stay, less blood loss and obtains a faster return to working life, without increasing costs or the postoperative recurrence of cysts or symptoms [65]. These results can be extrapolated to patients with polycystic liver disease. We stress again that, despite the low technical difficulty of laparoscopic fenestration and the good results obtained, it should only be performed in symptomatic patients.

Liver Hydatidosis (Figure 8)

The first report of laparoscopic surgery for HCL was published in 1992 [13]. However, the number of patients that have undergone laparoscopic surgery for liver hydatidosis remains low; only around 750 cases have been reported and conservative surgery has almost always been used. The fear of spillage and anaphylaxis has probably discouraged surgeons from using laparoscopy in this indication [51,66,67].

The theoretical advantages of the laparoscopic approach to hydatid disease of the liver are similar to those of LLR [12,51]. The disadvantages are the difficulty of access to certain segments, embolism, and control of hemorrhage [51].

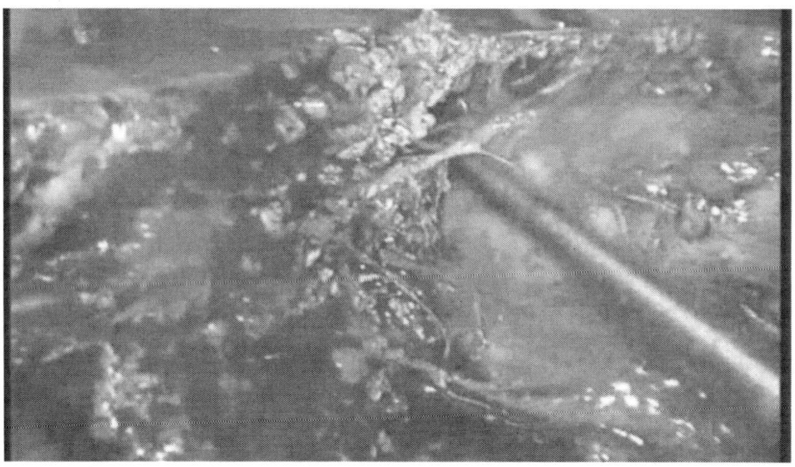

Figure 8. Liver hydatidosis. Laparoscopic total closed perycystectomy.

Classical contraindications for laparoscopy in liver hydatidosis include disseminated hydatid disease, intraparenchymal cysts, complicated cysts with cystobiliary communication, ruptured or infected cysts, cysts with thick and/or calcified walls, recurrent cysts and proximity to large vessels. Today, however, most of these conditions can be approached via laparoscopy [51,67-69]. Certainly, the laparoscopic approach is more complex in the presence of large or multiple cysts or when the cysts are in the central posterior segments [69]. The real feasibility of LLS in liver hydatidosis is not known [51].

2. Malignant (Primary and Metastasic) Lesions

LLR was initially performed only in benign lesions because of doubts regarding possible tumor dissemination, implants in trocars, poor identification of lesions, incomplete tumor resection and positive margins [1,5,12,18,20,21,33,34,52]. In 1994, two years after the first LLR for benign disease, the technique was applied to a malignant case for the first time [13,21]. In Nguyen's review published in 2009, 50% of the LLR reported were already performed in liver metastases and other malignancies, and this figure rose to 60% in the Korean multicenter study by Park et al. [3,12]. Theoretically, LLR in malignant disease has a number of advantages over the laparotomy approach, including the reduction of immunological alterations and surgical stress which are both promoters of tumor recurrence [1,6,26].

Although no RCTs have been performed, the efficiency of the LLR in cancer patients has been totally confirmed. The results for overall and disease-free survival in malignant disease and R0 resection rates in the approaches are similar, although the risk of a margin lower than 1 cm is greater in the LLR approach [1,4,5,15,16,21,26,35]. The most common criticisms are that patients undergoing LLR are a selected subgroup of straightforward cases, and the absence of randomized controlled trials comparing the two approaches [1,12,19,33-35]. In patients with malignant tumors, intraoperative laparoscopic ultrasound is mandatory to rule out other lesions and to obtain a negative margin [13,34].

Hepatocellular Carcinoma (HCC)

There are multiple treatment options for HCC (resection, transplantation, chemotherapy or ablative therapies). The number of patients with HCC who are candidates for surgical resection is low because HCC usually occurs in cirrhotic patients and the functional reserve limits the indications [60,70]. Traditionally, surgery was performed by laparotomy, but LLR in HCC has been shown to be a feasible, safe and efficient approach [4,13,25]. LLR for HCC is usually performed at specialized centers, and its use has not yet become widespread [16,19,20].

LLR is particularly useful in cirrhotic patients with HCC. It achieves better results than open surgery because it preserves abdominal collateral circulation, diminishes ascitic decompensation and reduces postoperative adhesions in these patients who may later require further surgery such as liver transplantation [13,16,18-20,25,26].

LLR is the best approach for small and peripheral HCC in cirrhotic liver [20]. The first cases treated were single HCC, but some authors claim that LLR is appropriate for up to three nodules or even more [19,20]. LLR can also be used prior to liver transplantation as a bridge method [21]. Laparoscopic RFA is another treatment option for HCC with low morbidity and mortality when resection or percutaneous RFA is not feasible [60,61].Two meta-analyses have compared open and LLR in HCC. LLR has shown better results in terms of reducing postoperative bleeding, transfusion requirements and morbidity, especially ascitic decompensation and postoperative stay [25,70]. The results for total and disease-free survival, positive margin percentage, mortality and recurrence are similar to those obtained with laparotomic surgery [21,25,70]. The decrease in intraoperative bleeding observed in LLR may be important in cancer because transfusion has been associated with poor survival and higher recurrence rate [25].

Liver Metastases from Colo-Rectal Cancer

Surgical resection is the treatment of choice in LM if it is feasible [6,13,21,24]. The review of Qiu et al. in 2013 included about 800 LM operated by LLR, but there are currently no RCTs comparing surgery of LM by LLR or laparotomy [71]. LLR has been performed as a first or second hepatectomy for LM [6,26]. The results of LLR treating LM as regards positive margin, total and disease-free survival are equal to or better than results obtained with laparotomic surgery. These findings confirm LLR's safety and oncological efficiency, along with the added benefits described above. Of course a certain bias in the selection of patients cannot be ruled out [4,13,16,17,34].

Other Malignant Tumors

Patients with LM from other tumors (neuroendocrine tumors, breast, GIST,...) and intrahepatic cholangiocarcinoma have been operated upon using a laparoscopic approach, but the published series are small [6].

3. Liver Transplantation

LLR has two main applications in the world of transplantation. The first is in the treatment of HCC as a bridge technique before liver transplant. LLR offers the following advantages: fewer intraabdominal adhesions during transplantation, and maintenance of the parietal integrity [4,6].The other is in the harvesting of the liver from the living donor [6]. In 2002, Cherqui published the first case of laparoscopic liver harvesting for adult-to-child living-donor transplantation [6,12,28,72,73]. Since then a number of cases have been performed. Most of them, especially adult-to-adult transplantation, were performed using the hybrid technique or hand-port [26,72-74]. In the last year, some reports of adult-to-adult right and left hemihepatectomies using a pure LLR approach have been published [4,12,28,72,73]. The drawbacks of LLR for harvesting are its technical complexity and the need to ensure total safety for the donor and the graft [28,72,73]. The advantage is the faster recovery in the donor [28,72,73].

Conclusion

Retrospective case-control studies have shown several advantages for LLR over laparotomy in surgical treatment of benign and malignant tumors: lower blood loss, less postoperative pain and analgesic consumption, earlier oral intake, shorter hospital stay, fewer adhesions and better postoperative aesthetic results without increased morbidity or worse oncologic outcomes. LLR therefore seems to be a safe, feasible and oncologically efficient option. Laparoscopic hepatectomy in the "favorable" segments (II to VI) may soon become the approach of choice despite the current absence of RCT studies. Major hepatectomy and resection of the posterior segments is not currently performed at many centers because of its technical difficulty.

References

[1] Croome KP, Yamashita MH Laparoscopic vs open hepatic resection for benign and malignant tumors. An updated meta-analysis *Arch Surg* 2010; 145: 1109-1118.

[2] Slakey DP, Simms E, Drew B, Yazdi F, Roberts B Complications of liver resection: laparoscopic versus open procedures *JSLS* 2013; 17: 46-55.

[3] Park JS, Han HS, Hwang DW, Yoon YS, Cho JY, Koh YS et al. Current status of laparoscopic liver resection in Korea. *JKMS* 2012; 27: 767-771.

[4] Mostaedi R, Milosevic Z, Han HS, Khatri VP Laparoscopic liver resection: current role and limitations *World J Gastrointest Oncol* 2012, 4: 187-han2.

[5] Lee KF, Cheung YS, Chong CN, Tsang YY, Ng WWC, Ling E et al. Laparoscopic versus open hepatectomy for liver tumors. A case control study *Hong Kong Med J* 2007;13.442-8.

[6] Edwin B, Nordin A, Kazaryan AM. Laparoscopic liver surgery: new frontiers. Scand J Surg 2011; 100: 54-65 7. Spencer L, Metcalfe MS, Strickland AD, Elsey EJ, Robertson GS, Lloyd DM Lessons from laparoscopic liver surgery: a nine-year case series. *HPB Surgery* 2008; doi: 10.1155/2008/458137.

[7] Salit Y, Bitterman A, Lefel O, Eisenberg D, Eden A, Barzelai M et al. Hand Assisted Laparoscopic Surgery for liver tumors *IMAJ* 2010; 12: 424-427.

[8] Reggiani P, Antonelli B, Rossi G Robotic surgery of the liver: italian experience and review of the literature *eCancer* 2013, 7: 358 DOI. 10.3332/ecancer.2013.358.

[9] Sanchez B, Aranda JM, Suarez MA, El-Adel M, Fernandez JL, Perez-Daga JA et al. Fast-track program in laparoscopic liver surgery *World J Gastrointest Surg* 2012; 4:246-250

[10] Machado MA, Makdissi FF, Surjan RC, Kappaz GT, Yamaguchi N. Two-stage laparoscopic liver resection for bilateral colorectal liver metastasis. *Surg Endosc* 2010, 24: 2044-47

[11] Nguyen KT, Gamblin TC, Geller DA World review of laparoscopic liver resection-2804 patients *Ann Surg* 2009; 250: 831-841

[12] Cannon RM, Scoggings CR, Callender GG, Quillo A, Mcmasters K, Martin II RCG Financial comparison of laparoscopic versus open hepatic resection using deviation-based cost modeling *Ann Surg Oncol* 2013; 20: 2887-2892.

[13] Dagher I, Di Giuro G, Dubrez J, Lainas P, Smadja C , Franco D Laparoscopic versus open right hepatectomy: a comparative study *Am J Surg* 2009; 198:173-177

[14] Tsung A, Geller DA, Sukato DC, Sabbaghian S, Tohme S, Steel J et al. Robotic versus Laparoscopic Hepatectomy. *A matched comparison Ann Surg* 2013; epub

[15] Hwang DW, Han HS, Yoon YS, Cho JY Laparoscopic liver resection. Future perspectives *GH Surgery* 2012; 2: 13-han

[16] Gueorguiev AL, Mackey R, Kowdley GC, Esquivel j, Cunningham SC Minimally invasive evaluation and treatment of colorrectal liver metastases *Int J Surg Oncol* 2011; 2011:686030. doi: 10.1155/2011/686030. Epub 2011 Jul 7. ID 686030.

[17] Herrero E, Cugat E, Garcia-Domingo MI, Rivero J, Camps J, Rodriguez A et al. Seccionectomia lateral izquierda por laparoscopia. Presentación de nuestra técnica *Cir Esp* 2011; 89: 650-656.

[18] Han HS, Yoon YS, Cho JY, 16 DW Laparoscopic liver resection for hepatocellular carcinoma. *Korean experiences Liver Cancer* 2013; 2. 25-30.

[19] Casaccia M, Andorno E, Di Domenico S, Nardi I, Bottino G, Nelli M, Valente U Laparoscopic liver resection for hepatocellular carcinoma in cirrhotic patients. Feasibility of non-anatomic resection in difficult tumor locations. *J Minim Access Surg* 2011; 7: 222-226.

[20] Kirchberg J, Reissfelder C, Weitz J, Koch M Laparoscopic surgery of liver tumors *Langenbecks Arch Surg* 2013; 398:931-938.

[21] M Goergen, O Facy, V Blasi, L Arru, V Lens, JS Azagra Right portal vein ligation and in-situ splitting by laparoscopy for two-stage hepatectomy. *Acta Chir Belg* 2014 In press.

[22] Brustia R, Scatton O, Perdigao F, El-Mouhadi S, Cauchy F, Soubrane O. Vessel identifications tags for open or laparoscopic associating liver partition and portal vein ligation for staged hepatectomy. *J Am Coll Surg* 2013;217:e51-5. doi: 10.1016/j.jamcollsurg.2013.08.020.

[23] Lin NC, Nitta H, Wakabayashi G Laparoscopic major hepatectomy. A systematic review and comparison of 3 techinuqes *Ann Surg* 2013; 257:205-213.

[24] Dagher I, Belli G, Fantini C, Laurent A, Tayat C, Lainas P, Tranchart H, Franco D, Cherqui D Laparoscopic hepatectomy for hepatocellular carcinoma. A european experience *J Am Coll Surg* 2010; 211:16-23.

[25] Shafaee Z, Kazaryan A, Marvin MR, Cannon R, Buell JF, Edwin B, Gayet B Is laparoscopic repeat hepatectomy feasible? A Tri-institutional analysis *J Am Coll Surg* 2011; 212: 171-179.

[26] Tzanis D, Shivathirtan N, Laurent A, Abu Hilal M, Soubrane O, Kazaryan AM et al. European experience of laparoscopic major hepatectomy. *J Hepatobiliary Pancreat Sci* 2013; 20: 120-124.

[27] Soubrane O, Perdigao Cotta F, Scatton O Pure laparoscopic right hepatectomy in a living donor *Am J Transplant* 2013; 13: 2467-2471.

[28] Milone L, Daskalaki D, Fernandes E, Damoli I, Giulanotti PC State of art in robotic hepatobiliary surgery *World J Surg* 2013; 37:2747-55.

[29] Kandil E, Naureline SI, Buell JF Robotic liver resection: inicial experience with three-arm robotic and single-port robotic technique *JSLS* 2013; 17:56-62.

[30] Van Dam RM, Wong Lun Hing EM, Van Breukelen GJP, Stoot JHMB, Van der Vorst JR, Bemelmans MHA et al. Open versus laparoscopic left lateral hepatic sectionectomy within an enhanced recovery ERAS programme (ORANGE II. Trial): study protocol for a randomised control trial *Trials* 2012; 13: 54-65.

[31] Belli G, Gayet B, Han HS, Wakabayashi G, Kim KH, Cannon R et al. Laparoscopic left hepatectomy a consideration for acceptance as standard of care *Surg Endosc* 2013; 27: 2721-2726.

[32] Abu-Hilal M, Di Fabio F, Salameh MA, Pearce NW Oncological efficiency analysis of laparosocopic liver resection for primary and metastastic cancer. *Arch Surg* 2012; 147:42-48.

[33] Bueno A, Rotellar F, Benito A, Martí-Cruchaga P, Zozaya G, Hermida J, Pardo F. Laparoscopic limited liver resection decreases morbidity irrespective of the hepatic segment resected. *HPB* (Oxford) 2013 Aug 22. doi: 10.1111/hpb.12147. [Epub ahead of print]

[34] Simillis C, Constantinides VA, Tekkis PP, Darzi A, Lovegrove R, Jiao L, Antoniou A.Laparoscopic versus open hepatic resections for benign and malignant neoplasms--a meta-analysis. *Surgery* 2007;141(2):203-211.

[35] Soyama A, Takatsuki M, Adachi T, Kitasato A, Torashima Y, Natsuda K et al. A hybrid method of laparoscopic-assisted open liver resection through a short upper

midline laparotomy can be applied for all types of hepatectomies *Surg Endosc* 2014; 28: 203-211.

[36] Ramia JM, De La Plaza R, Quiñones JE, Veguillas P, García-Parreño J. Resecciones menores laparoscopicas por tres trocares *Cir Esp* 2012; 90(10):670-672.

[37] Kobayashi S, Nagano H, Marubashi S, Wada H, Eguchi H, Takeda Y et al. A single incision laparoscopic hepatectomy for hepatocellular carcinoma. *Minim Invasive Ther Allied Technol* 2010; 19:367-71

[38] Shibao K, Higure A, Yamaguchi K Case report: laparoendoscopic single-site fenestration of giant hepatic cyst *Surg Technol Int* 2010; 20:133-6.

[39] Gaujoux S, Kingham TP, Jarnagin W, D´Angelica M, Allen PJ, Fong Y Single-incision laparoscopic liver resection. *Surg Endosc* 2011; 25:1489-1494.

[40] Cai XJ, Zhu ZY, Liang X, Yu H, Wang F, He JK, Li ZY Single incision laparoscopic liver resection: a case report *Chin Med J* 2010; 123:2619-20.

[41] Aldrighetti L, Guzzetti E, Ferla G Laparoscopic hepatic left lateral sectionectomy using the LaparoEndoscopic Single Site approach: evolution of minimally invasive liver surgery. *J Hepatobiliary Pancreat Sci* 2011; 18:103-105.

[42] Patel AG, Belgaumkar AP, James J, Singh UP, Carswll KA, Murgatroyd B Single incision laparoscopic left lateral segmentectomy of colorectal liver *metastases Surg Endosc* 2011; 25: 649-650.

[43] Toyama Y, Miyake R, Son K, Yoshida S, Usuba T, Nojiri et al. Three-port laparoscopic partial hepatectomy using an ultrasonically activated device. J Hepatobiliary Pancreat Surg 2006; 13:317-322. 45. Rotellar F, Pardo F, Benito A, Marti P, Zozaya G, Pedano N A novel extra-glissonian approach for totally laparoscopic left hepatectomy *Surg Endosc* 2012; 26: 2617-2622.

[44] Rotellar F, Pardo F, Bueno A, Marti P, Zozaya G Extracorporeal tourniquet method for intermittent hepatic pedicle clamping during laparoscopic liver surgery: an easy, cheap an effective technique Langenbecks *Arch Surg* 2012; 397: 481-485.

[45] Azagra S, Goergen M, Gilbart E, Jacobs D. Laparoscopic anatomical (hepatic) left lateral segmentectomy - technical aspects *Surg Endosc* 1996; 110: 758-761.

[46] Cannon RM, Brock GN, Marvin MR, Buell JF Laparoscopic liver resection: an examination of our first 300 patients. *J Am Coll Surg* 2011; 213: 501-507.

[47] Carswell KA, Sagias FG, Murgatroyd B, Rela M, Heaton N, Patel AG. Laparoscopic versus open left lateral segmentectomy *BMC Surgery* 2009; 9:14 doi: 10.1186/1471-2482.

[48] Rao A, Rao G, Ahmed I Laparoscopic left lateral liver resection should be a standard operation *Surg Endosc* 2011; 25: 1603-1610.

[49] Radical laparoscopic treatment for liver hydatidosis Ramia JM, Poves I, Castellón C, Diez-Valladares L, Loinaz C, Serrablo A, Suarez MA *World J Surg* 2013;37:2387-92.

[50] Nguyen KT, Laurent A, Dagher I, Geller D, Steel J, Thomas MT et al. Minimally invasive liver resection for metastasic colorectal cancer *Ann Surg* 2009; 250: 842-848

[51] Jain G, Parmar J, Mohammed MM, Bryant T, Kitteringham L, Pearce N, Abu-Hilal M Strecthing the limits of laparoscopic surgery: two stage laparoscopic liver resection *J Laparaendosc Adv Surg Tech* 2010; 20: 51-54.

[52] Robles R, Marín C, Lopez-Conesa A, Capel A, Perez-Flores D, Parrilla P. Comparative study of right portal vein ligation versus embolisation for induction of hypertrophy in

two-stage hepatectomy for multiple bilateral colorectal liver metastases. *Eur J Surg Oncol*. 2012 Jul;38(7):586-93.

[53] Di Fabio F, Whistance R, Rahman S, Primrose JN, Pearce NW, Abu Hilal M. Exploring the role of laparoscopic surgery in two-stage hepatectomy for bilobar colorectal liver metastases. *J Laparaendosc Adv Surg Tech* 2012; 22: 647-650.

[54] Ayiomamitis GD, Low JK, Alkari B, 5 SH, Ammori BJ Role of laparoscopic right portal vein ligation in planning staged or major liver resection *J Laparaendosc Adv Surg Tech* 2009; 19: 409-13.

[55] Ramia JM, Adel F, De la Plaza R, Veguillas P, García-Parreño J. *Primer tiempo laparoscopico en una cirugia hepatica en dos tiempos Cir Esp 2013 Oct 1.* doi:pii: S0009-739X(13)00266-2. 10.1016/j.ciresp.2013.05.013. [Epub ahead of print]

[56] Polignano FM, Quyn AJ, Sanjay P, Henderson NA, Tait IS. Totally laparoscopic strategies for the management of colorectal cancer with synchronous liver metástasis. *Surg Endosc* 2012; 26: 2571-2578.

[57] Aliyev S, Agcaoglu O, Aksoy E, Taskin HE; Vogt D, Fung J et al. Efficacy of laparoscopic radiofrequency ablation for the treatments of patients with small solitary colorectal liver metastasis *Surgery* 2013; 151:556-562.

[58] Herbold T, Wahba R, Bangard C, Demir M, Drebber U, Stippel DL The laparoscopic approach for radiofrequency ablation of hepatocellular carcinoma. Indication, technique, and results. *Langenbecks Arch Surg* 2013; 398: 47-53

[59] Cillo U, Vitale A, Dupuis D, Corso S, Neri D, D´Amico F et al. Laparoscopic ablation of hepatocellular carcinoma in cirrhotic patients unsuitable for liver resection or percutaneous treatment: a cohort study *PLos One* 2013; 8: e57249.

[60] Alvarez FA, Ardiles V, 10 Claria R et al. Associating liver partition and portal vein ligation for staged hepatectomy (ALPPS): tips and tricks. *J Gastrointest Surg* 2013; 17: 814-21.

[61] Schnitzbauer AA, Lang SA, Goessmann H et al. Right portal vein ligation combined with in situ splitting induces rapid left lateral liver lobe hypertrophy enabling 2-staged extended right hepatic resection in small-for-size settings. *Ann Surg* 2012; 255: 405-14.

[62] Buell JF, Cherqui D, Geller DA, O´Rourke N, Iannitti D, Dagher I et al. The Intenational position on laparoscopic liver surgery. The Louisville Statement 2008. *Ann Surg* 2009; 250:825-830.

[63] Qiu JG, Wu H, Jiang H, Huang JW, Pankaj P, Xu YL et al. Laparoscopic fenestration vs open fenestration in patients with congenital hepatic cysts. A meta-analysis. *World J Gastroenterol* 2011; 17: 3359-3365.

[64] Yaghan R, Heis H, Bani-hani K, Matalka I, Shatanawi N,Ghraibeh K, Bani-hani A. Is fear of anaphylactic shock discouraging surgeons from more widely adopting percutaneous and laparoscopic techniques in the treatment of liver hydatid cyst? *Am J Surg* 2004; 187:533-537.

[65] Muqim R, Kamran K, Khalil J, Gul T, Farid S Laparoscopic treatment of hepatic hydatid cyst. *J Coll Phys Surg Pak* 2011; 21: 468–471.

[66] Manterola C, Fernandez O, Muñoz S, Vial M, Losada H, Carrasco R et al. Laparoscopic pericystectomy for liver hydatid cysts. *Surg Endosc* 2002; 16: 521-524.

[67] Ertem M, Karahasanoglu T, Yavuz N, Erguney S. Laparocopically treated liver hydatid cysts. *Arch Surg* 2002; 137: 1170-1173.

[68] Xiong JJ, Altaf K, Javed MA, Huang W, Mukherjee R, Mai G et al. Meta-analysis of laparoscopic vs open liver resection for hepatocellular carcinoma *World J Gastroenterol* 2012; 18: 6657-6668.

[69] Qiu J, Chen S, Pankaj P, Wu H Laparoscopic hepatectomy for hepatic colorrectal metastases. A retrospective comparative chort analysis and literature review. *PLos One* 2013; 8: e60153.

[70] Rotellar F, Pardo F, Benito A, Marti P, Zozaya G, Lopez L et al. Totally laparoscopic right-lobe hepatectomy for adult living donor liver transplantation: useful strategies to enhance safety *Am J Transplant* 2013, 13: 3269-3273.

[71] Samstein B, Cherqui D, Rotellar F, griesemer A, Halazun KJ, Kato T et al. Totally laparoscopic full left hepatectomy for living donor liver transplantation in adolescent and adults *Am J Transplant* 2013; 13: 2462-2466.

[72] Marubashi S, Wada H, Kawamoto K, Kobayashi S, Eguchi H, Doki Y, Mori M, Nagano H. Laparoscopy-assisted hybrid left-side donor hepatectomy. *World J Surg* 2013;37:2202-10.

In: Laparoscopy
Editor: Christos Iavazzo
ISBN: 978-1-63321-404-0

Chapter 5

Single Incision Laparoscopic Hepatectomy

Ioannis D. Gkegkes, M.D.[1] ***and Christos Iavazzo, M.D., Ph.D.***[2]
[1]First Department of Surgery, General Hospital of Attica "KAT", Athens, Greece
[2]Gynaecological Oncology Department, Christie Hospital, Manchester, United Kingdom

Abstract

Single site port laparoscopic technique represents a promising minimally invasive procedure in the field of surgical oncology. The potential advantages of this method, such as less port-associated complications, better cosmesis and earlier recovery, could also be applied on liver surgery. The initial clinical outcomes of single incision laparoscopic procedure are encouraging and increase the expectations of this rather innovative surgical technique on hepatic resections.

The evolution of minimal invasive surgery has currently rendered laparoscopic techniques a useful alternative to open access surgery. The first laparoscopic liver resection was taken place in the early nineties.[1] The progression of major hepatectomies performed by the laparoscopic approach has been much slower due to the technical difficulties of the procedure and the absence of means to face the probability of an uncontrolled haemorrhage. Fortunately, the evolution of minimally invasive surgery and the progress on medical technology as well allowed the achievement of major laparoscopic hepatectomies with satisfying results.[2,3] Lately, technical novelties in the field of single incision laparoscopic surgery (SILS) permitted the realisation of single incision laparoscopic hepatectomy (SILH) expanding the frontiers of minimally invasive surgery.

Laparo-endoscopic single site surgery (LESS) is considered to be on of the recent surgical methods.[4] Since 1992, when the first laparoscopic appendectomy was performed by the use of a single umbilical incision,[5] various others surgical operations have been achieved including nephrectomies,[6], colostomies,[7] hernias,[8] cholecystectomies,[9] and splenectomies.[10] The major technical issues, such as the absence of specific port systems, the loss of instrumental triangulation, the effect of crowding and clashing between the instruments, the absence of high definition laparoscope, the lack of articulating instruments, have hold back the extensive utilization of single port-surgical technique while the lack of training programmes have made such operations difficult in the aspect of technique.

The last ten years have been made steps ahead and many technical issues have resolved. Presently, numerous multi-channel port devices are available. The single incision ports are usually made by flexible materials in order to increase the range of movements among the instruments, while the insertion of single site ports necessitate an incision of a diameter that range from 18 to 70 mm. In case of large hepatic resections, the limited dimensions of the port require its removal with the aim to pass the resected specimen through the incision. Apart the use of multi-channel port devices, the utilization of laparoscopic surgical ports combined with conventional wound retractors does not limit the diameter of the applied ports as well as the dimension of the single incision. Due to the fact that the position of the ports can be variable and greater manipulation of the instruments is permitted, while on the other hand, the removal of resected specimens needs a new incision at fascia, resulting in the loss of pneumoperitoneum. Last but not least, the coaxial presence of both the camera and the instruments at the multi-channel port systems eliminate the effect of triangulation. The utilization of proximally curved instruments with double bending (such as S-Portal curved instruments, Karl Storz GmbH & Co. KG) permits the crossing over of the laparoscopic instruments and allows their proper triangulation.

Single incision laparoscopic hepatic surgery represents an innovative alternative for the management of liver diseases. At present, the available clinical evidence on single incision hepatic surgery and particular on hepatectomy are scarce due to the novelty of the technique. According to a latest review, there is complete absence of large case series.[11] Reduced morbidity, less postoperative pain, shorter hospital stay and the better cosmetic outcome represent some of the potential benefits of single-port-access surgery. The effect of the limited surgical trauma at the abdominal wall caused by single incision technique may be particularly beneficial by reducing the events of bleeding, wound infections, ascites or incisional hernias, especially in patients with chronic liver diseases. In addition, the choice of the single incision during the placement of the trocars is in relationship with the patient's body type and the position of the lesions at the hepatic parenchyma.[12] Furthermore, the most frequent reasons for conversion to open laparotomy can be the poor localization of the neoplasia, the bleeding that can not otherwise treated and the slow progression during the liver parenchymal transection. From the available literature, the rates of conversion in open or in multiple laparoscopic surgery are considered relatively low,[12] while the absence of complications or deaths associated to the single port technique are relatively similar to the low incidence at the traditional laparoscopy.[13,14]

The application of SILS technique is also combined by some patient associated limits. The selection of umbilicus as the entry point of the multi-channel port devices restricts the number of patients who are suitable candidates for SILS in correlation to the patient's BMI. This problem can be resolved by using 8-mm as an alternative to 5-mm ports while the manipulation of the camera at 30 degree up or down can avoid the crowding the laparoscopic instruments. Regarding the visualisation of the surgical field can as well be assisted by the possible use of flexible endoscopes.[15] Furthermore, the various movements of the instruments may create gas leaking from some port systems, reducing the necessary pneumoperitoneum to carry out the operation.

Surgical Technique

The patient is placed in a reverse Trendelenburg position with his/her legs open while the surgeon is placed among them. A supraumbilical vertical incision is performed, the fascia is exposed and two absorbable stay sutures are applied into the fascia. A single-port device (which allows the entrance in the abdominal cavity a high definition camera, two assistant ports and an insufflator cannula) is safely and easily inserted into the abdomen through peritoneum by using a Mayo-Guyon clamp. Pneumoperitoneum is established by inducing carbon dioxide through the specific single-port cannula, at a constant pressure of <12 mmHg in order to prevent gas embolism. The high definition laparoscope is inserted throughout the single-port device with the aim to visualize the peritoneal cavity and then to introduce the rest of the instruments. Then, through an assistant port (10 mm access port), an intra-operative ultrasonography is performed, with the intention to valuate intraoperatively the extension of the surgical resection and the width of its safe resection margin. With the utilization of bipolar forceps and harmonic shears can be performed hepatic parenchymal transection. During the process of the hepatic transection, intra-operative ultrasonography is advisable to be repeated with the intention to guide the resection. With the completion of the transaction, the resected specimen is extracted from the abdominal cavity in a plastic bag, through the supraumbilical hole after removing the single-port device. Meticulous haemostasis is performed and both fascia and skin are closed.

In conclusion, the application of SILS technique, in liver surgical practice, appears to be promising. The continuous evolution and improvement of the laparoscopic instruments, as well as the increasing clinical experience on this field, can define the limitations and the real potentials of SILS technique on hepatobiliary surgery.

References

[1] Gagner M, Rheault M, Dubuc J. Laparoscopic partial hepatectomy for liver tumor. *Surg Endosc* 1992;6:97-8.

[2] Tzanis D, Shivathirthan N, Laurent A, Abu Hilal M, Soubrane O, Kazaryan AM, et al. European experience of laparoscopic major hepatectomy. *J Hepatobiliary Pancreat Sci* 2013;20:120-24.

[3] Pearce NW, Di Fabio F, Teng MJ, Syed S, Primrose JN, Abu Hilal M. Laparoscopic right hepatectomy: A challenging, but feasible, safe and efficient procedure. *Am J Surg* 2011;202:e52-8.

[4] Rao PP, Rao PP, Bhagwat S. Single-incision laparoscopic surgery-current status and controversies. *J Minim Access Surg* 2011;7:6-16.

[5] Pelosi MA, Pelosi MA 3rd. Laparoscopic appendectomy using a single umbilical puncture (minilaparoscopy). *J Reprod Med* 1992;37:588-94.

[6] Tam YH, Sihoe JD, Cheung ST, Lee KH, Chan KW, Pang KK. Single-incision laparoscopic nephrectomy and heminephroureterectomy in young children using conventional instruments: First report of initial experience. *Urology* 2011;77:711-15.

[7] Pietrasanta D, Romano N, Prosperi V, Lorenzetti L, Basili G, Goletti O. Single-incision laparoscopic right colectomy for cancer: A single-centre preliminary experience. *Updates Surg* 2010;62:111-15.
[8] Surgit O. Single-incision Laparoscopic surgery for total extraperitoneal repair of inguinal hernias in 23 patients. *Surg Laparosc Endosc Percutan Tech* 2010;20:114-18.
[9] Roberts KE, Solomon D, Duffy AJ, Bell RL. Single-incision laparoscopic cholecystectomy: A surgeon's initial experience with 56 consecutive cases and a review of the literature. *J Gastrointest Surg* 2010;14:506-10.
[10] Targarona EM, Pallares JL, Balague C, Luppi CR, Marinello F, Hernández P, et al. Single incision approach for splenic diseases: A preliminary report on a series of 8 cases. *Surg Endosc* 2010;24:2236-240.
[11] Gkegkes ID, Iavazzo D. Single incision laparoscopic hepatectomy: A systematic review. *Journal of Minimal Access Surgery* 2014; 10: 34-39.
[12] Pan M, Jiang Z, Cheng Y, Xu X, Zhang Z, Zhou C, et al. Single-incision laparoscopic hepatectomy for benign and malignant hepatopathy: Initial experience in 8 Chinese patients. *Surg Innov* 2012;19:446-51.
[13] Lin NC, Nitta H, Wakabayashi G. Laparoscopic major hepatectomy: A systematic literature review and comparison of 3 techniques. *Ann Surg* 2013;257:205-13.
[14] Rao A, Rao G, Ahmed I. Laparoscopic vs. open liver resection for malignant liver disease. A systematic review. Su*r*geon 2012;10:194-201.
[15] Jung YW, Kim SW, Kim YT. Recent advances of robotic surgery and single port laparoscopy in gynecologic oncology. *J Gynecol Oncol* 2009;20:137-44.

In: Laparoscopy
Editor: Christos Iavazzo

ISBN: 978-1-63321-404-0

Chapter 6

Laparoscopic Colorectal Surgery

***Victor H. Barnica, M.D.*[1]**
***and Assar A. Rather, M.D., F.A.C.S.*[2]**
[1]Mercy Catholic Medical Center, Darby, PA, US
[2]Bayhealth Medical Center, Dover, DE, US

Abstract

Laparoscopy was first described at the beginning of 20th century. The interface of creative surgeons and novel technology has resulted in significant advances and has radically transformed the landscape of operative surgery. In almost a century of gastrointestinal surgery, few advances can compare to the revolution engendered by the advent of minimally invasive surgery. Minimally invasive surgery has become the standard of care for a number of gastrointestinal afflictions.

Refinement of laparoscopic techniques has been the biggest contributor to the increase in the number of procedures performed in the last decade. The associated shorter length of stay, quicker recovery, less pain and large reduction in wound related problems has led to an increase in patient demand. Physiological basis for the benefits ascribed to minimally invasive surgery resides in the theoretic reduction in the inflammatory and immune responses when compared with conventional open approach. Pain caused by laparoscopic surgery is variable in duration, intensity and character. A combination of simple measures such as evacuating the insufflated gas, use of local anesthetic, preoperative use of paracetamol and use of moderately short acting intraoperative opioid reduces the immediate and referred pain. As in all aspects of medicine, Laparoscopic surgery requires experience on the part of surgeon in order to afford patients the best possible outcome and deal with the unique complications associated with its approach. In general laparoscopic approach should be considered for operations if same or similar procedure can be performed as would be done with open surgery with more benefits and less complications.

Introduction

The first laparoscopic colonic resections, which were described in the early 1990's, [1, 2] revolutionized and changed paradigms in the way surgery and more specifically, colorectal surgery is performed in the current surgical era. The initial skepticism within the surgical community, arose from early reports in the literature mentioning a high incidence in port site metastases and perhaps a suboptimal oncological resection, potentially compromising outcomes and survival. The proposed hypothesis for a higher incidence of metastases went from cancer cell growth stimulation by insufflation of the abdominal cavity, contaminated instruments and direct implantation at the site of extraction. More recent data suggests that the incidence of port metastases was just comparable to those seen at the incision site after open surgical resections [3-6]. It was not until 2004, when a large prospective randomized controlled trial. The Clinical Outcomes of Surgical Therapy, (COST) study [3], which randomized almost 900 patients to laparoscopic or open colectomy for primary colonic malignancies, presented solid evidence that laparoscopic colectomy had comparable outcomes to open surgery, it was then, when laparoscopy for colonic malignancies gained wide acceptance. Laparoscopy for benign colorectal pathology, such as rectal prolapse, inflammatory bowel disease (IBD) and diverticulosis has been largely proven to offer at least, comparable results as with open surgery in terms of functional outcomes in addition to the well-known superior short term outcomes, which are discussed later in this chapter. As technology has moved forward and laparoscopic instruments and energy devises have been perfected, the different techniques have also evolved into more refined and precise techniques minimizing blood loss and operative time. Currently, laparoscopy has been adopted for the management of a variety of gastrointestinal pathological entities, including benign, malignant, inflammatory and even re operative surgery, in well selected cases.

In this chapter, we will discuss the most popular colorectal laparoscopic procedures and their indications, as well as different techniques with a particular focus on outcomes.

A) Laparoscopic segmental colectomy which includes:

- Right colectomy
- Left/Sigmoid colectomy

B) Total /Subtotal colectomy with and without anastomosis
C) Proctectomy/Proctocolectomy with and without anastomosis
D) Low anterior resection of the rectum

A) Laparoscopic Segmental Colectomy

Right Colectomy

Indications:

- Malignancies of the ascending colon or proximal transverse colon
- Polyps that are not amenable to endoscopic removal

- Cecal volvulus
- Crohn's disease

Operating Room Setup and Patient Position

For right hemicolectomy or ileocolic resection, the surgeon typically stands on the patient's left side. Position the patient supine on the operating room table with at least left, if not both arms tucked, and properly padded and protected alongside the body to prevent injuries to the ulnar nerve or brachial plexus. A moldable bean bag may be placed under the torso to secure the patient to the operating table. This helps to keep the patient's body from sliding during the steep changes in position required for laparoscopic colectomy. Two monitors are placed at the right side of the patient (one at the head and one at the bottom of the table). The camera person should stand next to the surgeon so that the operating team views the monitor from the same angle and facilitate guidance of the laparoscope.

Trocar Placement

The first trocar is typically placed in the supraumbilical region however, in some cases infraumbilical initial trocar placement may be utilized. This allows a vertical midline extraction of the specimen. It is recommended that the initial trocar is placed with an open technique, particularly for reoperative surgery, but a Veress needle may be used based on surgeon's preference. A 30 degree laparoscope is used in all procedures. Two 10 to 12 millimeter ports are placed on the left side about a handbreadth apart. Additional 5mm trocars can be placed in the suprapubic area or right lower quadrant, which may facilitate the lateral mobilization of the ascending colon and hepatic flexure. Clearly 10 to 12 millimeter ports offer more versatility as compared to 5 millimeter ports, but with the availability of 5 millimeter vessel sealing devices, laparoscopes, and other instrumentation, small trocars may be used at the surgeon's discretion.

Technique

A thorough inspection of the liver and the peritoneal cavity is required for patients with cancer to exclude metastatic disease. A combination of Trendelenburg position and tilt towards the left is utilized (Right side up) to expose the cecum. The small bowel is carefully placed towards the left upper quadrant to complete our exposure. Different techniques have been described to perform the mobilizations of the colon and ligation of the vascular pedicles. The most commonly used techniques are medial to lateral approach and lateral to medial. We prefer lateral to medial technique.

Lateral-to-Medial Technique

Once the terminal ileum and cecum have been exposed. The cecum is grasped with atraumatic graspers and retracted medially and towards the left upper quadrant. The white line of Toldt is opened just lateral to the cecum with a 5-mm energy device or electrocautery scissors and this dissection continued cephalad towards the hepatic flexure.

The cecum and ascending colon are reflected medially, exposing the right ureter, Gerota's fascia, and duodenum .Once the duodenum is visualized the dissection is complete.

The patient is repositioned in reverse Trendelenburg and the transverse colon is retracted caudad and towards the abdominal wall by grasping the greater omentum in proximity to the colon, this maneuver applies tension over the gastrocolic ligament facilitating its division. The division of the gastrocolic ligament is started slightly distal to the middle colic vessels, dissection is continued towards the hepatic flexure completing the mobilization of the transverse colon. Inferior traction on the latter, allows mobilization of the posterior transverse mesocolon, exposing the duodenum further, this can be done bluntly and with minimal use of an energy devise.

The mobilization is complete if the ascending colon and ileocecal junction can easily reach the extraction site.

After a complete mobilization of the colon, ligate the vessels intracorporeally. Anterolateral retraction of the colon facilitates the identification of ileocolic trunk. Isolate the vessel close to the root by scoring the mesentery on both sides of the vessel and creating a window. The vessels are typically divided by using a vessel sealing device or endoscopic linear stapler with a white vascular cartridge. Mesenteric dissection on the small bowel side is accomplished with a vessel sealer and the bowel is transected with an endoscopic GIA stapler. The Right branch of the middle colic artery and vein are divided with a vessel sealing device.

A grasper is left on the cecum or terminal ileum to bring the specimen to the extraction site. The pneumoperitoneum is released and the supra umbilical trocar site extended up to four centimeters. A wound protector is placed and the specimen is then carefully delivered.

The ileocolonic anastomosis is completed utilizing a GIA stapler in a side to side, functional end to end fashion and returned into the peritoneal Cavity. The pneumoperitoneum is restored by closing the wound protector and the anastomosis is inspected to ensure hemostasis, as well as proper orientation of the terminal ileum. The fascia is closed with absorbable # 1 PDS and the skin is closed with interrupted subcuticular sutures.

Medial-to-Lateral Technique

This technique follows the same steps as the lateral to medial approach, except that the order of the steps is completely opposite, starting with mesenteric and vascular dissection and finishing with the mobilization of the colon from the lateral attachments. Using atraumatic graspers, superior and medial traction is applied to the right mesocolon in proximity to the cecum. The ileocolic pedicle is identified under the mesentery. Utilizing monopolar shears or any energy devise, a window is created in the mesentery by scoring the peritoneum along the axis of the pedicle. The artery and vein are dissected circumferentially and divided utilizing a bipolar vessel sealing devise, vascular endoscopic clips or stapler, applied just distal to the takeoff from the mesenteric vessels. Once the vessels are divided, blunt dissection under the mesentery is carried out in a cephalad fashion, until the duodenum is visualized and gently dissected off the posterior aspect of the transverse mesocolon, utilizing blunt technique with any atraumatic blunt tipped endoscopic instrument. The right branch of the middle colic artery and vein are divided as described above. Once the medial (mesenteric) dissection is completed, the lateral mobilization of the colon is performed as described in the previous section.

Left Colectomy and Sigmoid Resection

Indications

- Diverticular disease
- Segmental Crohn's colitis
- Endoscopically unresectable polyps
- Colon cancer
- Volvulus
- Endometriosis
- Rectal prolapse

Operating Room Set up and Patient Position

The patient is placed in a modified lithotomy position, the pelvis should be just above the break at the lower end of the operating table to provide adequate access to the anus for stapled anastomosis, intraoperative endoscopy, and/or perineal dissection if required. Place the legs in a 20 to 25 degree abducted position with the thighs at a lower level than that of the abdominal wall. The surgeon generally stands on the opposite side of the pathology, but may stand between the patient's legs for mobilization of the splenic flexure. The first assistant should stand opposite the surgeon, on the same side as the pathology. The second assistant (the camera person) should stand next to the surgeon.

Trocar Placement

The first trocar is typically placed in the supraumbilical region however, in some cases infraumbilical initial trocar placement may be utilized. This allows a vertical midline extraction of the specimen. A 30 degree laparoscope is used in all procedures. Two 10 to 12 millimeter ports are placed on the right side about a handbreadth apart. A third trocar may be placed in the left lower quadrant to aid in the mobilization of the splenic flexure. A left upper quadrant trocar placed lateral to the rectus muscle may be used for additional retraction, this site also provides an excellent vantage point for visualization of the anastomosis.

Technique

With the patient placed in a steep Trendelenburg position and a tilt towards the right, the small bowel is carefully brought to the right upper quadrant to gain proper exposure to the descending and sigmoid colon mesentery.

Lateral-to-Medial Technique

The sigmoid colon is retracted medially utilizing atraumatic graspers, the lateral attachments are divided up to the splenic flexure, using monopolar cautery or any other energy devise. As this dissection is carried out, the posterior aspect of the left mesocolon is carefuly dissected off the retroperitoneum, properly exposing the left ureter and Gerota's fascia. The splenic flexure is then mobilized, this may be facilitated by placing the patient in steep reverse Trendelenburg. The transverse colon is mobilized by diving the gastrocolic ligament with the energy devise of choice. This maneuver is facilitated by lifting the transverse colon towards the abdominal wall and gentle traction towards the pelvis. Divide the attachments of the body and tail of pancreas to the colonic mesentery obtaining a full splenic flexure release. Once complete mobilization has been accomplished, the vascular dissection is carried out. Of note, if colectomy is being performed in the setting of benign disease, the vascular dissection can be done at the level of the superior hemorrhoidal and left colic arteries. In the setting of malignant disease, a high ligation of the inferior mesenteric artery (IMA) is performed, just distal to the takeoff from the aorta. It is imperative to once again, confirm the location of the left ureter prior to vessel ligation. The vessels are divided either using bipolar energy devise, vascular endoscopic clips or stapler. Our preference is to perform the vascular ligation utilizing endoscopic stapler. Division of the mesentery is continued cephalad and the inferior mesenteric vein is identified at the base of the ligament of Treitz, this is isolated and ligated using any of the devises above mentioned. The distal margin of colonic resection is chosen depending on the etiology and extent of disease. A window is created at the mesentery in proximity to the wall of the colon, and division is carried out utilizing an endoscopic 60mm linear stapler.

A small Pfannensteil incision is the preferred extraction site in our practice. A wound protector is utilized and the specimen is delivered. The proximal resection is done extracorporeally utilizing the same technique utilized for the distal margin. The staple line is removed from the proximal margin utilizing electrocautery, a purse-string suture is used and a circular stapler anvil is inserted into the proximal end of the colon. The purse-string suture is secured and the colon is reintroduced into the peritoneal cavity. The pneumoperitoneum is reestablished by closing the fascia at the ends and leaving the suture ends untied to facilitate placement of a Hasson trocar. The length of the colon is assessed to ensure the proximal end will reach the distal without tension. Further mobilization may need to be performed in order to avoid tension at the anastomosis. The circular stapler is inserted transanally and spiked through the distal colonic/rectal stump under direct visualization. Proper orientation of the colon is assured to avoid twisting of the mesentery. The anvil is engaged to the stapler's spike utilizing an atraumatic grasper to avoid damage to the anvil's mechanism. The stapler is closed, fired and removed carefully. Inspection of the resection margins (Donuts) inside the stapler is done on the back table. A leak test is performed by clamping the colon proximal to the anastomosis, utilizing a laparoscopic bowel clamp. Transanal air insufflation is used to test the anastomosis under water submersion. Flexible sigmoidoscope can also be used to leak test and also to rule out anastomotic bleeding. Integrity of the anastomosis is confirmed if no obvious bubbles are observed. Hemostasis is assured and the pneumoperitoneum is evacuated removing all trocars under direct visualization. The extraction site and the 12 mm trocar sites are closed at the fascia with absorbable sutures.

Medial-to-Lateral Technique

In this technique, the vascular approach is the first step of the dissection. The vessels are exposed opening the peritoneum at the base of the sigmoid mesocolon. With this approach, the surgeon is able to identify the left ureter and gonadal vessels prior to the mobilization, minimizing ureteral injuries.

Using an atraumatic grasper, the sigmoid mesocolon is retracted anteriorly towards the abdominal wall, exposing the base of the mesentery. The mesentery is scored starting at the sacral promontory and this dissection continued cephalad along the anterolateral aspect of the aorta, creating a window immediately under the inferior mesenteric artery (IMA) up to its origin in the aorta. The IMA is carefully skeletonized near its origin prior to its division, thus decreasing the risk of injury to the left sympathetic trunk and left ureter. The IMA is divided at its origin, utilizing either bipolar sealing devise, vascular endoscopic clips or linear stapler. The inferior mesenteric vein (IMV) is identified immediately to the left of the IMA, which is dissected and divided just lateral to the ligament of Treitz in a similar fashion as the IMA.

Once the vascular dissection is completed, the mesentery is dissected off the retroperitoneum utilizing blunt dissection in a medial to lateral fashion. The rest of the mobilization is done in a lateral to medial fashion, as it was described above.

B) Total and Subtotal Abdominal Colectomy

Indications

- Ulcerative colitis refractory to medical management
- Dysplasia in the setting of long standing Ulcerative colitis
- Familial adenomatous polyposis syndrome (FAP)
- Hereditary nonpolyposis colorectal cancer (HNPCC)

Trocar Placement

The first trocar is typically placed in the supraumblical region; however, in certain cases, an infraumbilical initial trocar may be utilized. This is typically done when a vertical midline extraction in the lower abdomen is possible (based on patients' body habitus and pathology) this site may be used. In general, four operating trocars are placed, one in each quadrant lateral to the rectus sheath [41]. The sizes of trocars vary based on the instruments used for dissection, vessel ligation and bowel transection. The dissection can begin on either side, beginning in the right or left iliac fossa.

Mobilization of Right Colon

Both medial-to-lateral and lateral-to-medial approaches can be utilized and the choice depends on surgeons' experience and preference. We describe the lateral to medical approach first. Position the patient in steep Trendelenburg position with the table tilted towards the left (right side up), facilitating the exposure by displacing the small bowel loops from right lower quadrant.

The mobilization of the ascending colon begins along the white line of Toldt while the assistant retracts the ascending colon medially. Dissection can be performed with a variety of energy devices including ultrasonic Scalpel, bipolar sealing devices or electrocautery using scissors or hooks. Once the ureter, Gerota's fascia, and duodenum are exposed, the dissection of the hepatic flexure is completed.

Continued mobilization medially exposes the third portion of the duodenum, thus completing the mobilization of the ascending colon.

Mobilization of Transverse Colon

The patient is placed in reverse Trendelenburg position to allow gravity play its role during this portion of the procedure. The Transverse colon is grasped with an atraumatic grasper and the gastrocolic ligament retracted towards the abdominal wall and superiorly to create some degree of countertraction. Utilizing an energy device, the gastrocolic ligament is divided at its full length, from hepatic to splenic flexure. Carefully identify and preserve the gastroepiploic vessels. Applying constant traction and countertraction on the omentum in cephalad direction and transverse colon in caudal direction exposes the lesser sac. Once in the lesser sac, lyse any adhesions from the stomach to transverse mesocolon and completely separate the omentum from the transverse colon until the splenic flexure is reached. In order to facilitate complete mobilization, the surgeon may need to change position and move to right side or in between the patient's legs.

Mobilization of Left Colon

The patient is placed in Trendelenburg position with a right side tilt (right side down) of the table. Mobilization on the left side along the white line of Toldt is carried out in a similar fashion to that on the right colon, starting at the left pelvic brim. Meticulously identify and preserve the left ureter and the gonadal vessels. Again, complete dissection of all attachments and clear identification of Gerota's fascia and completely mobilize the left mesocolon. The splenic flexure and the distal transverse colon are then mobilized, this dissection is made easier sometimes, if the surgeon stands between the patient's legs and uses left lower quadrant port site. Care should be taken as the splenic flexure is taken down to avoid injury to the spleen.

Transection of the Mesenteric Vessels

Once complete mobilization of the colon, the vessels are ligated intracorporeally. Anterolateral retraction of the colon facilitates this identification of major vascular pedicles. The vessels are isolated by scoring the mesentery over the vessel and creating windows in the mesentery on each side. These vessels are typically divided by using a vessel-sealing device or endoscopic linear stapler with a (white or gray) vascular cartridge. Again our preference is to use vascular stapler. In the medial-to-lateral approach, the major vascular pedicles are identified and divided first before the lateral mobilization of the colon. During this approach, the same principles are followed as if segmental resection is being done in a medial to lateral approach as described earlier in this chapter. Identify the distal end of resection and circumferentially expose the colonic or rectal wall. The bowel is divided using a 60-mm endoscopic stapler with a blue or green cartridge. A grasper is used to grab the proximal staple line to assist in specimen extraction. The skin incision is extended in the midline or a Pfannenstiel incision can be used for specimen extraction utilizing a wound protector. The small bowel should be inspected in its entirety to rule out the presence of crohn's disease. This can be done either intracorporeally or outside the peritoneal cavity. If an ileorectal anastomosis is to be constructed, this is done in the same fashion as it is done with the colorectal anastomosis described in the left/sigmoid colectomy section earlier in this chapter. As with conventional surgery, the integrity of the anastomosis is confirmed with a leak test as described earlier.

C) Proctectomy

With the patient in steep Trendelenburg position to allow for gravity retraction of the small bowel from the pelvis.

The uterus is retracted anteriorly by suspending it with a suture through the abdominal wall. Once the superior hemorrhoidal artery has been divided, the rectum is mobilized entering presacral space just posterior to the rectosigmoid junction at the sacral promontory in the avascular plane, often eluded to as the "Holy plane", the dissection is carried distally up to the levator muscles.

The ureters are identified as they cross the pelvic brim to enter the bladder and kept away from the dissection field. The dissection is continued laterally and subsequently anteriorly staying on the rectal side of the Denonvillier's Fascia. The rectum is separated from the vagina in females and prostrate/seminal vesicles in males. Once the rectum is circumferentially mobilized up to the level of levators, the perineal dissection is then carried out. This involves removal of anorectum with preservation of external sphincter. It is accomplished as in open surgery and the dissection is carried proximally in a circumferential manner to the level of levator ani muscle, where the dissection meets with the mobilized rectum from above. The entire specimen can be removed through the perineal incision. Then, place a moist sponge to temporarily seal the wound and reinstate pneumoperitoneum.

D) Low Anterior Resection

Indications:

- Resection of the rectosigmoid or rectum for both benign and malignant conditions.
- Rectal polyps not amenable to endoscopic or transanal resection.
- Low rectal cancer without sphincter invasion.

Operating Room Setup and Patient Positioning

The patient is placed on modified lithotomy position with both arms are placed alongside the body.

Trocar Placement

The trocar placement is similar to that utilized during left and sigmoid colectomy. The pneumoperitoneum is then established using a open technique with a Hasson trocar as described earlier in this chapter. Once the pneumoperitoneum is established to 15mmHg, a 30 degree camera is introduced, followed by the rest of the trocars as previously described.

The mobilization of the sigmoid and descending colon is performed in a medial-to-lateral approach (see left and sigmoid colectomy), the left ureter and gonadal vessels are identified in the retroperitoneum, followed by the vascular dissection, involving the IMA and IMV. The lateral mobilization of the sigmoid, descending colon and splenic flexure are carried out.

Once mobilization of the colon is satisfactorily completed, the rectal dissection is started. While the assistant retracts the rectum cephalad, the presacral space is opened utilizing electrocautery, careful blunt dissection may be helpful to identify the proper plane of dissection between the presacral fascia and mesorectum, this is oftentimes referred to as the “holy plane”. The hypogastric nerves should be identified and carefully pushed away from the dissection plane to avoid injury to them. The peritoneal reflection is opened following a counter clock wise direction, continuing the dissection towards the right of the rectum, division of the middle rectal vessels is done utilizing an energy devise as dissection progresses deeper into the pelvis. Continuing with the dissection circumferentially, the anterior dissection is carried at the rectovaginal space in women and Denonvillier’s fascia in men. Once the circumferential dissection is completed beyond the level of the tumor with sufficient distal margins, the mesorectum is thinned down at the transection margin, utilizing electrocautery or any energy device in order to facilitate the transection. Utilizing a linear 45mm or 60mm articulating stapler, introduced through the 12mm trocar on the right lower quadrant, the rectum is retracted cephalad and to the left and division is carried at the selected transection point. The umbilical trocar site is enlarged up to 4cm and the specimen is delivered and divided with a linear stapler. A circular stapler is used to create our anastomosis, utilizing the same technique described in the left and sigmoid colectomy section.

Decision to create a protective diverting loop ileostomy is based upon patient factors like nutrition status, preoperative radiation, technical difficulties and level of anastomosis among others.

Outcomes

The benefits that laparoscopic colorectal surgery offers are no different than what minimal access surgery offers over other traditional surgical procedures.

Several studies including randomized trials and meta-Analysis support the fact that patients who undergo laparoscopic colon resection have a shorter recovery time to first flatus and bowel movement, [4, 8-9] which in turn leads to shorter hospital stay ranging from 0.8 to 1.4 days less than open surgery [3, 4, 7, 8, 11-17, 21]. The benefits of laparoscopy in pain control after surgery have also been well documented by numerous randomized trials, showing decreased pain, narcotic requirements and faster recovery [3, 7, 9, 10, 12-15]. Another not so tangible but probable benefit from laparoscopic surgery, which translates into less patient trauma and less postoperative pain, may be the association with less immunosuppression, though the data remain a subject of debate and the clinical relevance of this effect remains unclear [18]. In a recent prospective randomized trial study by Veenhof et al. comparing the immunologic response to stress after laparoscopic or open colorectal surgery, expression of HLA-DR, levels of interleukin 6 (IL-6) and C reactive protein (CRP) where compared among groups utilizing repeated measures of 2 way ANOVA to ensure that the results were secondary to the operation performed and not to the perioperative care. Expression of HLA-DR was lower (P= 0.002), IL-6 (P= 0.001) and C reactive protein levels (P= 0.022) were the highest in the open surgery group when compared to laparoscopic group levels. The results suggest that immune response remained highest and may explain why patients in the laparoscopic arm present an accelerated recovery [19]. Another recent study by Wang et al. compared the immunologic response to stress of individuals undergoing laparoscopic versus open colorectal surgery, inflammatory reactions, based on interleukin-6 and C-reactive protein levels, were less intense following laparoscopic operation compared to open operation; however, there were no differences in specific immunity (CD3+ and CD4+ counts, and the CD4+/CD8+ ratio) during these two types of surgical procedures [20]. The afore mentioned results may suggest that a combination of reduction in surgery related stress and preservation of the postoperative immune function may contribute to better postoperative results, nonetheless, the precise clinical relevance of a preserved immune integrity in postoperative patients is yet to be elucidated.

One of the most notable advantages of laparoscopic colorectal surgery is the remarkable decrease, not only in pain and incisional hernias, but also the incidence on surgical site infections (SSI) when compared to open colorectal surgery [26,27]. A recent study utilizing NSQIP data, reviewed over 3,000 patients undergoing elective laparoscopic and open partial colectomy. After propensity score matching, those patients who underwent laparoscopic segmental colectomy presented a significantly lower incidence of SSI when compared to those in the open colectomy group (9.0% vs. 5.9%; p=0.003) [28].

As far as complications are concerned, there is a specific subset of complications directly related to the laparoscopic approach for colorectal procedures. Complications ranging from those related to access, for instance trocar related complications such as bleeding, bowel injury and trocar site hernias as well as intraoperative complications such as injury to solid organs, bleeding and bowel injury have also been described in numerous studies to different extents. The lack of a standardized trocar insertion technique in the current literature addressing laparoscopy in colorectal surgery, makes it difficult to draw conclusions as to what technique carries a higher incidence of complications. The majority of available data addressing this particular issue, come from laparoscopic surgery for other abdominal procedures and it involves a variety of patient-specific factors like previous abdominal surgeries, morbid obesity or a combination of both. That, in addition to the diverse preferences among surgeons in different circumstances makes it difficult to study this in a retrospective fashion. Hence, the reported complication rates in the literature are widely variable. For instance, in a recent review of 6000 cases [21] the reported incidence of visceral and vascular injuries utilizing open cut down technique (Hasson) for the insertion of the first trocar was 0%. Only 7.9% of patients had previous abdominal surgery which clearly suggesting its safety in virgin abdomens. In another study the incidence of bowel injury during a laparoscopic procedure was reported to be 0.13% to 0.22%. The small bowel was the most common site of injury 55% followed by the colon at 38%. The most common mechanism of injury was Veress needle insertion in 42% of cases, occurring even more often than thermal injuries during laparoscopic dissection and manipulation (26%). A history of prior abdominal surgery or adhesions was a significant risk factor for injury, accounting for 69% of the cases of bowel injury. [22]

A recent meta-Analysis by Ahmand et al. involving 4860 patients compared the use of open technique and close entry technique. Open technique had a reduced incidence in failed entry attempts when compared to a close entry technique, with no difference in the incidence of visceral or vascular injury. However, studies were limited to small numbers, excluding many patients with previous abdominal surgery and women with a raised body mass index who may have unusually high complication rates [23]. Bleeding from trocar sites has been equally described in the literature, however the true incidence is not known with certainty, since most of those bleeds are dealt with in the operating room, nonetheless, incidence has been reported within the range of 1% or less [24, 25]. Perhaps the reason for this issue being under reported is that only small portion of those bleeds go unrecognized and develop an abdominal wall hematoma, significantly increasing morbidity and perhaps requiring evacuation and control of the involved vessel. Bleeding from the abdominal wall may not become apparent until after the port is removed, stopping the tamponade effect over muscular or subcutaneous bleeding. Major bleeding from trocar sites, that require significant efforts to control is not very common and is usually due to injury to the inferior epigastric vessels while inserting secondary trocars. Placing and removing trocars carefully under direct visualization may reduce the risk of injury to major abdominal wall vessels and increase the chances to identify it prior to leaving the operating room. Significant bleeding may necessitate extension of the incision at the trocar site and the use of hemostatic sutures to the fascia or muscle. Minor trocar related bleedings can usually be controlled with electrocautery.

The literature is less clear-cut when talking about the incidence of major intraoperative complications like bowel injury, hemorrhage and solid organ injury comparing open and laparoscopic approaches. Two recent meta-Analyses focusing on short and long term outcomes between laparoscopic and open colorectal surgery showed conflicting results [29, 30]. The incidence of ureteral injury during colorectal surgery is overall relatively low and has been reported to be 0.3 to 1.5 % across the literature. [31-35] However, over the past two decades there has been an increase in such injures, presumably due to the increase in the popularity of laparoscopic surgery, as suggested by Palaniappa et al. [36], whose data demonstrated a slight but significant increased incidence of iatrogenic ureteral injuries (0.15% vs 0.66%, P= 0.007) when comparing open versus laparoscopic approach.

Perhaps the most dreaded and potentially fatal complication in colorectal surgery is an anastomotic leak. The risk of anastomosis leak may differ based on the technique and anatomic location, which may carry differences in vascular supply arrangement, mesenteric mobility, bacterial loads and consistency of the fecal matter. The incidence of anastomotic complications between total laparoscopic and laparoscopic assisted colectomies has been assessed in multiple studies including different types of resections, invariably showing comparable rates of anastomotic complications between the two techniques, applied to different segments of the colon [37, 38]. The most significant differences found between the two approaches are the length of extraction site, which tends to be smaller in those with intracorporeal anastomosis and longer operative times [39, 40].

Conclusion

Laparoscopic colorectal procedures are becoming more popular as the technology improves and the body of evidence proving its benefits continues to grow. Although the learning curve its quite steep, more and more surgical trainees are completing their training with a fair amount of complex laparoscopic cases, including basic segmental colonic resections. The laparoscopic approach is associated with longer operating-room times, however as surgeons become more proficient with the different techniques, operative times continue to drop. Laparoscopic colorectal surgery in experienced hands is just as safe as the traditional open approaches and it is significantly superior in terms of short-term outcomes, such as faster recovery, less pain, earlier return of bowel function and shorter hospital stays with a faster return to work, which translates into meaningful advantages for patients. Although minimally invasive, it is paramount to understand that the laparoscopic approach has a very unique set of complications related to the technique itself, the surgeon should be cognizant of those and be prepared to deal with them. The long term outcomes, including the appropriateness of oncological resections with comparable survival rates, make laparoscopy the preferred method of bowel resection and perhaps will soon become the standard of care approach in colorectal surgery.

References

[1] Jacobs M., Verdeja J. C., Goldstein H. S. Minimally invasive colon resection (laparoscopic colectomy). *Surg. Laparosc. Endosc.*, 1991;1:144–50.

[2] Schlinkert R. T. Laparoscopic-assisted right hemicolectomy. *Dis. Colon. Rectum.*, 1991 Nov;34(11):1030-1.

[3] Clinical Outcomes of Surgical Therapy Study Group. A comparison of laparoscopically assisted and open colectomy for colon cancer. *N. Engl. J. Med.*, 2004 May 13;350 (20): 2050–9.

[4] Lacy A. M., García-Valdecasas J. C., Delgado S., et al. Laparoscopy- assisted colectomy versus open colectomy for treatment of non-metastatic colon cancer: a randomised trial. *Lancet,* 2002 Jun. 29;359 (9325): 2224–9.
[5] Allardyce R. A. Is the port site really at risk? Biology, mechanisms and prevention: a critical review. *Aust. N. Z. J. Surg.,* 1999;69:479–85.
[6] Zmora O., Gervaz P., Wexner S. D. Trocar site recurrence in laparoscopic surgery for colorectalcancer: myth or real concern? *Surg. Endosc.*, 2001;15:788–93.
[7] Kaiser A. M., Kang J. C., Chan L. S., et al. Laparoscopic-assisted versus open colectomy for colon cancer: a prospective randomized trial. *J. Laparoendosc. Adv. Surg. Tech. A.,* 2004;14: 329–34.
[8] Schwenk W., Haase O., Neudecker J., et al. Short term benefits of laparoscopic colorectal resection. *Cochrane Database Syst. Rev.*, 2005;(3):CD003145.
[9] The Colon Cancer Laparoscopic or Open Resection Study Group. Laparoscopic surgery versus open surgery for colon cancer: short-term outcomes of a randomized trial. *Lancet Oncol.*, 2005;6:477–84.
[10] Milsom J. W., Bo¨hm B., Hammerhofer K. A., et al. A prospective, randomized trial comparing laparoscopic versus conventional techniques in colorectal cancer surgery: a preliminary report. *J. Am. Coll. Surg.*, 1998;187:46–57.
[11] Weeks J. C., Nelson H., Gelber S., et al. Short-term quality-of-life outcomes following laparoscopically- assisted colectomy vs open colectomy for colon cancer: a randomized trial. *JAMA,* 2002;287:321–8.
[12] Stage J. G., Schulze S., Moller P., et al. Prospective randomized study of laparoscopic versus open colonic resection for adenocarcinoma. *Br. J. Surg.*, 1997;84:391–6.
[13] Hasegawa H., Kabeshima Y., Watanabe M., et al. Randomized controlled trial of laparoscopic versus open colectomy for advanced colorectal cancer. *Surg. Endosc.,* 2003;17:636–40.
[14] Schwenk W., Böhm B., Müller J. M. Postoperative pain and fatigue after laparoscopic or conventional colorectal resections: a prospective randomized trial. *Surg. Endosc.*, 1998;12:1131–6.
[15] Hewitt P. M., Ip S. M., Kwok S. P., et al. Laparoscopic-assisted versus open surgery for colorectal cancer: comparative study of immune effects. *Dis. Colon. Rectum,* 1998;41: 9019.
[16] Curet M. J., Putrakul K., Pitcher D. E., et al. Laparoscopically assisted colon resection for colon carcinoma: perioperative results and long-term outcome. *Surg. Endosc.*, 2000; 14: 1062–6.
[17] Guillou P. J., Quirke P., Thorpe H., et al. Short-term endpoints of conventional versus laparoscopic-assisted surgery in patients with colorectal cancer (MRC CLASICC trial): multicentre, randomized controlled trial. *Lancet,* 2005;365:1718–26.
[18] Ng C. S. H., Whelan R. L., Lacy A. M., Yim A. P. Is minimal accesssurgery for cancer associated with immunologic benefits? *World J. Surg.*, 2005 Aug.; 29(8):975–81.
[19] Veenhof A. A., Vlug M. S., van der Pas M. H., Sietses C., van der Peet D. L., de Lange-de Klerk E. S., Bonjer H. J., Bemelman W. A., Cuesta M. A. Surgical stress response and postoperative immune function after laparoscopy or open surgery with fast track or standard perioperative care: a randomized trial. *Ann. Surg.*, 2012 Feb.;255 (2): 216-21.

[20] Wang G., Zhiwei Jiang, Kun Zhao, Guoli Li, Fengtao Liu, Huafeng Pan, Jieshou Li Immunologic response after laparoscopic colon cancer operation within an enhanced recovery program. *J. Gastrointest. Surg.*, 2012 Jul.;16(7):1379-88.

[21] Lal P., Vindal A., Sharma R., et al. Safety of open technique for first-trocar placement in laparoscopic surgery: a series of 6,000 cases. *Surg. Endosc.*, 2012; 26(1): 182–8.

[22] Van der Voort M., Heijnsdijk E. A., Gouma D. J. Bowel injury as a complication of laparoscopy. *Br. J. Surg.*, 2004; 91: 16538.

[23] Ahmad G., O'Flynn H., Duffy J. M., Phillips K., Watson A. Laparoscopic entry techniques. *Cochrane Database Syst. Rev.*, 2012 Feb. 15; 2:CD006583.

[24] Karthik S., Augustine A. J., Shibumon M. M., Pai M. V. Analysis of laparoscopic port site complications: A descriptive study. J. Minim. Access Surg., 2013 Apr.;9(2): 59-64.

[25] Azevedo J. L., Azevedo O. C., Miyahira S. A., Miguel G. P., Becker O. M. Jr., Hypólito O. H., Machado A. C., Cardia W., Yamaguchi G. A., Godinho L., Freire D., Almeida C. E., Moreira C. H., Freire D. F. Injuries caused by Veress needle insertion for creation of pneumoperitoneum: a systematic literature review. *Surg. Endosc.*, 2009, Jul. ;23(7): 1428-32.

[26] Kiran R. P., El-Gazzaz G. H., Vogel J. D., Remzi F. H. Laparoscopic approach significantly reduces surgical site infections after colorectal surgery: data from national surgical quality improvement program. *J. Am. Coll. Surg.*, 2010; 211: 232-8.

[27] Bilimoria K. Y., Bentrem D. J., Merkow R. P., Nelson H., Wang E., Ko C. Y., Soper N. J. Laparoscopic-assisted vs. open colectomy for cancer: comparison of short-term outcomes from 121 hospitals. *J. Gastrointest. Surg.*, 2008; 12: 2001-9.

[28] Wilson M. Z., Hollenbeak C. S., Stewart D. B. Laparoscopic colectomy is associated with a lower incidence of postoperative complications compared with open colectomy: a propensity score-matched cohort analysis. *Colorectal Dis.*, 2013 Dec. 21 doi: 10.1111/ codi.12537. (accepted not published).

[29] Ohtani H., Tamamori Y., Arimoto Y., et al. A meta-analysis of the short- and long-term results of randomized controlled trials that compared laparoscopy-assisted and conventional open surgery for colorectal cancer. *J. Cancer*, 2011;2:425–34.

[30] Sammour T., Kahokehr A., Srinivasa S., et al. Laparoscopic colorectal surgery is associated with a higher intraoperative complication rate than open surgery. *Ann. Surg.*, 2011; 253(1): 35–43.

[31] Dowling R. A., Corriere J. N. Jr., Sandler C. M. Iatrogenic ureteral injury. *J. Urol.*, 1986; 135(5): 912-915.

[32] Parpala-Spårman T., Paananen I., Santala M., Ohtonen P., Hellström P. Increasing numbers of ureteric injuries after the introduction of laparoscopic surgery. *Scand. J. Urol. Nephrol.*, 2008; 42(5): 422-427.

[33] Selzman A. A., Spirnak J. P. Iatrogenic ureteral injuries: a 20-year experience in treating 165 injuries. *J. Urol.*, 1996; 155(3): 878-881

[34] Liu C. Laparoscopic Ureteral Surgery: Prevention and Management of Laparoscopic Surgical Complications. Miami, FL: Society of Laparoscopic Surgeons, Inc; 1999.

[35] Gomel V., James C. Intraoperative management of ureteral injury during operative laparoscopy. *Fertil Steril.*, 1991; 55(2): 416-419.

[36] Nam Y. S., Wexner S. D. Clinical value of prophylactic ureteral stent indwellingduring laparoscopic colorectal surgery. *J. Korean Med. Sci.*, 2002; 17(5): 633–5.

[37] Ko¨ckerling F., Rose J., Schneider C., et al. Laparoscopic colorectal anastomosis: risk of postoperative leakage. Results of a multicenter study. Laparoscopic Colorectal Surgery Study Group (LCSSG). *Surg. Endosc.*, 1999; 13(7): 639–44.

[38] Scatizzi M., Kro¨ning K. C., Borrelli A., et al. Extracorporeal versus intracorporeal anastomosis after laparoscopic right colectomy for cancer: a case-control study. *World J. Surg.,* 2010; 34(12): 2902–8.

[39] Lee K. H. , Ho J., Akmal Y., Nelson R., Pigazzi A., Short- and long-term outcomes of intracorporeal versus extracorporeal ileocolic anastomosis in laparoscopic right hemicolectomy for colon cancer, *Surg. Endosc.*, (2013) 27:1986–1990.

[40] Magistro C., Di Lernia S., Ferrari G., Zullino A., Mazzola M., De Martini P., De Carli S., Forgione S., Bertoglio C. L. and Pugliese R. Totally laparoscopic versus laparoscopic-assisted right colectomy for colon cancer: is there any advantage in short-term outcomes? A prospective comparative assessment in our center, *Surg. Endosc.,* (2013) 27:2613–2618.

[41] Rather A. A., Weiss E. G., Laparoscopy for Crohn's colitis. Nguyen N. T.; Scott-Conner C. E, The SAGES manual Vol. 2: Advanced Laparoscopy and Endoscopy, Third edition, Springer New York, 2012, p 515-530.

In: Laparoscopy
Editor: Christos Iavazzo
ISBN: 978-1-63321-404-0

Chapter 7

Role of Diagnostic Laparoscopy in Gastric Cancer Staging

***Abraham El-Sedfy*[1,2], *Matthew Dixon*[1,4], *Savtaj S. Brar*[2,3], *John G. Cannon*[1] and *Natalie G. Coburn*[1,3]**

[1]Sunnybrook Research Institute, Toronto, Ontario, Canada
[2]Department of Surgery, Saint Barnabas Medical Center, Livingston, New Jersey, US
[3]Department of Surgery, University of Toronto, Toronto, Ontario, Canada
[4]Department of Surgery, Maimonides Medical Center, Brooklyn, New York, US

Abstract

Despite declining incidence, gastric cancer remains one of the most common cancers worldwide and one of the most common causes of cancer-related mortality. Accurate staging forms the basis for making appropriate decisions on treatment strategies for patients with gastric cancer; whether to select curative intent resection, palliative resection and/or referral for neo-adjuvant therapies. The importance of pre-operative staging is highlighted by the significant morbidity and mortality rates associated with an exploratory laparotomy for unresectable disease. Radiological investigations are performed preoperatively, however, there is a reported considerable rate of under-staging by non-invasive imaging modalities. The addition of diagnostic laparoscopy for certain patients improves clinical staging of patients with gastric cancer as it enables better detection of peritoneal seeding, tumor deposits to non-local lymph nodes and liver metastasis, which may not be detected by available imaging modalities. A complete staging laparoscopy should include the inspection of the stomach, diaphragm, liver and ovaries. Peritoneal washings for cytological analysis during staging laparoscopy have been advocated for the identification of free intraperitoneal cancer cells, despite the absence of any evidence of gross peritoneal disease, as the length of time added to the procedure is not significant. Positive cytology of peritoneal washings is a poor prognostic indicator and a strong predictor of recurrence even after an R0 resection and may impact treatment decisions with regards to perioperative therapy. This chapter will discuss the role of diagnostic laparoscopy in the staging of gastric cancer.

Introduction

Despite decreasing incidence, gastric cancer remains the third most common cause of cancer-related death worldwide [1]. In Korea and Japan, where the incidence of gastric cancer is high, population based screening by contrast barium radiography and/or endoscopy results in a greater proportion of cases being detected in the early stage [2]. However, late stage presentation of the disease is common in Europe and North America [3].

Surgical resection with curative intent remains the best treatment modality for patients with gastric cancer [4]. However, the presence of metastatic disease is associated with very poor outcomes and is currently considered, by most, a contraindication to curative resection [5, 6]. Patients with metastatic disease may be better treated with palliative modalities such as chemotherapy, radiation therapy, or stenting, reserving surgery for those with significant symptoms [4, 7, 8]. Accurate preoperative staging is therefore critical for determining the treatment strategy for patients with gastric cancer.

Understaging by Radiological Modalities

The management and treatment of gastric cancer is complex and resource intensive [9]. Once the diagnosis of gastric cancer is confirmed on esophagogastroduodenoscopy (EGD), accurate staging of tumor depth (T), regional lymph node involvement (N) and distant metastases (M) provides clinicians with information required to establish treatment strategies. Conventionally, staging of gastric cancer has been done by radiological imaging, primarily computed tomography (CT), abdominal ultrasound (AUS), and more recently magnetic resonance imaging (MRI) [10]. Despite advances in radiological imaging, there remains sub-optimal identification of advanced disease [11].

In gastric cancer patients, metastatic disease is most often found in the peritoneum, liver, or lymph nodes [12]. Multiple studies have shown that preoperative staging by radiological imaging is insufficient for the accurate staging of advanced gastric cancer [13]. A significant limitation is the inability of standard radiological imaging to detect small metastatic lesions (<1 cm), subcapsular liver metastases, peritoneal carcinomatosis, or free intraperitoneal cancer cells [4].

Conventional imaging studies fail to detect peritoneal seeding in about 13% to 37% of patients with advanced gastric adenocarcinoma [14-17]. Recent advances in CT scanning technology have not significantly improved these results. Burbidge et al., reported a sensitivity and specificity of current generation CT scanning for detecting peritoneal metastases as 25% and 99%, respectively [18]. Failure of radiologic staging, to identify occult metastases, results in a high rate of unnecessary laparotomies in patients with incurable gastric cancer.

Improved Accuracy with Diagnostic Laparoscopy on Staging of Patients with Gastric Cancer

Diagnostic laparoscopy has shown to improve detection of peritoneal carcinomatosis in patients with gastric cancer that would be undetected by CT or AUS [19]. With thorough laparoscopic inspection, the accuracy for detecting intra-abdominal M1 disease is 94% to 100% [11, 14]. A recent study found that almost one third of patients who were preoperatively identified as M0 by conventional imaging modalities, had radiologically occult intra-abdominal metastases to the liver, peritoneum and para-aortic lymph nodes, which were discovered by diagnostic laparoscopy [20]. Sarela et al., evaluated 657 patients with potentially resectable gastric cancer over a 10 year period and discovered that 31% had M1 disease [20]. Increased accuracy by diagnostic laparoscopy alters the staging results obtained by CT and ultrasound imaging. Nakagawa et al., report corrected staging following diagnostic laparoscopy in 47% of patients [21].

Effects of Diagnostic Laparoscopy on Management of Gastric Cancer

Although diagnostic laparoscopy has been demonstrated to improve staging accuracy, it is only significant if the management of patients with gastric cancer is affected [22]. The imperative is to identify patients with metastatic disease who would neither benefit from surgical resection nor would require neoadjuvant chemotherapy, but who may be candidates for non-curative treatment or best supportive care [11]. A systematic review evaluating the accuracy and role of diagnostic laparoscopy in patients with gastric cancer revealed that up to 60% of patients had a change in their treatment course after diagnostic laparoscopy and up to 44% of patients avoided an unnecessary laparotomy [11]. In patients with advanced gastric cancer, this study found that diagnostic laparoscopy changed management in 25% to 54% of patients with advanced gastric cancer while only 3.8% in early gastric cancer [11].

The importance of sparing patients from unnecessary laparotomy is highlighted by the significant complications, physical and psychological stresses associated with this invasive procedure, particularly in late stage gastric cancer patients [23, 24]. Morbidity and mortality rates following exploratory laparotomies in patients for which a curative resection is not feasible have been reported to range from 13% to 23% and from 10% to 36%, respectively [14, 16, 25-27]. Karanicolas et al., in study using the SEER database, found the in-hospital mortality of patients undergoing a staging laparoscopy is 5.3%, compared to 13.1% for patients who underwent a futile laparotomy ($p<0.001$) [28]. This study also showed the median hospital length of stay is shorter with staging laparoscopy compared to a negative laparotomy (2 days vs. 10 days, $p <0.001$) [28]. Another study also of diagnostic laparoscopy found significantly shorter hospital stays when compared to negative laparotomy (1.4 days vs. 6.5 days, $p < 0.5$) [14]. The shorter recovery time achieved by avoiding futile laparotomy is particularly important as it may lead to quicker referral to oncology and initiation of chemotherapy [13, 16, 29-32].

Given its diagnostic accuracy, its ability to change management in appropriately selected patients, and the benefits to the patient in terms of reduction in hospital length of stay and mortality, staging laparoscopy should be utilized in the staging of all patients with advanced gastric cancer.

Indications for Diagnostic Laparoscopy in Patients with Gastric Cancer

Although diagnostic laparoscopy has been incorporated in treatment guidelines for gastric cancer [33, 34], it still is not universally performed preoperatively [35, 36]. In the United States, based on the analysis of the Surveillance, Epidemiology and End Results Database, only 8.3% of patients with gastric cancer underwent a diagnostic laparoscopy [36]. In Canada, based on provincial data from Ontario, only 5.1% of patients with gastric cancer underwent a diagnostic laparoscopy before curative-intent resection [35].

Deciding which patients should undergo diagnostic laparoscopy has been debated, and variation exists amongst treatment guidelines. The European Society for Medical Oncology (ESMO) recommends performing a staging laparoscopy in any patient believed to have resectable disease [37].

In the United Kingdom, the National Health Service (NHS) recommends performing a laparoscopy in all patients with gastric cancer [34]. Other practice guidelines have recommended that staging laparoscopy be reserved for advanced gastric cancer, where there is a higher likelihood of metastases [38, 39]. The Society of Gastrointestinal and Endoscopic Surgeons (SAGES) guidelines recommend that a diagnostic laparoscopy be performed in advanced (T3 and T4) cancers and against its use in early gastric (T1 and T2) cancer [40]. The Scottish Intercollegiate Guidelines Network (SIGN) indicate that laparoscopy should be considered in patients with suspected full thickness gastric wall tumor involvement [38]. In the United States, the National Comprehensive Cancer Network (NCCN) guidelines recommend diagnostic laparoscopy for patients considered for surgical resection without pre-operative therapy and in patients with suspected T3 or T4 tumors [33].

Results from an international multidisciplinary RAND/UCLA expert panel suggest that a diagnostic laparoscopy be performed for all patients undergoing resection of cT3-cT4 lesions [9]. Furthermore, diagnostic laparoscopy is indicated prior to multivisceral resection [9]. Diagnostic laparoscopy may also be useful for staging hepatic metastases if current generation CT, MRI or ultrasound is unavailable [16]. Complications that mandate immediate surgical intervention are a contraindication to diagnostic laparoscopy [41].

For patients with early gastric cancer, surgical resection alone is recommended. If a diagnostic laparoscopy is performed for early gastric cancer, it can be performed immediately prior to resection as a one-stage procedure. Gotoda et al., performed a study of 5265 patients with EGC who underwent a gastrectomy and D2 lymphadenectomy, which revealed that these patients had no risk or a lower risk of lymph node metastasis than risks of mortality from the gastrectomy [42].

Furthermore, Sarela et al., analyzed data from CT scan staged M0 gastric cancer patients who were found to have M1 disease on diagnostic laparoscopy and revealed that M1 disease was significantly more prevalent in patients with T3/T4 stage gastric cancer (63%) in comparison to patients with non-visible tumors or T1/T2 stage (17%; P=0.001) [20].

Role of Peritoneal Lavage Cytology during Diagnostic Laparoscopy

In gastric cancer, peritoneal dissemination is one of the most common patterns of metastasis and recurrence [43]. Peritoneal lavage for cytological analysis have been advocated for the identification of free intra-peritoneal cancer cells, despite the absence of any evidence of gross peritoneal disease. The etiology of these free intra-peritoneal cancer cells is not fully understood, however, they are thought to arise where the primary tumor invades the serosa [44]. Supporting this hypothesis, positive cytology is associated with advanced T stage, but has no association with N stage [45]. The presence of free intra-peritoneal cancer cells suggests a poor prognosis [45, 46] and is a strong predictor of recurrence even after complete resection of tumor with microscopic examination of margins revealing no tumor cells (R0 resection) [47]. Reported recurrence rates for patients with positive cytology range from 11% to 100% [48], but appear to be dependent upon the method used to detect cancer cells in peritoneal washings and the length of time that the patients are observed for recurrence. Diagnostic laparoscopy provides an excellent opportunity to perform a peritoneal lavage that would yield a cytological sample for analysis [21].

The treatment implications of positive peritoneal cytology are debated. Although the Union Internationale Contre le Cancer (UICC) / American Joint Committee on Cancer (AJCC) have recently defined positive peritoneal cytology as M1 disease [49], the third edition of the Japanese gastric cancer guidelines classifies a macroscopically curative resection with positive cytology as an R1 resection and not as metastatic disease [50]. The rationale to include positive peritoneal cytology as metastatic disease derives from multiple studies revealing that patients with an R0 resection and positive peritoneal washings had median survival rates similar to those with M1 disease and long-term survival was rare [47, 51-55].

While some authors state that positive cytology is a contra-indication to resection [33, 56], others feel that positive peritoneal cytology is useful for identifying patients who are unlikely to benefit from resection alone, and would require additional treatment in order to improve survival [53]. Some authors have suggested that early detection and eradication of intra-peritoneal cancer cells may improve patient survival [57, 58]. Lorenzen et al., reported that 37% of gastric cancer patients with positive peritoneal cytology had no free intraperitoneal cancer cells in repeat washings after a minimum of six weeks of chemotherapy [59]. These patients had improved median survival (36.1 vs. 9.2 months; p= 0.002) and 2-year survival (71.4 vs. 25%; p = 0.002) compared to patients who had persistently positive cytology [59]. However, the 5-year survival of patients converted from positive to negative peritoneal cytology was only 14.3% [59].

The role of surgery in patients with positive peritoneal cytology is not clear. In a study of patients with gastric cancer and positive peritoneal cytology, Mezhir et al., found that surgery is not associated with improved survival [57]. Patients who were initially cytology positive and underwent gastrectomy after conversion to cytology negative with neoadjuvant chemotherapy had similar median disease specific survival (DSS) when compared to those, in a historical cohort, that had no resection after conversion to cytology negative (2.5 years [range 0.6-4.5] vs. 2.3 years [range 0.4-3.1], respectively [log rank P=0.76]) [57]. Due to low power of the study, there was no statistically significant difference in median DSS between patients with repeat negative cytology who underwent gastrectomy in comparison to those who underwent a gastrectomy despite persistent positive cytology (2.2 years [range 0.02-4.2] vs. 1.4 years [range 0.60-4.0], respectively [log rank P=0.14]) [57].

Some have also suggested that the prognosis of patients with positive peritoneal cytology may be improved with intra-peritoneal chemotherapy. A systematic review and meta-analysis was recently performed by Coccolini et al., comparing intra-peritoneal chemotherapy and surgery in comparison to radical resection alone [60]. They revealed an incremental improvement in overall survival in the first 3 years following intra-peritoneal chemotherapy and surgery over surgery alone, however no difference was observed between the two groups at 5 years [60]. Furthermore, recent studies have shown the use of extensive peritoneal lavage followed by intra-peritoneal chemotherapy to improve 5-year survival of patients with positive peritoneal cytology over those with intra-peritoneal therapy alone (43.8% vs. 4.6%, $p < 0.0001$) [61]. Intra-peritoneal chemotherapy has been demonstrated to be prophylactic against peritoneal recurrence and results in improved survival [62, 63]. Although it remains investigational at this point, as we await the results from a Japanese phase III trial (CCOG 1102) evaluating the efficacy of extensive intra-operative peritoneal lavage in the treatment of resectable advanced gastric cancer [64]. Identification of intra-peritoneal cancer cells may have an impact on intra-operative treatment strategies.

Current guidelines are inconsistent in their recommendations for peritoneal washings. In Japan, obtaining peritoneal washings for the local staging of gastric cancer has been recommended by the Japanese Gastric Cancer Association [65]. In addition, SAGES recommends obtaining peritoneal washings at the time of diagnostic laparoscopy [20]. Conversely, ESMO does not consider obtaining peritoneal washings a necessary practice [37]. The NCCN do not explicitly incorporate peritoneal washings into their gastric cancer treatment guidelines, though do consider positive peritoneal cytology a criterion of unresectable disease [33]. Results from an international multidisciplinary RAND/UCLA expert panel thought that performing peritoneal lavage is appropriate, but not necessary [9].

Although the time necessary to perform a peritoneal lavage is insignificant when added to a diagnostic laparoscopy, there is no reliable mechanism for intra-operative assessment of cytology. Therefore, the addition of peritoneal lavage to a diagnostic laparoscopy must be planned prior to scheduled resection, necessitating two separate procedures if resection is performed.

Confirmation of M0 Status Following Neo-Adjuvant Chemotherapy

Management of gastric cancer includes tissue diagnosis by EGD and the use of imaging modalities for determination of presence of locoregional and distant disease. Patients with early stage gastric cancer undergo resection alone. Patients with advanced stage disease often relapse with local or systemic recurrence following curative intent resection [66]. For patients with advanced gastric cancer, randomized trials have established the use of multimodality therapy in conjunction with surgical resection as standard of care [67-70]. If there is no evidence of occult gross or cytological metastatic disease, then patients either begin neoadjuvant therapy or proceed to surgical resection followed by chemoradiotherapy.

In patients undergoing neo-adjuvant chemotherapy, a diagnostic laparoscopy may be useful if equivocal response is revealed radiographically.

As a proportion of patients following neoadjuvant therapy progress to develop radiological occult metastatic disease, several authors have advocated for a repeat diagnostic laparoscopy before surgical intervention [14, 30, 71]. The Medical Research Adjuvant Gastric Cancer (MAGIC) phase III trial revealed that 6% of patients in the neoadjuvant treatment group did not come to a surgical resection and that 18% underwent a palliative resection following intra-operative findings of unresectable disease [67]. Cardona et al., reported similar results in their study where 11% of the patients in their treatment arm did not come to a surgical resection and that 7% of patients of patients that received neoadjuvant chemotherapy developed metastases that were not recognized with repeat imaging [71]. Of patients who had occult metastasis, 75% had clearly visible disease on repeat diagnostic laparoscopy, with the remainder with positive cytology only [71]. Repeat diagnostic laparoscopy following neoadjuvant chemotherapy may be a valuable tool in selecting those patients with advanced gastric cancer for curative resection and sparing those with occult metastases and disease progression from an unnecessary laparotomy [71].

Performing a Complete Diagnostic Laparoscopy

Diagnostic laparoscopy may be performed either immediately prior to surgery (one-stage) or as an independent procedure (two-stage), allowing for thorough evaluation of results, including biopsies and cytology, by a multidisciplinary team with the goal of devising the best treatment strategy [72].

Patient Preparation, Position and Room Setup

After risks and benefits of diagnostic laparoscopy are explained to the patient and informed consent is obtained, the patient is brought to the operating room and positioned supine on the operating room table with the arms tucked. (Figure 1) The patient undergoes the procedure under general anesthesia. The surgeon is positioned on the left side of the patient, and the first assistant and scrub nurse are positioned on the right side. For optimal visualization, the monitors are generally placed at the head of the operating room table, however this can be modified to improve ergonomics. Patient positioning can be adjusted during the procedure. Patients may be placed in Trendelenburg position for evaluation of the lower abdomen, reverse Trendelenburg position for evaluation of the upper abdomen and may be tilted right side up or left side up for evaluation of the right and left sides, respectively.

Trocar Position, Laparoscope and Systematic Approach to Performing a Diagnostic Laparoscopy with Peritoneal Washings

With the patient in the supine position, initial entry can be approached with an open laparoscopic (Hasson) technique or in closed laparoscopic entry with Veress needle. Entry into the abdomen usually occurs through the umbilicus with placement of a 10 to 12 mm port [47]. (Figure 2) Generally a 30 degree (10mm) laparoscope is used for exploration and better visualization [47]

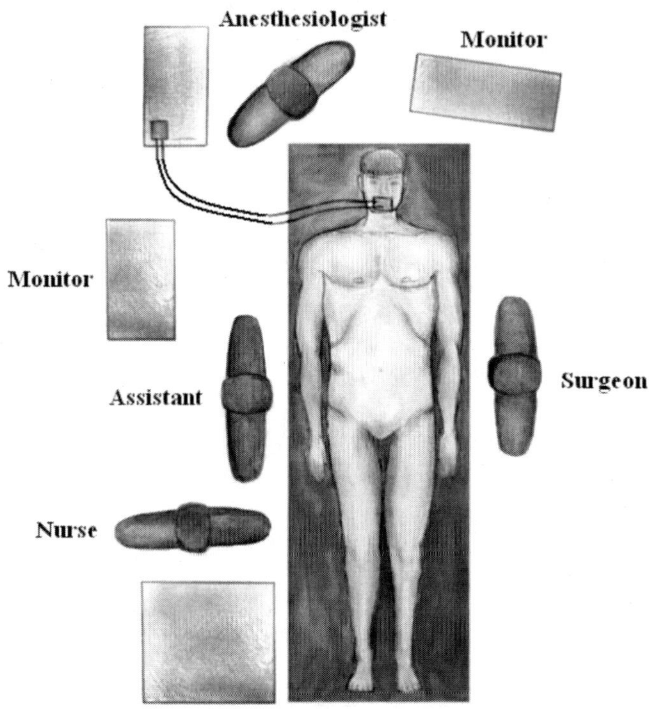

Figure 1. Patient positioning and room setup for diagnostic laparoscopy.

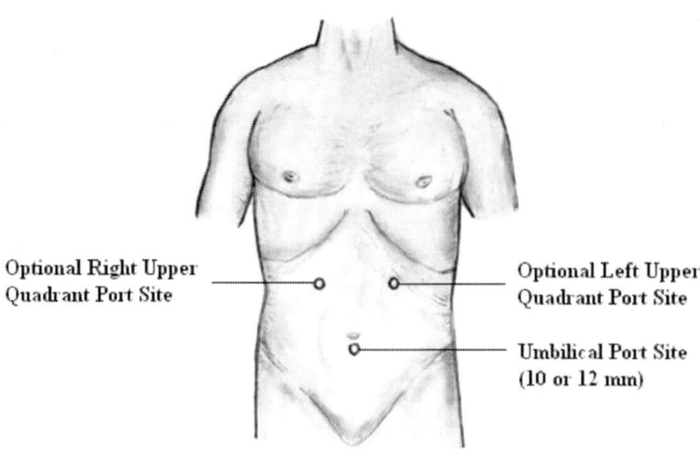

Figure 2. Port placement for diagnostic laparoscopy.

A complete staging laparoscopy should include a systematic inspection of the entire abdominal cavity to minimize the chance of missing critical or subtle findings [72]. At first entry through the umbilical port with the laparoscope, the surgeon should provide a panoramic view of the entire abdominal cavity with evaluation of the anterior abdominal wall and peritoneum, which may provide clues in terms of the disease process, but may also help for deciding on subsequent port positioning. Additional 5 mm trocars can be placed under direct visualization in the right and/or left upper quadrant, as needed [71, 72]. These 5 mm ports may be upsized if necessary. A systematic approach begins with evaluation of the omentum and root of the mesentery, pelvis (ovaries in females), right and left paracolic gutters, left hemidiaphragm and spleen and right hemidiaphragm [72]. Following this initial inspection, attention is directed to a thorough examination of all hepatic lobes of the liver, gallbladder, hepatic hilum [47, 72]. If concerns for invasion of the pancreas exist, then examination of the lesser sac is performed; however this is not routinely done due to disruption/violation of fascial planes [16, 72]. Finally, the stomach, as well as the perigastric nodes along the greater and lesser curvature, are inspected [47, 72]. Peritoneal, serosal, or greater omental or lesser omental deposits should always be biopsied, while needle or core biopsy should be used on large masses [72]. (Figure 3 and 4) While the primary goal is to detect the presence of unresectable disease, it is also useful to assess the primary tumor (size, location, and invasion) and anatomy that may aid in future surgical planning [72].

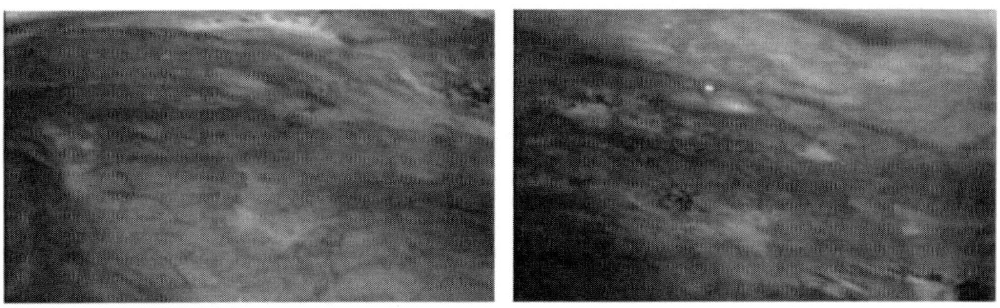

Figure 3. Carcinomatosis.

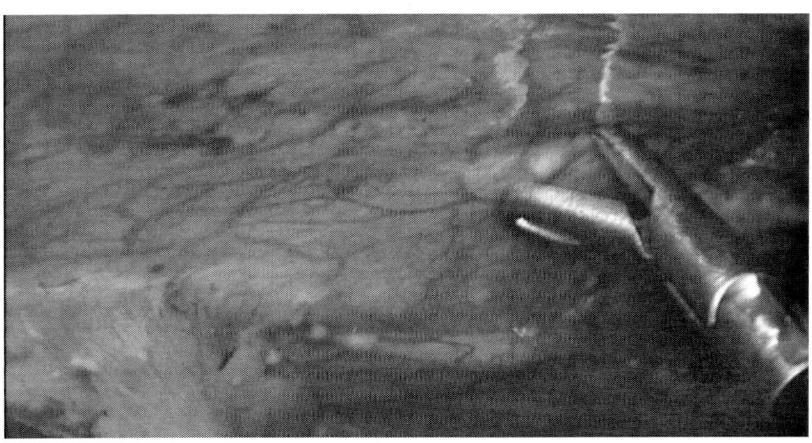

Figure 4. Biopsy of Peritoneal Deposit.

During a diagnostic laparoscopy, suction and irrigation should be set up to aspirate ascitic fluid, which should be sent for cytological analysis [71]. If no ascitic fluid can be aspirated, peritoneal washing can be performed by instilling 100 to 200 ml of normal saline into the right and left upper quadrants and pelvis, which is then aspirated after gentle agitation [71]. (Figure 5)

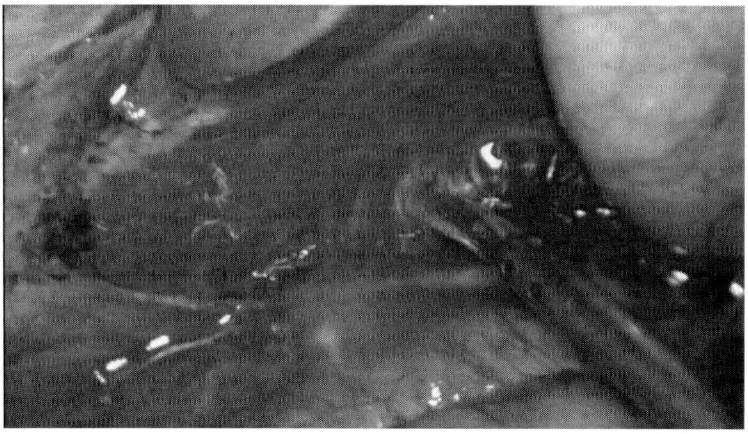

Figure 5. Peritoneal Lavage.

At completion of the diagnostic laparoscopy and before removal of the laparoscope, a final survey of the abdominal cavity should be performed to ensure hemostasis and the absence of injury to any visceral organs. Additional cannula ports should be removed under direct vision to ensure no bleeding from port sites. Pneumoperitoneum should be evacuated to minimize the risks of referred pain and port sites larger than 10 mm should undergo fascial closure [72].

Addition of Laparoscopic Ultrasonography

Laparoscopic ultrasonography has become a valuable adjunct to diagnostic laparoscopy. Laparoscopic ultrasound provides the surgeon with the improved ability to determine tumor depth and local extension, as well as detection of small liver lesions and lymph node metastases [72]. Anderson et al., reported that laparoscopic ultrasonography detected liver metastases (2%), lymph node metastases (25%) and advanced local tumor invasion (9%) in a group of 44 patients who were deemed resectable by radiographic staging [73]. Bemelman et al., reported that laparoscopic ultrasonography found metastatic disease in 28% of patients with gastric cancer [74]. Although it shows an advantage to detecting metastatic disease, it did not reveal an advantage to local tumor staging over existing imaging modalities [75].

In staging for gastric cancer, laparoscopic ultrasonography is useful in evaluation of the liver. As in the performance of a diagnostic laparoscopy, a systematic approach to evaluation with laparoscopic ultrasonography minimizes the chance of missing a critical finding [72]. Most probes pass through a 10 mm port and use 5-7.5 MHz frequencies. Initial evaluation should begin with the lateral right lobe, moving medially towards the falciform ligament [72]. As the probe is moved towards the falciform ligament, transhepatic views of the retroperitoneum, gallbladder, vena cava and porta hepatis can be accomplished [72]. Following this evaluation, the left lateral segment of the liver is evaluation from the falciform ligament laterally and with transhepatic views of the celiac plexus, periaortic nodes, and portal vein [72]. If a suspicious lesion is encountered, it must biopsied either by excision for superficial lesions or needle biopsy for deep lesions.

Risks and Complications Associated with Diagnostic Laparoscopy

Diagnostic laparoscopy in patients with advanced gastric cancer is considered safe, with multiple studies showing morbidity in less than 2% of patients and few, to no, incidences of mortality [21, 76, 77]. A retrospective analysis of 389 diagnostic laparoscopies performed by Hunerbein et al., reported severe laparoscopy-associated complications in 4% of patients (including wound infection, intestinal perforation, lung embolism and myocardial infarction) and mortality from multiple organ failure in 1 patient following laparoscopic tumor biopsy [78]. Complications required conversion from diagnostic laparoscopy to open surgery in 5% of their cases secondary to adhesions, hemorrhage, intestinal perforation and technical problems not otherwise specified [78]. Diagnostic laparoscopy has the added risk of performing an additional surgery, which may incur additional costs and delay definitive treatment as scheduling is subject to operating room availability.

Port-site metastases following diagnostic laparoscopy have been identified as a possible risk of diagnostic laparoscopy [79]. However, evidence has shown that port site metastases are a rare occurrence even during staging of advanced gastric tumors [80]. Incidences of port site metastases most often occur following diagnostic laparoscopy revealing widespread disease progression [76]. Based on the rarity and limitation to patients already presenting with widespread dissemination, Shoup et al., argues that the danger of port site metastases should not dissuade the use of diagnostic laparoscopy for gastrointestinal tumor staging [81]

Future Directions

The role of a diagnostic laparoscopy as a staging modality has been established. Novel methods to increase diagnostic laparoscopy's ability to detect metastatic disease are currently being described in multiple recent studies, which have explored the use of fluorescent laparoscopy as a method to increase diagnostic laparoscopy's sensitivity to detect small metastases missed by white-light laparoscopy [82-84]. These studies are performed using fluorescent light following sensitization by 5-aminolevulinic acid (5-ALA). 5-ALA acts by triggering protoporphyrin IX synthesis and accumulate in malignant cells by overwhelming the heme production pathway in tumor cells [82]. Initial studies performed in model organisms have shown increased detection of peritoneal metastases by 5-ALA sensitization followed by fluorescent detection [82, 85]. Comparison of fluorescent and white-light diagnostic laparoscopy by Zöpf et al., in 30 patients with gastrointestinal malignancies, reported that examination by fluorescent laparoscopy yielded the discovery of a greater number of metastatic lesions. However, fluorescent light laparoscopy did not identify peritoneal metastases in any patients previously staged free of peritoneal disease by white light [86]. Current limitations of fluorescent light laparoscopy include its inability for deep observations as penetration of light is low, making it difficult to be used in the detection of micrometastases in lymph nodes without excision [87]. Therefore, further research is necessary to develop cancer specific probes, increasing sensitivity by using fluorescent laparoscopy, which may one day yield results that may alter clinical decision-making [87].

Conclusion

Accurate staging is critical to make informed therapeutic strategy decisions in cases of advanced gastric cancer. Non-invasive radiological imaging by computed tomography and ultrasound has traditionally been used to stage gastric cancer however these imaging modalities may understage metastatic disease. Diagnostic laparoscopy provides significantly greater sensitivity to detect peritoneal metastases than either ultrasound or computed tomography and does not result in significantly increased risk to the patient. Increased accuracy by diagnostic laparoscopy affects clinical decision-making and spares patients from unnecessary and dangerous exploratory laparotomy. Diagnostic laparoscopy should be considered an essential addition to radiological imaging for staging patients presenting with cT3-cT4 stage gastric cancer.

References

[1] World Health Organization, International Agency for Research on Cancer. GLOBOCAN 2012: Estimated Cancer Incidence, Mortality and Prevalence Worldwide in 2012. Available at: http://globocan.iarc.fr/Default.aspx.

[2] Tan YK, Fielding JW. Early diagnosis of early gastric cancer. *Eur J Gastroenterol Hepatol.* 2006 Aug;18(8):821-9.

[3] Thrumurthy SG, Chaudry MA, Hochhauser D, Mughal M. The diagnosis and management of gastric cancer. *BMJ.* 2013;347:f6367.

[4] Meyer HJ, Wilke H. Treatment strategies in gastric cancer. *Dtsch Arztebl Int.* 2011 Oct;108(41):698-705; quiz 6.

[5] Fujitani K, Yang HK, Kurokawa Y, et al. Randomized controlled trial comparing gastrectomy plus chemotherapy with chemotherapy alone in advanced gastric cancer with a single non-curable factor: Japan Clinical Oncology Group Study JCOG 0705 and Korea Gastric Cancer Association Study KGCA01. *Jpn J Clin Oncol.* 2008 Jul;38(7):504-6.

[6] Kerkar SP, Kemp CD, Duffy A, et al. The GYMSSA trial: a prospective randomized trial comparing gastrectomy, metastasectomy plus systemic therapy versus systemic therapy alone. *Trials.* 2009;10:121.

[7] Brar S, Law C, McLeod R, et al. Defining Surgical Quality in Gastric Cancer: A RAND/UCLA Appropriateness Study. *J Am Coll Surg*. 2013 May 8.

[8] Mahar AL, Coburn NG, Singh S, Law C, Helyer LK. A systematic review of surgery for non-curative gastric cancer. *Gastric Cancer.* 2012 Sep;15 Suppl 1:S125-37.
[9] Dixon M, Cardoso R, Tinmouth J, et al. What studies are appropriate and necessary for staging gastric adenocarcinoma? Results of an international RAND/UCLA expert panel. *Gastric Cancer.* 2013 Apr 30.
[10] Hallinan JT, Venkatesh SK. Gastric carcinoma: imaging diagnosis, staging and assessment of treatment response. *Cancer Imaging.* 2013;13:212-27.
[11] Leake PA, Cardoso R, Seevaratnam R, et al. A systematic review of the accuracy and indications for diagnostic laparoscopy prior to curative-intent resection of gastric cancer. *Gastric Cancer.* 2012 Sep;15 Suppl 1:S38-47.
[12] Esaki Y, Hirayama R, Hirokawa K. A comparison of patterns of metastasis in gastric cancer by histologic type and age. *Cancer.* 1990 May 1;65(9):2086-90.
[13] Blackshaw GR, Barry JD, Edwards P, Allison MC, Thomas GV, Lewis WG. Laparoscopy significantly improves the perceived preoperative stage of gastric cancer. *Gastric Cancer.* 2003;6(4):225-9.
[14] Burke EC, Karpeh MS, Conlon KC, Brennan MF. Laparoscopy in the management of gastric adenocarcinoma. *Ann Surg.* 1997 Mar;225(3):262-7.
[15] Kriplani AK, Kapur BM. Laparoscopy for pre-operative staging and assessment of operability in gastric carcinoma. *Gastrointest Endosc.* 1991 Jul-Aug;37(4):441-3.
[16] Lowy AM, Mansfield PF, Leach SD, Ajani J. Laparoscopic staging for gastric cancer. *Surgery.* 1996 Jun;119(6):611-4.
[17] Possik RA, Franco EL, Pires DR, Wohnrath DR, Ferreira EB. Sensitivity, specificity, and predictive value of laparoscopy for the staging of gastric cancer and for the detection of liver metastases. *Cancer.* 1986 Jul 1;58(1):1-6.
[18] Burbidge S, Mahady K, Naik K. The role of CT and staging laparoscopy in the staging of gastric cancer. *Clin Radiol.* 2013 Mar;68(3):251-5.
[19] D'Ugo DM, Coppola R, Persiani R, Ronconi P, Caracciolo F, Picciocchi A. Immediately preoperative laparoscopic staging for gastric cancer. *Surg Endosc.* 1996 Oct;10(10):996-9.
[20] Sarela AI, Lefkowitz R, Brennan MF, Karpeh MS. Selection of patients with gastric adenocarcinoma for laparoscopic staging. *Am J Surg.* 2006 Jan;191(1):134-8.
[21] Nakagawa S, Nashimoto A, Yabusaki H. Role of staging laparoscopy with peritoneal lavage cytology in the treatment of locally advanced gastric cancer. *Gastric Cancer.* 2007;10(1):29-34.
[22] Shandall A, Johnson C. Laparoscopy or scanning in oesophageal and gastric carcinoma? *Br J Surg.* 1985 Jun;72(6):449-51.
[23] Schwarz RE. Factors influencing change of preoperative treatment intent in a gastrointestinal cancer practice. *World J Surg Oncol.* 2007;5:32.
[24] Smith BR, Stabile BE. Gastric adenocarcinoma: reduction of perioperative mortality by avoidance of nontherapeutic laparotomy. *J Gastrointest Surg.* 2007 Feb;11(2):127-32.
[25] D'Ugo DM, Persiani R, Caracciolo F, Ronconi P, Coco C, Picciocchi A. Selection of locally advanced gastric carcinoma by preoperative staging laparoscopy. *Surg Endosc.* 1997 Dec;11(12):1159-62.
[26] Lehnert T, Rudek B, Kienle P, Buhl K, Herfarth C. Impact of diagnostic laparoscopy on the management of gastric cancer: prospective study of 120 consecutive patients with primary gastric adenocarcinoma. *Br J Surg.* 2002 Apr;89(4):471-5.

[27] Yano M, Tsujinaka T, Shiozaki H, et al. Appraisal of treatment strategy by staging laparoscopy for locally advanced gastric cancer. *World J Surg.* 2000 Sep;24(9):1130-5; discussion 5-6.

[28] Karanicolas PJ, Elkin EB, Jacks LM, et al. Staging laparoscopy in the management of gastric cancer: a population-based analysis. *J Am Coll Surg.* 2011 Nov;213(5):644-51, 51 e1.

[29] Asencio F, Aguilo J, Salvador JL, et al. Video-laparoscopic staging of gastric cancer. A prospective multicenter comparison with noninvasive techniques. *Surg Endosc.* 1997 Dec;11(12):1153-8.

[30] Feussner H, Omote K, Fink U, Walker SJ, Siewert JR. Pretherapeutic laparoscopic staging in advanced gastric carcinoma. *Endoscopy.* 1999 Jun;31(5):342-7.

[31] Sarela AI, Miner TJ, Karpeh MS, Coit DG, Jaques DP, Brennan MF. Clinical outcomes with laparoscopic stage M1, unresected gastric adenocarcinoma. *Ann Surg.* 2006 Feb;243(2):189-95.

[32] Smith A, Finch MD, John TG, Garden OJ, Brown SP. Role of laparoscopic ultrasonography in the management of patients with oesophagogastric cancer. *Br J Surg.* 1999 Aug;86(8):1083-7.

[33] Ajani JA, Bentrem DJ, Besh S, et al. Gastric cancer, version 2.2013: featured updates to the NCCN Guidelines. *J Natl Compr Canc Netw.* 2013 May 1;11(5):531-46.

[34] Allum WH, Blazeby JM, Griffin SM, Cunningham D, Jankowski JA, Wong R. Guidelines for the management of oesophageal and gastric cancer. *Gut.* 2011 Nov;60(11):1449-72.

[35] Coburn NG, Lourenco LG, Rossi SE, et al. Management of gastric cancer in Ontario. *J Surg Oncol.* 2010 Jul 1;102(1):54-63.

[36] Karanicolas PJ, Elkin EB, Jacks LM, Strong VE, Brennan MF, Coit DG. Underuse of staging laparoscopy for gastric cancer results in a high rate of futile laparotomy in the USA. *Journal of the American College of Surgeons.* 2012;211(3):S106.

[37] Van Cutsem E, Dicato M, Geva R, et al. The diagnosis and management of gastric cancer: expert discussion and recommendations from the 12th ESMO/World Congress on Gastrointestinal Cancer, Barcelona, 2010. *Ann Oncol. 2011* Jun;22 Suppl 5:v1-9.

[38] Alderson D. Scottish Intercollegiate Guidelines Network (SIGN) 87--the management of oesophageal and gastric cancer. *Clin Oncol* (R Coll Radiol). 2008 Sep;20(7):530-1.

[39] Society of American Gastrointestinal and Endoscopic Surgeons. Guidelines for Diagnostic Laparoscopy. http://www.sages.org/publications/guidelines/guidelines-for-diagnostic-laparoscopy/. Available at.

[40] Hori Y. Diagnostic laparoscopy guidelines : This guideline was prepared by the SAGES Guidelines Committee and reviewed and approved by the Board of Governors of the Society of American Gastrointestinal and Endoscopic Surgeons (SAGES), November 2007. *Surg Endosc.* 2008 May;22(5):1353-83.

[41] Shelat VG, Thong JF, Seah M, Lim KH. Role of staging laparoscopy in gastric malignancies - our institutional experience. *World J Gastrointest Surg.* 2012 Sep 27;4(9):214-9.

[42] Gotoda T, Yanagisawa A, Sasako M, et al. Incidence of lymph node metastasis from early gastric cancer: estimation with a large number of cases at two large centers. *Gastric Cancer.* 2000 Dec;3(4):219-25.

[43] Boku T, Nakane Y, Minoura T, et al. Prognostic significance of serosal invasion and free intraperitoneal cancer cells in gastric cancer. *Br J Surg.* 1990 Apr;77(4):436-9.
[44] Abe N, Watanabe T, Toda H, et al. Prognostic significance of carcinoembryonic antigen levels in peritoneal washes in patients with gastric cancer. *Am J Surg.* 2001 Apr;181(4):356-61.
[45] Creasman WT, Rutledge F. The prognostic value of peritoneal cytology in gynecologic malignant disease. *Am J Obstet Gynecol.* 1971 Jul 15;110(6):773-81.
[46] Moore GE, Sako K, Kondo T, Badillo J, Burke E. Assessment of the exfoliation of tumor cells into the body cavities. *Surg Gynecol Obstet.* 1961 Apr;112:469-74.
[47] Bentrem D, Wilton A, Mazumdar M, Brennan M, Coit D. The value of peritoneal cytology as a preoperative predictor in patients with gastric carcinoma undergoing a curative resection. *Ann Surg Oncol.* 2005 May;12(5):347-53.
[48] Leake PA, Cardoso R, Seevaratnam R, et al. A systematic review of the accuracy and utility of peritoneal cytology in patients with gastric cancer. *Gastric Cancer.* 2011 Sep;15 Suppl 1:S27-37.
[49] American Joint Committee on Cancer. Chapter 11: Stomach. In: Edge S, Byrd D, Compton C, et al., eds. *AJCC Cancer Staging Manual 7th ed.* New York: Springer.
[50] Japanese Gastric Cancer Association. Japanese classification of gastric carcinoma: 3rd English edition. *Gastric Cancer.* 2011;14:101-12.
[51] Bando E, Yonemura Y, Takeshita Y, et al. Intraoperative lavage for cytological examination in 1,297 patients with gastric carcinoma. *Am J Surg.* 1999 Sep;178(3):256-62.
[52] Bonenkamp JJ, Songun I, Hermans J, van de Velde CJ. Prognostic value of positive cytology findings from abdominal washings in patients with gastric cancer. *Br J Surg.* 1996 May;83(5):672-4.
[53] Burke EC, Karpeh MS, Jr., Conlon KC, Brennan MF. Peritoneal lavage cytology in gastric cancer: an independent predictor of outcome. *Ann Surg Oncol.* 1998 Jul-Aug;5(5):411-5.
[54] Kodera Y, Yamamura Y, Shimizu Y, et al. Peritoneal washing cytology: prognostic value of positive findings in patients with gastric carcinoma undergoing a potentially curative resection. J Surg Oncol. 1999 Oct;72(2):60-4; discussion 4-5.
[55] Mezhir JJ, Shah MA, Jacks LM, Brennan MF, Coit DG, Strong VE. Positive peritoneal cytology in patients with gastric cancer: natural history and outcome of 291 patients. *Indian J Surg Oncol.* 2011 Mar;2(1):16-23.
[56] Badgwell B, Cormier JN, Krishnan S, et al. Does neoadjuvant treatment for gastric cancer patients with positive peritoneal cytology at staging laparoscopy improve survival? *Ann Surg Oncol.* 2008 Oct;15(10):2684-91.
[57] Mezhir JJ, Shah MA, Jacks LM, Brennan MF, Coit DG, Strong VE. Positive peritoneal cytology in patients with gastric cancer: natural history and outcome of 291 patients. Ann Surg Oncol. 2010 Dec;17(12):3173-80.
[58] Vogel I, Kalthoff H. Disseminated tumour cells. Their detection and significance for prognosis of gastrointestinal and pancreatic carcinomas. *Virchows Arch.* 2001 Aug;439(2):109-17.
[59] Lorenzen S, Panzram B, Rosenberg R, et al. Prognostic significance of free peritoneal tumor cells in the peritoneal cavity before and after neoadjuvant chemotherapy in

patients with gastric carcinoma undergoing potentially curative resection. *Ann Surg Oncol.* 2010 Oct;17(10):2733-9.

[60] Coccolini F, Cotte E, Glehen O, et al. Intraperitoneal chemotherapy in advanced gastric cancer. Meta-analysis of randomized trials. *Eur J Surg Oncol.* 2014 Jan;40(1):12-26.

[61] Kuramoto M, Shimada S, Ikeshima S, et al. Extensive intraoperative peritoneal lavage as a standard prophylactic strategy for peritoneal recurrence in patients with gastric carcinoma. *Ann Surg.* 2009 Aug;250(2):242-6.

[62] Yonemura Y, Ninomiya I, Kaji M, et al. Prophylaxis with intraoperative chemohyperthermia against peritoneal recurrence of serosal invasion-positive gastric cancer. *World J Surg.* 1995 May-Jun;19(3):450-4; discussion 5.

[63] Yu W, Whang I, Suh I, Averbach A, Chang D, Sugarbaker PH. Prospective randomized trial of early postoperative intraperitoneal chemotherapy as an adjuvant to resectable gastric cancer. *Ann Surg.* 1998 Sep;228(3):347-54.

[64] Misawa K, Mochizuki Y, Ohashi N, et al. A Randomized Phase III Trial Exploring the Prognostic Value of Extensive Intraoperative Peritoneal Lavage in Addition to Standard Treatment for Resectable Advanced Gastric Cancer: CCOG 1102 Study. *Jpn J Clin Oncol.* 2014 Jan;44(1):101-3.

[65] La Torre M, Rossi Del Monte S, Ferri M, Cosenza G, Mercantini P, Ziparo V. Peritoneal washing cytology in gastric cancer. How, when and who will get a benefit? A review. *Minerva Gastroenterol Dietol.* 2011 Mar;57(1):43-51.

[66] Jain VK, Cunningham D, Chau I. Preoperative and postoperative chemotherapy for gastric cancer. *Surg Oncol Clin N Am.* 2012 Jan;21(1):99-112.

[67] Cunningham D, Allum WH, Stenning SP, et al. Perioperative chemotherapy versus surgery alone for resectable gastroesophageal cancer. *N Engl J Med.* 2006 Jul 6;355(1):11-20.

[68] Macdonald JS, Smalley SR, Benedetti J, et al. Chemoradiotherapy after surgery compared with surgery alone for adenocarcinoma of the stomach or gastroesophageal junction. *N Engl J Med.* 2001 Sep 6;345(10):725-30.

[69] Stahl M, Walz MK, Stuschke M, et al. Phase III comparison of preoperative chemotherapy compared with chemoradiotherapy in patients with locally advanced adenocarcinoma of the esophagogastric junction. *J Clin Oncol.* 2009 Feb 20;27(6):851-6.

[70] Ychou M, Boige V, Pignon JP, et al. Perioperative chemotherapy compared with surgery alone for resectable gastroesophageal adenocarcinoma: an FNCLCC and FFCD multicenter phase III trial. *J Clin Oncol.* 2011 May 1;29(13):1715-21.

[71] Cardona K, Zhou Q, Gonen M, et al. Role of repeat staging laparoscopy in locoregionally advanced gastric or gastroesophageal cancer after neoadjuvant therapy. *Ann Surg Oncol.* 2013 Feb;20(2):548-54.

[72] Greene FL, Heniford BT. Minimally Invasive Cancer Management. Second ed. New York: Springer; 2010.

[73] Anderson DN, Campbell S, Park KG. Accuracy of laparoscopic ultrasonography in the staging of upper gastrointestinal malignancy. *Br J Surg.* 1996 Oct;83(10):1424-8.

[74] Bemelman WA, van Delden OM, van Lanschot JJ, et al. Laparoscopy and laparoscopic ultrasonography in staging of carcinoma of the esophagus and gastric cardia. *J Am Coll Surg.* 1995 Nov;181(5):421-5.

[75] van Delden OM, de Wit LT, Nieveen van Dijkum EJ, Reeders JW, Gouma DJ. Laparoscopic ultrasonography for abdominal tumor staging. *Eur Radiol.* 1998;8(8):1405-8.

[76] McCulloch P, Johnson M, Jairam R, Fischer W. Laparoscopic staging of gastric cancer is safe and affects treatment strategy. *Ann R Coll Surg Engl.* 1998 Nov;80(6):400-2.

[77] Muntean V, Mihailov A, Iancu C, et al. Staging laparoscopy in gastric cancer. Accuracy and impact on therapy. *J Gastrointestin Liver Dis.* 2009 Jun;18(2):189-95.

[78] Hunerbein M, Rau B, Hohenberger P, Schlag PM. The role of staging laparoscopy for multimodal therapy of gastrointestinal cancer. *Surg Endosc.* 1998 Jul;12(7):921-5.

[79] Cook TA, Dehn TC. Port-site metastases in patients undergoing laparoscopy for gastrointestinal malignancy. *Br J Surg.* 1996 Oct;83(10):1419-20.

[80] Deogracias ML, Rodriguez-Sanjuan JC, de la Torre F, et al. Absence of port-site metastases following staging laparoscopy for gastric carcinoma. *Rev Esp Enferm Dig.* 2006 Oct;98(10):755-9.

[81] Shoup M, Brennan MF, Karpeh MS, Gillern SM, McMahon RL, Conlon KC. Port site metastasis after diagnostic laparoscopy for upper gastrointestinal tract malignancies: an uncommon entity. *Ann Surg Oncol.* 2002 Aug;9(7):632-6.

[82] Gahlen J, Prosst RL, Pietschmann M, et al. Laparoscopic fluorescence diagnosis for intraabdominal fluorescence targeting of peritoneal carcinosis experimental studies. *Ann Surg.* 2002 Feb;235(2):252-60.

[83] Gahlen J, Stern J, Laubach HH, Pietschmann M, Herfarth C. Improving diagnostic staging laparoscopy using intraperitoneal lavage of delta-aminolevulinic acid (ALA) for laparoscopic fluorescence diagnosis. *Surgery.* 1999 Sep;126(3):469-73.

[84] Kishi K, Fujiwara Y, Yano M, et al. Staging laparoscopy using ALA-mediated photodynamic diagnosis improves the detection of peritoneal metastases in advanced gastric cancer. *J Surg Oncol.* 2012 Sep 1;106(3):294-8.

[85] Canis M, Botchorishvili R, Berreni N, et al. 5-aminolevulinic acid-induced (ALA) fluorescence for the laparoscopic diagnosis of peritoneal metastasis. AST An experimental study. *Surg Endosc.* 2001 Oct;15(10):1184-6.

[86] Zopf T, Schneider AR, Weickert U, Riemann JF, Arnold JC. Improved preoperative tumor staging by 5-aminolevulinic acid induced fluorescence laparoscopy. *Gastrointest Endosc.* 2005 Nov;62(5):763-7.

[87] Murayama Y, Ichikawa D, Koizumi N, et al. Staging fluorescence laparoscopy for gastric cancer by using 5-aminolevulinic acid. *Anticancer Res.* 2012 Dec;32(12): 5421-7.

In: Laparoscopy
Editor: Christos Iavazzo

ISBN: 978-1-63321-404-0

Chapter 8

Role of Laparoscopic Resection in Gastric Cancer Treatment

Abraham El-Sedfy[1,2], Savtaj S. Brar[1,3], Matthew Dixon[1,4], John G. Cannon[2] and Natalie G. Coburn[1,3]
[1]Sunnybrook Research Institute, Toronto, Ontario, Canada
[2]Department of Surgery, Saint Barnabas Medical Center, Livingston, New Jersey, US
[3]Department of Surgery, University of Toronto, Toronto, Ontario, Canada
[4]Department of Surgery, Maimonides Medical Center, Brooklyn, New York, US

Abstract

Increasingly, laparoscopic resection has been used in treatment of early gastric cancer. Laparoscopic approaches that have been described for the treatment of early gastric cancer include: 1) Laparoscopic intragastric mucosal resections; 2) Laparoscopic wedge resection; and 3) Laparoscopic assisted gastrectomy. Furthermore, combining endoscopic resection with laparoscopic lymphadenectomy has also been investigated in cases where lymph node involvement cannot be excluded. In recent randomized controlled trials and meta-analyses, laparoscopic resection has been shown to improve post-operative pain, bleeding, length of hospitalization and cosmesis, when compared with open gastrectomy. Despite few studies reporting oncologic outcomes, indications have expanded from early gastric cancer to locally advanced gastric cancer in some centers. Multicenter randomized controlled trials are currently ongoing in Korea to evaluate oncologic outcome for laparoscopic resections for advanced gastric cancer (KLASS II trial). This chapter will discuss the role of laparoscopic resection in the treatment of gastric cancer.

Introduction

Although rates of incidence have decreased worldwide, gastric cancer remains the fifth most common cancer overall, and the third most common cause of cancer-related death [1]. The epidemiology of gastric cancer is diverse, with over 10-fold differences in incidence between low and high-risk regions [2]. Population-based screening by double contrast barium radiography and/or endoscopy is common in East Asian countries, where rates of gastric cancer remain high [3, 4]. Screening in Japan and Korea allows for earlier detection of gastric cancer, where analysis of a Japanese registry demonstrated that early stage disease makes up approximately 50% of currently treated cases [5]. In the western world, where incidences of gastric cancer are lower and large-scale screening is not employed, the majority of gastric cancer cases present as late stage disease [6].

Laparoscopic surgery first emerged in the 1930s, with most operations restricted to the lysis of benign abdominal adhesions and biopsy of abdominal organs [7]. It was not until the technological advancements in the 1980s, giving us the ability to project intra-abdominal images onto screens, that laparoscopic assisted surgery truly became an integral part of general surgery [7]. In Japan, Kitano et al. performed the first laparoscopic gastrectomy with a Billroth I reconstruction for gastric cancer in 1991 [8]. In 1992, Goh et al., from Singapore, performed the first laparoscopic distal gastrectomy with Billroth II reconstruction on a patient for chronic gastric ulcers [9]. Soon thereafter, laparoscopic surgery as a treatment modality for gastric cancer emerged, as Ohgami et al. performed the first laparoscopic wedge resection via intragastric mucosal resection for early gastric cancer in 1992 [10]. Ohashi et al. is also credited for pioneering the intragastric mucosal resection for posterior wall tumors [11]. In Europe, Azagra et al., also recognized as pioneers in the minimally invasive field, performed the first laparoscopic resection for gastric cancer in 1993 [12].

Laparoscopic techniques for gastric cancer were initially slow to be adopted. In1997, a worldwide survey of advanced laparoscopic surgeons found only 118 instances of laparoscopic gastrectomy [13]. More recently, the role of laparoscopic surgery for gastric cancer has increased significantly. Much of this growing interest is due to improvements in laparoscopic technology and developments in minimally invasive surgical techniques, along with growing experience and dissemination of evidence supporting the use of laparoscopic gastrectomy. The aim of this chapter is to describe and discuss the role of laparoscopic resection as a surgical modality for the treatment of gastric cancer.

Indications

Laparoscopic Resection for Early Gastric Cancer

Laparoscopic resection for gastric cancer has emerged as a minimally invasive surgical modality for the resection of early gastric cancer, especially in East Asian countries where resection of early gastric cancer is more frequently performed [12, 14, 15]. Early gastric cancer is defined as cases in which tumor invasion is confined to the mucosa or submucosa, irrespective of lymph node involvement (T1 cancer, any N) [16]. Increased interest in minimally invasive operations for the treatment of early gastric cancer stems from the favorable outcomes for resection. Long-term survival data from Japan revealed 5-year survival rates of 99% for early gastric cancer limited to the mucosa and 96% for early gastric cancer showing submucosal invasion [17, 18]. Based on information from the Korean Laparoscopic Gastrointestinal Surgery Study Group (KLASS), 3783 laparoscopic gastric cancer operations were performed in Korea in 2009, a five-fold increase over the number reported in 2004 [19].

Initially, laparoscopic resection was reserved for early gastric cancer with a low risk of perigastric lymph node involvement because of the difficulty in completing an adequate lymphadenectomy [20]. The depth of cancer invasion plays a role in the risk of lymph node metastasis. When gastric cancer is limited to the mucosa, the incidence of lymph node metastasis is less than 3%, but rises to approximately 20% with invasion of the submucosa [17, 18]. As techniques and instruments evolved, giving surgeons the ability to complete an extended lymphadenectomy, in most Asian centers, the indication has expanded to include all early gastric cancer with risk of lymph node involvement that is not indicated for endoscopic submucosal dissection [20].

Despite the increase in its application, laparoscopic assisted gastrectomy (LAG) is still considered controversial due to a lack of large-scale study data on short and long-term outcomes [21]. In Japan and Korea, early gastric cancer is considered the only indication for LG. It is interesting to note that Western guidelines (SIGN, ESMO, NCCN) highlight the potential for laparoscopic resection but state that further study of this approach is required [22-25]. Recently, a multidisciplinary expert panel from a RAND/UCLA study agreed that it was appropriate to perform a laparoscopic distal gastrectomy for patients with distal T1-2 N0 gastric cancer [26]. The expert panel agreed that it was appropriate to perform a laparoscopic total gastrectomy on patients with proximal T1 N0 disease but indeterminate for T2 N0 disease [26]. Furthermore, the panel disagreed about performing laparoscopic gastric resections on patients with advanced gastric cancer [26].

A number of small RCTs and retrospective studies comparing open gastrectomy vs. LG for early gastric cancer treatment have favorably supported the use of LG [27-30]. These studies have identified reduced operative blood loss, decreased post-operative pain, and earlier discharge time as benefits associated with LG in comparison to open gastrectomy. In a recent meta-analysis of 782 LG and 380 open gastrectomies performed from 2000 to 2012 by Sun et al., the LG group had shorter wound lengths, fewer instances of surgical morbidity, and more rapid bowel recovery and first food intake [31]. However, the LG group also had increased operative times and less extensive lymph node harvest [31]. Operative duration for LG are operator dependent, and studies addressing the learning curve for LG have found significantly decreased procedure length after completion of 50 LG operations [32, 33]. Large-scale retrospective analysis of 1294 patients who underwent LG for early gastric cancer by Kitano et al. reported 5-year disease-free survival rates of 99.8% for stage IA, disease, 98.7% for stage IB disease, and 85.7% for stage II disease [34].

Recently, Kim et al. published a large-scale case-control and case matched retrospective study comparing curative intent laparoscopic and open gastrectomy in 2976 patients [35]. Their case-control study revealed no statistical difference in overall survival, disease-specific survival and recurrence-free survival between the two groups for stages IB to IV [35]. However, the laparoscopic group was associated with an increased overall survival for stage IA patients treated by laparoscopic resection in comparison to open resection (95.3% vs. 90.3%, $p<0.001$; respectively) [35]. However, no significant difference in overall survival was observed for all stages in their case-matched series after the propensity scoring system was applied [35]. Furthermore, prospective RCTs to determine differences in oncological outcomes following LG compared to open gastrectomy are currently ongoing, to confirm comparable results that have been demonstrated in the large scale retrospective studies. Both the Japan Clinical Oncology Group (JCOG 0912 study) and the Korean Laparoscopic Gastrointestinal Surgery Study Group (KLASS I Study) are conducting large multi-center RCT's to compare differences in long-term survivorship following LG and open gastrectomy for early gastric cancer [28, 36].

Laparoscopic Resection for Advanced Gastric Cancer

Following the first report of laparoscopy-assisted gastrectomy with D2 lymphadenectomy by Uyama et al. in 1999, laparoscopic resection has emerged as a potential surgical modality for advanced gastric cancer [37]. However, laparoscopic surgery for advanced gastric cancer remains a subject of significant debate. Concerns arise from the technical challenge and uncertainty associated with performing a complete D2 lymph node dissection by laparoscopy [38]. If the extent of resection and lymph node dissection normally performed during open surgery could be replicated laparoscopically, oncological safety would theoretically be equivalent between open and laparoscopic treatment [19].

The use of LG for disease resection in cases of advanced gastric cancer is still under investigation due to the technical challenge of laparoscopic lymph node retrieval [39]. Large-scale retrospective studies from China and Korea have reported LG as a safe alternative to open gastrectomy for advanced gastric cancer [38, 39]. A RCT performed by Huscher et al. comparing laparoscopic and open surgery for advanced gastric cancer in 59 patients reported no significant difference in disease-free survival [28], however with only 59 patients with advanced gastric cancer, this study was under powered to determine oncologic equivalence. However, adequately powered RCT comparing LG and open gastrectomy are necessary to affirm LG as a safe alternative for resection of advanced gastric cancer. A phase III study (KLASS 02) has been initiated to evaluate LG for use in advanced gastric cancer patients [40], with results expected in September of 2015.

Performing Laparoscopic Gastric Resections for Patients with Gastric Cancer

Patient Position and Room Setup

After risks and benefits are explained to the patient and informed consent is obtained, the patient is brought to the operating room and positioned supine on the operating room table with the arms and legs abducted. The patient undergoes the procedure under general anesthesia. The surgeon is positioned on the right or left side of the patient depending on the operative field with the first assistant standing opposite [20]. The laparoscope assistant is positioned between the patient's abducted legs [20]. This position offers the laparoscopist an advantage in terms of maneuverability; however, some surgeon's may elect to not have the patient's legs abducted. For optimal visualization, the monitors are generally placed at the head of the operating room table, however this can be changed as to improve ergonomics. (Figure 1) Patient positioning during the procedure can be changed by adjustments to the operating room table. Patient can be placed in Trendelenburg position for evaluation of the lower abdomen, reverse Trendelenburg position for evaluation of the upper abdomen and the patient can be tilted right side up or left side up for evaluation of the right and left sides, respectively. In general, the operation is performed with the patient supine in 10-degree reverse Trendelenburg position [20].

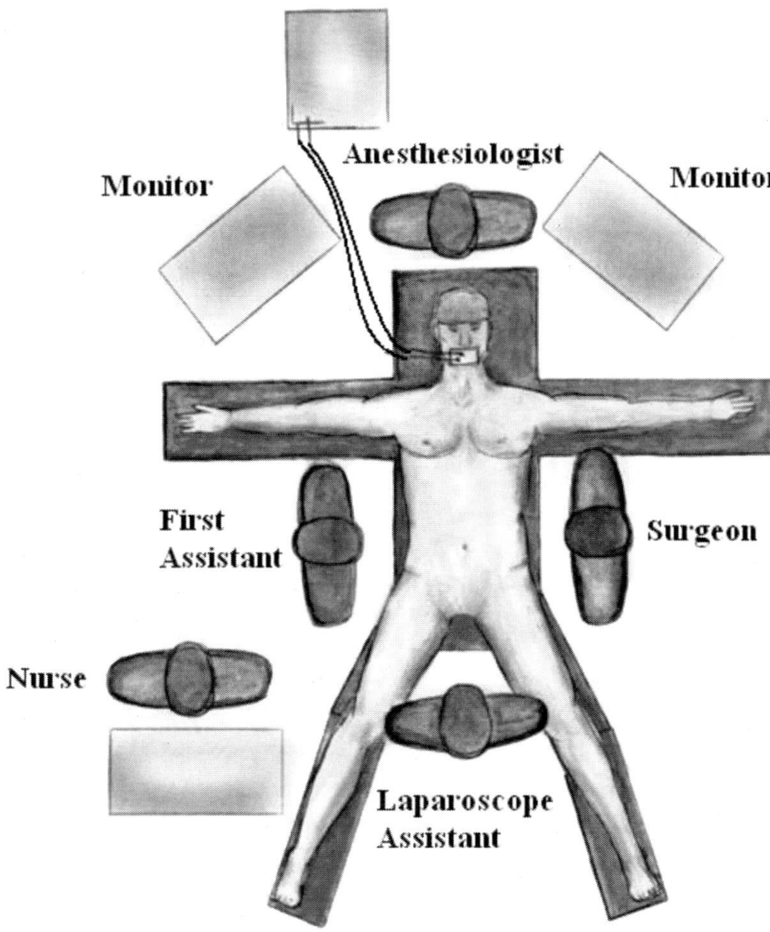

Figure 1. Patient positioning and room setup for laparoscopic gastrectomy.

Cannula Position and Choice of Laparoscope

With the patient in the supine position allowing access to all four quadrants of the abdomen, initial entry into the abdomen usually occurs through the umbilicus with placement of a 10 to 12 mm port [20]. Entry can be approached with an open laparoscopic (Hasson) technique or in closed laparoscopic entry with Veress needle. Generally a 30-degree (10mm) laparoscope is used for exploration for better visualization. At first entry through the umbilical port with the laparoscope, the surgeon should provide a panoramic view of the entire abdominal cavity with evaluation of the anterior abdominal wall and peritoneum, which may provide clues in terms of the disease process but also may help for deciding on port positioning. Two additional 10 mm trocars are then placed under direct visualization just above the level of the umbilicus on the right and left side (20). Then two additional trocars are placed in the right and left upper quadrants of the abdomen under direct visualization [20]. (Figure 2)

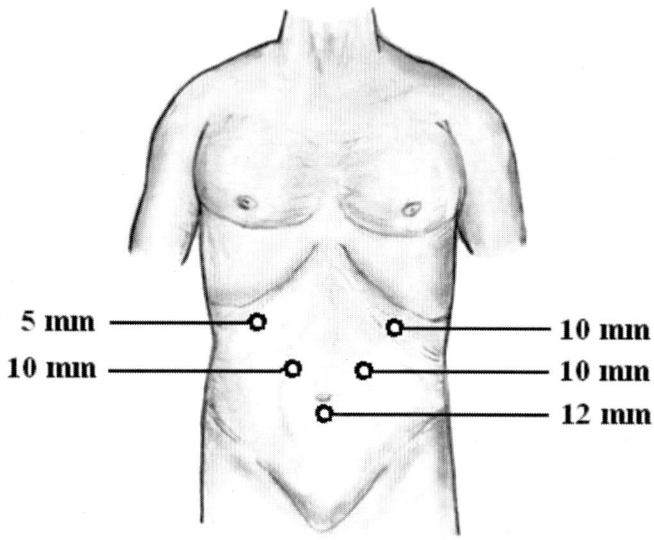

Figure 2. Port placement for laparoscopic gastrectomy.

Types of Laparoscopic Resections and Techniques

This chapter will examine 3 laparoscopic approaches for the treatment of EGC: (1) laparoscopic intragastric mucosal resection (LIGMR), (2) Laparoscopic wedge resection (LWR), and (3) laparoscopic assisted gastrectomy (LAG).

Laparoscopic Intragastric Mucosal Resection

First described by Ohashi et al. in 1995 for the resection of gastric mucosal tumors, LIGMR involves the placement of 3 balloon trocars in the gastric lumen, penetrating both the abdominal and stomach wall [11]. (Figure 3) The use of balloon-equipped ports prevents air leak while also stabilizing the instrumentation on the gastric wall [11]. LIGMR allows mucosal resection of any part of the stomach except the anterior wall while also preserving the muscularis propria [11]. LIGMR is a useful surgical option for resection of gastric submucosal tumors located near the esophagogastric junction or pyloric junction not easily accessed by other laparoscopic resection techniques [41]. There have been no published randomized comparison studies of LIGMR versus other resection techniques, however multiple single center studies have reported successful resection of gastric lesions using LIGMR [41-43]. Use of LIGMR has largely decreased following the establishment of endoscopic techniques as safe and effective for resection of tumors confined to the mucosa [44].

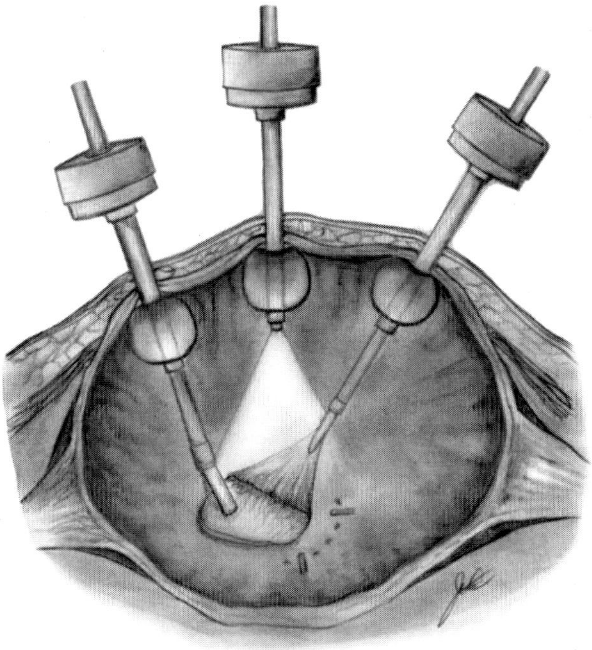

Figure 3. Laparoscopic intragastric mucosal resection. (Adapted from Ohgami et al. 1999 (10)).

Laparoscopic Wedge Resection

Laparoscopic wedge resection has also emerged as a laparoscopic treatment that allows for full-thickness resection of lesions from the anterior wall of the stomach. LWR is preceded by endoscopic confirmation of lesion accessibility, as it is suitable for resection of gastric lesions <5cm in diameter that are not located near the cardia or pylorus [45]. Two LWR techniques have been developed for gastric lesion resection, the "lesion lifting method", and a second method that involves an incision made in the seromuscular layer of the anterior stomach wall.

The "lesion lifting method" entails the use of a hollow needle at the lesion site for application of a T-tack in the lumen of the stomach. The T-tack lifts the lesion and allows resection with suitable margins by laparoscopic stapler [46]. (Figure 4) Tumors located at the posterior wall of the stomach or near the esophagogastric junction present an operative challenge for the "lesion lifting" LWR method, but may be resected using traction sutures [47]. The second method of LWR, first described by Kitano et al., involves making an incision into the seromuscular layer of the anterior stomach wall over the tumor. The incision causes the mucosal lesion to bulge through the anterior stomach wall, facilitating lesion resection [48]. Despite advances made in both the "lesion lifting" and "anterior seromuscular incision" LWR methods, advancements of endoscopic resection techniques for early gastric cancer resection has significantly reduced LWR use [44].

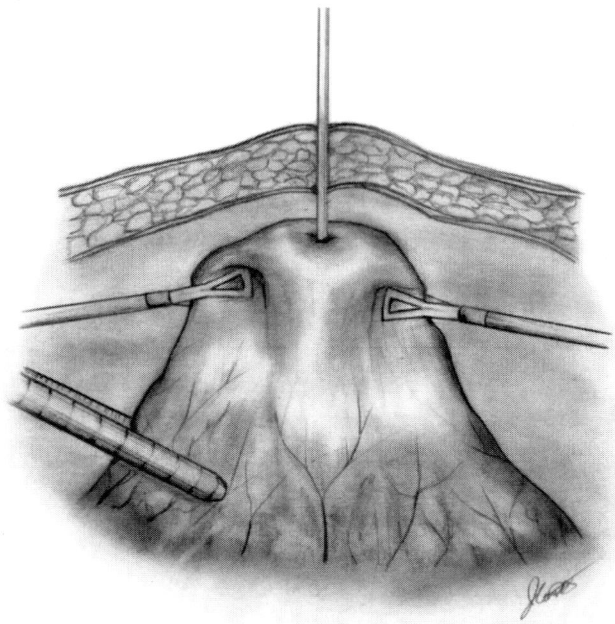

Figure 4. Laparoscopic wedge resection. (Adapted from Ohgami et al. 1999 (10)).

Laparoscopic Assisted Gastrectomy

Laparoscopic assisted gastrectomy as a surgical option is increasingly being utilized for treatment of early gastric cancer in which lymph node involvement is suspected [44]. After the patient is positioned and ports are placed, laparoscopic assisted distal gastrectomy is started by dissection of the greater omentum and gastrocolic ligament from the inferior pole of the spleen to the infrapyloric area, which allows dissection of station 4d lymph nodes [20]. The left gastroepiploic vessels are then clipped and divided, allowing for dissection of station 4sd lymph nodes [20]. This is followed by careful dissection of the greater omentum and gastrocolic ligament in the infrapyloric region, which exposes the head of the pancreas and the right gastroepiploic vessels which are clipped and divided [20]. This allows for dissection of station 6 lymph nodes [20]. The liver is then retracted caudally, allowing for dissection of the lesser omentum and lymph node station 3 [20]. The right gastric artery is then clipped and divided which allows dissection of station 5 lymph nodes [20]. The duodenum is transected with a linear staple at the bulbus before dissection of the left gastric vessels [20]. Then dissection of lymph nodes along the common hepatic artery and celiac artery (stations 8 and 9) is performed, followed by division of the left gastric vessels, providing dissection of lymph node station 7 [20]. Dissection of the left cardiac and superior gastric lymph nodes (stations 1 and 3) is then performed. To complete a D2 lymphadenectomy, though technically challenging, involves dissection and skeletonisation of the splenic artery from its origin to obtain station 11 lymph nodes and skeletonisation of the proper hepatic artery to obtain station 12a lymph nodes [49]. A 5 cm mini-laparotomy may be made in the upper midline to complete the gastrectomy and Roux-en-Y reconstruction. For distal gastrectomy, a Billroth II reconstruction is acceptable. The abdomen is then thoroughly irrigated and a closed-suction Jackson-Pratt drain is placed near the duodenal stump and the operative wounds are then closed.

Totally laparoscopic distal gastrectomies have been performed without the need for exteriorization through a mini laparotomy. Song et al. performed a prospective non-randomized multicenter study comparing totally laparoscopic distal gastrectomy and laparoscopic assisted distal gastrectomy and showed that totally laparoscopic distal gastrectomy provided faster bowel recovery but was associated with higher operative costs [50].

Evolution of Function Preserving Resections

Recent advances have been made in developing minimally invasive surgical techniques to improve quality of life following radical gastric resections, by reducing the burden of dumping syndrome, reflux gastroesophagitis and weight loss [51]. Minimally invasive procedures combining laparoscopic resection with function-preserving gastric surgery include: 1) pylorus-preserving gastrectomy (PPG) for distal lesions; 2) proximal gastrectomy (PG) for proximal lesions; and 3) laparoscopic subtotal Gastrectomy with small remnant gastric pouch for proximal lesions.

Laparoscopic Pylorus-Preserving Gastrectomy

Pylorus-Preserving Gastrectomy (PPG), originally used for the resection of benign gastric diseases such as gastric ulcers [52], has emerged as an increasingly utilized treatment strategy for early gastric cancer patients. Preservation of pyloric function following gastric resection has been shown to reduce sequelae of gastric resection including dumping syndrome [53], bile reflux [54], and post-operative weight loss [55]. Laparoscopic-assisted PPG (LAPPG), which combines the benefits of PPG with the benefits of laparoscopic procedures, has been implemented as a treatment modality in numerous institutions in Japan and Korea [56].

LAPPG entails preservation of the pyloric branch of the vagal nerve and of the right gastric artery to the pyloric cuff, therefore maintaining pyloric circulation and motility [55, 57]. Concerns have been raised that LAPPG does not allow for adequate lymph node dissection, especially of the suprapyloric lymph node basin (58). Studies evaluating the rate of lymph node metastasis following distal gastrectomy for early gastric cancer have found a 4% rate of metastases to the suprapyloric lymph nodes, however 29-24% of patients showing lymph node metastases had T2-T3 gastric cancer [58]. Retrospective analysis of 3646 cases of T1 tumors located in the body of the stomach from the Gastric Cancer Data Base in Japan, performed by Nakajima et al., showed a 0.2% metastatic rate to the suprapyloric lymph nodes [59]. Indications for LAPPG include (1) Intramucosal or submucosal gastric adenocarcinoma without lymph node involvement (cT1, cN0) and (2) Tumor located in the mid stomach (at least 5cm proximal to the pyloric ring) [56, 58].

Multiple retrospective studies have been performed evaluating survival following treatment by either LAPPG or PPG for gastric cancer. Morita et al. evaluated 611 patients following PPG for T1 gastric cancer and revealed a 5-year OS rate of 96.3% [60]. Hiki et al. evaluated 305 cases treated by PPG and revealed a 5-year OS rate of 98% [61]. Jiang et al. analyzed 188 patients following LAPPG and revealed a 3-year OS rate of 97.8% and a disease-specific survival rate of 99.3% [62].

Recently, Kumagai et al. performed a feasibility and safety evaluation of totally laparoscopic pylorus-preserving gastrectomy (TLPPG) using an intracorporeal gastrogastrostomy and revealed that it was a safe procedure, but required longer operative time than performing a LAPPG [63]. Short term outcomes of 60 patients with early gastric cancer in the middle stomach were evaluated following TLPPG, where there were no intraoperative complications or conversions to open surgery during their study and only one patient required return to the operating room secondary to bleeding [63].

Laparoscopic Assisted Proximal Gastrectomy and Laparoscopic Assisted Subtotal Gastrectomy with Small Remnant Pouch

With technological advancements in laparoscopy and improved surgical training, many different types of gastrectomies have been developed, namely laparoscopic total gastrectomy and laparoscopic proximal gastrectomy. Resection by total gastrectomy is the most common treatment strategy for proximal gastric tumors [64]. Laparoscopy-assisted total gastrectomy (LATG) is feasible, but more technically challenging relative to laparoscopy assisted distal gastrectomy (LADG) [65, 66].

Furthermore, LATG is associated with higher rates of patient morbidity, increased operative blood loss and increased post-operative hospital stays [65, 66]. In addition, LATG is also associated with a higher rate of anastomotic stricture when compared to LADG as shown by Lee et al. (26.9% vs. 8.0%, respectively) [66].

Laparoscopic proximal gastrectomy has been suggested as a function-preserving surgical strategy for proximal third early gastric cancer [58]. Due to the association with markedly higher rates of complications including anastomotic stenosis, reflux esophagitis and no change in nutritional status in comparison to total gastrectomies, An et al. concluded that PG are not a better option than total gastrectomy for proximal third early gastric cancer [67]. There has been no apparent advantage with laparoscopic-assisted PG (LAPG) [68].

To improve post-operative quality of life, Jiang et al. have developed a novel approach for selected patient with proximal early gastric cancer, laparoscopy-assisted subtotal gastrectomy (LAsTG), which involves preserving a small proximal gastric pouch [69]. LAsTG carries some concerns pertaining to oncological and reconstruction safety with the preservation of a limited remnant stomach [58]. The indications for LAsTG include 1) a pre-operative diagnosis of T1N0 early gastric cancer; 2) tumor location is in the proximal third of the stomach; 3) distance between tumor and gastroesophageal junction (GEJ) of at least 5cm and 4) remnant gastric stump measuring 2-3 cm from GEJ [58].

Combined Laparoscopic and Endoscopic Resection

Laparoscopic and endoscopic cooperative surgery (LECS) technique was developed by Hiki et al. for the dissection of submucosal tumors of the stomach [70, 71]. The LECS technique involves initial endoscopic identification and confirmation of tumor location followed by endoscopic submucosal dissection [70, 71].

Laparoscopic serosal dissection is performed and a stapling device is applied to close the incision line [70, 71]. LECS is indicated in the treatment of early gastric cancers larger than 3 cm in diameter located at the greater curvature of the stomach or for lesions with extensive ulcerations that may not be amenable to endoscopic submucosal dissection [71]. Importantly, LECS does not involve lymphadenectomy.

Combining endoscopic resection with laparoscopic lymphadenectomy has also been investigated in cases where lymph node involvement cannot be disregarded [72, 73]. However, Abe et al. noted early and delayed gastric ischemia of the preserved stomach secondary to division of major feeding arteries during lymphadenectomy, which resulted in gastric perforation in 1 of 21 patients [73]. In addition, 2 out of 21 patients exhibited gastric emptying problems, although preoperative quality of life was maintained with no dietary restrictions [73]. Further studies are necessary before this becomes an acceptable alternative to gastrectomy without compromising oncologic principles [73].

Future Directions

Novel surgical approaches, including natural orifice transluminal endoscopic surgery (NOTES) and single-incision laparoscopic surgery (SILS), are currently being investigated as minimally invasive treatment options for EGC [74]. NOTES entails incision-less surgery to access the peritoneal cavity through natural orifices [75]. Although it has been applied sporadically in bariatric surgery, Nakajima et al. has shown that transvaginal NOTES may represent an option for performing partial gastrectomy for patients with gastric submucosal tumors [59].

Hybrid procedures are being developed including NOTES with SLN biopsy and NOTES with laparoscopy with the goal of expanding indications for its application [75, 76]. In comparison to NOTES, which is still in early stages of development, SILS shows earlier promise in the treatment of gastric cancer. SILS is applied in appendix, gallbladder, colon and bariatric surgery [74]. With favorable cosmetic results, Omori et al. demonstrated SILS distal gastrectomy as a feasible and safe approach for EGC [77], while Ahn et al. performed the first SILS total gastrectomy with D1 lymphadenectomy for proximal EGC [74]. As instrumentation improves and surgeon experience increases, these novel approaches show potential in improving cosmesis and reducing post-operative pain in comparison to the current laparoscopic approaches.

Conclusion

Laparoscopic surgical techniques have emerged as an attractive alternative to open surgical procedures for cases of early gastric cancer that are not amenable to endoscopic resection. Recent results from RCT have shown that laparoscopic resection leads to reduced rates of operative complication and reduces the average duration of post-operative stay. These RCT have also shown that laparoscopic resection has favorable patient outcomes; however further, large-scale and multi-center RCT are necessary to affirm oncological safety following laparoscopic resection in cases of advanced gastric cancer. Laparoscopic resection has also been implemented for treatment of advanced gastric cancer however the results are less clear in this instance, as there are significant concerns about oncological safety. Implementation of laparoscopic technique offers significant possible benefit to operative safety and post-operative recovery; however further work is necessary to ensure these benefits do not come at the cost of patient safety.

References

[1] World Health Organization, International Agency for Research on Cancer. GLOBOCAN 2012: Estimated Cancer Incidence, Mortality and Prevalence Worldwide in 2012. Available at: http://globocan.iarc.fr/Default.aspx.

[2] Parkin DM. International variation. *Oncogene*. 2004 Aug 23;23(38):6329-40.

[3] Jung KW, Park S, Kong HJ, et al. Cancer statistics in Korea: incidence, mortality, survival, and prevalence in 2008. *Cancer Res. Treat*. 2011 Mar;43(1):1-11.

[4] Whiting JL, Sigurdsson A, Rowlands DC, Hallissey MT, Fielding JW. The long term results of endoscopic surveillance of premalignant gastric lesions. *Gut*. 2002 Mar;50(3):378-81.

[5] Maruyama K, Kaminishi M, Hayashi K, et al. Gastric cancer treated in 1991 in Japan: data analysis of nationwide registry. *Gastric. Cancer*. 2006;9(2):51-66.

[6] Strong VE, Song KY, Park CH, et al. Comparison of gastric cancer survival following R0 resection in the United States and Korea using an internationally validated nomogram. *Ann. Surg*. 2010 Apr;251(4):640-6.

[7] Spaner SJ, Warnock GL. A brief history of endoscopy, laparoscopy, and laparoscopic surgery. *J. Laparoendosc. Adv. Surg. Tech. A*. 1997 Dec;7(6):369-73.

[8] Kitano S, Iso Y, Moriyama M, Sugimachi K. Laparoscopy-assisted Billroth I gastrectomy. *Surg. Laparosc. Endosc*. 1994 Apr;4(2):146-8.

[9] Goh P, Tekant Y, Isaac J, Kum CK, Ngoi SS. The technique of laparoscopic Billroth II gastrectomy. *Surg. Laparosc. Endosc*. 1992 Sep;2(3):258-60.

[10] Ohgami M, Otani Y, Kumai K, Kubota T, Kim YI, Kitajima M. Curative laparoscopic surgery for early gastric cancer: five years experience. *World J. Surg*. 1999 Feb;23(2):187-92; discussion 92-3.

[11] Ohashi S. Laparoscopic intraluminal (intragastric) surgery for early gastric cancer. A new concept in laparoscopic surgery. *Surg. Endosc*. 1995 Feb;9(2):169-71.

[12] Azagra JS, Goergen M, De Simone P, Ibanez-Aguirre J. Minimally invasive surgery for gastric cancer. *Surg. Endosc*. 1999 Apr;13(4):351-7.

[13] Goh PM, Alponat A, Mak K, Kum CK. Early international results of laparoscopic gastrectomies. *Surg. Endosc.* 1997 Jun;11(6):650-2.

[14] Dikken JL, van de Velde CJ, Coit DG, Shah MA, Verheij M, Cats A. Treatment of resectable gastric cancer. *Therap. Adv. Gastroenterol.* 2012 Jan;5(1):49-69.

[15] Hartgrink HH, Jansen EP, van Grieken NC, van de Velde CJ. Gastric cancer. *Lancet.* 2009 Aug 8;374(9688):477-90.

[16] Japanese Gastric Cancer A. Japanese Classification of Gastric Carcinoma - 2nd English Edition. *Gastric. Cancer.* 1998 Dec;1(1):10-24.

[17] Gotoda T. Endoscopic resection of early gastric cancer. *Gastric Cancer.* 2007;10(1): 1-11.

[18] Sano T, Kobori O, Muto T. Lymph node metastasis from early gastric cancer: endoscopic resection of tumour. *Br. J. Surg.* 1992 Mar;79(3):241-4.

[19] Kim HH, Ahn SH. The current status and future perspectives of laparoscopic surgery for gastric cancer. *J. Korean Surg. Soc.* 2011 Sep;81(3):151-62.

[20] Kitano S, Shiraishi N. Laparoscopic Approaches to Gastric Cancer. In: Greene FL, Heniford BT, eds. Minimally Invasive Cancer Management. Second ed. New York: Springer; 2010. p. 113-24.

[21] Zeng YK, Yang ZL, Peng JS, Lin HS, Cai L. Laparoscopy-assisted versus open distal gastrectomy for early gastric cancer: evidence from randomized and nonrandomized clinical trials. *Ann. Surg.* 2012 Jul;256(1):39-52.

[22] Ajani JA, Bentrem DJ, Besh S, et al. Gastric cancer, version 2.2013: featured updates to the NCCN Guidelines. *J. Natl. Compr. Canc. Netw.* 2013 May 1;11(5):531-46.

[23] Alderson D. Scottish Intercollegiate Guidelines Network (SIGN) 87--the management of oesophageal and gastric cancer. *Clin. Oncol.* (R Coll Radiol). 2008 Sep;20(7):530-1.

[24] Allum WH, Blazeby JM, Griffin SM, Cunningham D, Jankowski JA, Wong R. Guidelines for the management of oesophageal and gastric cancer. *Gut.* 2011 Nov;60(11):1449-72.

[25] Van Cutsem E, Dicato M, Geva R, et al. The diagnosis and management of gastric cancer: expert discussion and recommendations from the 12th ESMO/World Congress on Gastrointestinal Cancer, Barcelona, 2010. *Ann. Oncol.* 2011 Jun;22 Suppl 5:v1-9.

[26] Brar S, Law C, McLeod R, et al. Defining Surgical Quality in Gastric Cancer: A RAND/UCLA Appropriateness Study. *J. Am. Coll Surg.* 2013 May 8.

[27] Hayashi H, Ochiai T, Shimada H, Gunji Y. Prospective randomized study of open versus laparoscopy-assisted distal gastrectomy with extraperigastric lymph node dissection for early gastric cancer. *Surg. Endosc.* 2005 Sep;19(9):1172-6.

[28] Huscher CG, Mingoli A, Sgarzini G, et al. Laparoscopic versus open subtotal gastrectomy for distal gastric cancer: five-year results of a randomized prospective trial. *Ann. Surg.* 2005 Feb;241(2):232-7.

[29] Kitano S, Shiraishi N, Fujii K, Yasuda K, Inomata M, Adachi Y. A randomized controlled trial comparing open vs laparoscopy-assisted distal gastrectomy for the treatment of early gastric cancer: an interim report. *Surgery.* 2002 Jan;131(1 Suppl):S306-11.

[30] Lee JH, Han HS. A prospective randomized study comparing open vs laparoscopy-assisted distal gastrectomy in early gastric cancer: early results. *Surg. Endosc.* 2005 Feb;19(2):168-73.

[31] Sun J, Li J, Wang J, et al. Meta-analysis of randomized controlled trials on laparoscopic gastrectomy vs. open gastrectomy for distal gastric cancer. *Hepatogastroenterology.* 2012 Sep;59(118):1699-705.

[32] Fujiwara M, Kodera Y, Miura S, et al. Laparoscopy-assisted distal gastrectomy with systemic lymph node dissection: a phase II study following the learning curve. *J. Surg. Oncol.* 2005 Jul 1;91(1):26-32.

[33] Kim MC, Jung GJ, Kim HH. Learning curve of laparoscopy-assisted distal gastrectomy with systemic lymphadenectomy for early gastric cancer. *World J. Gastroenterol.* 2005 Dec 21;11(47):7508-11.

[34] Kitano S, Shiraishi N, Uyama I, Sugihara K, Tanigawa N. A multicenter study on oncologic outcome of laparoscopic gastrectomy for early cancer in Japan. *Ann. Surg.* 2007 Jan;245(1):68-72.

[35] Kim HH, Han SU, Kim MC, et al. Long-Term Results of Laparoscopic Gastrectomy for Gastric Cancer: A Large-Scale Case-Control and Case-Matched Korean Multicenter Study. *J. Clin. Oncol.* 2014 Jan 27.

[36] Kim HH, Han SU, Kim MC, et al. Prospective randomized controlled trial (phase III) to comparing laparoscopic distal gastrectomy with open distal gastrectomy for gastric adenocarcinoma (KLASS 01*). J. Korean Surg. Soc.* 2013 Feb;84(2):123-30.

[37] Uyama I, Sugioka A, Fujita J, Komori Y, Matsui H, Hasumi A. Laparoscopic total gastrectomy with distal pancreatosplenectomy and D2 lymphadenectomy for advanced gastric cancer. *Gastric. Cancer.* 1999 Dec;2(4):230-4.

[38] Chen K, Xu XW, Mou YP, et al. Systematic review and meta-analysis of laparoscopic and open gastrectomy for advanced gastric cancer. *World J. Surg. Oncol.* 2013;11:182.

[39] Choi YY, Bae JM, An JY, Hyung WJ, Noh SH. Laparoscopic gastrectomy for advanced gastric cancer: Are the long-term results comparable with conventional open gastrectomy? A systematic review and meta-analysis. *J. Surg. Oncol.* 2013 Sep 24.

[40] Miura S, Kodera Y, Fujiwara M, et al. Laparoscopy-assisted distal gastrectomy with systemic lymph node dissection: a critical reappraisal from the viewpoint of lymph node retrieval. *J. Am. Coll. Surg.* 2004 Jun;198(6):933-8.

[41] Tagaya N, Mikami H, Kogure H, Kubota K, Hosoya Y, Nagai H. Laparoscopic intragastric stapled resection of gastric submucosal tumors located near the esophagogastric junction. *Surg. Endosc.* 2002 Jan;16(1):177-9.

[42] Sahm M, Pross M, Lippert H. Intraluminal resection of gastric tumors using intragastric trocar technique. *Surg. Laparosc. Endosc. Percutan. Tech.* 2011 Aug;21(4):e169-72.

[43] Uchikoshi F, Ito T, Nishida T, Kitagawa T, Endo S, Matsuda H. Laparoscopic intragastric resection of gastric stromal tumor located at the esophago-cardiac junction. *Surg. Laparosc. Endosc. Percutan. Tech.* 2004 Feb;14(1):1-4.

[44] Koeda K, Nishizuka S, Wakabayashi G. Minimally invasive surgery for gastric cancer: the future standard of care. *World J. Surg.* 2011 Jul;35(7):1469-77.

[45] Mochizuki Y, Kodera Y, Fujiwara M, et al. Laparoscopic wedge resection for gastrointestinal stromal tumors of the stomach: initial experience. *Surg. Today.* 2006;36(4):341-7.

[46] Ohgami M, Otani Y, Kumai K, Kubota T, Kitajima M. [Laparoscopic surgery for early gastric cancer]. *Nihon Geka Gakkai Zasshi.* 1996 Apr;97(4):279-85.

[47] Kiyozaki H, Saito M, Chiba H, Takata O, Rikiyama T. Laparoscopic wedge resection of the stomach for gastrointestinal stromal tumor (GIST): non-touch lesion lifting method. *Gastric. Cancer.* 2013 Jun 7.
[48] Kitano S, Shimoda K, Miyahara M, et al. Laparoscopic approaches in the management of patients with early gastric carcinomas. *Surg Laparosc Endosc.* 1995 Oct;5(5):359-62.
[49] Cui M, Xing JD, Yang W, et al. D2 dissection in laparoscopic and open gastrectomy for gastric cancer. *World J. Gastroenterol.* 2012 Feb 28;18(8):833-9.
[50] Song KY, Park CH, Kang HC, et al. Is totally laparoscopic gastrectomy less invasive than laparoscopy-assisted gastrectomy?: prospective, multicenter study. *J. Gastrointest. Surg.* 2008 Jun;12(6):1015-21.
[51] Park do J, Lee HJ, Jung HC, Kim WH, Lee KU, Yang HK. Clinical outcome of pylorus-preserving gastrectomy in gastric cancer in comparison with conventional distal gastrectomy with Billroth I anastomosis. *World J. Surg.* 2008 Jun;32(6):1029-36.
[52] Maki T, Shiratori T, Hatafuku T, Sugawara K. Pylorus-preserving gastrectomy as an improved operation for gastric ulcer. *Surgery.* 1967 Jun;61(6):838-45.
[53] Sasaki I, Fukushima K, Naito H, Matsuno S, Shiratori T, Maki T. Long-term results of pylorus-preserving gastrectomy for gastric ulcer. *Tohoku J. Exp. Med.* 1992 Dec;168(4):539-48.
[54] Tomita R, Fujisaki S, Tanjoh K. Pathophysiological studies on the relationship between postgastrectomy syndrome and gastric emptying function at 5 years after pylorus-preserving distal gastrectomy for early gastric cancer. *World J. Surg.* 2003 Jun;27(6):725-33.
[55] Isozaki H, Okajima K, Momura E, et al. Postoperative evaluation of pylorus-preserving gastrectomy for early gastric cancer. *Br. J. Surg.* 1996 Feb;83(2):266-9.
[56] Hiki N, Kaminishi M. Pylorus-preserving gastrectomy in gastric cancer surgery--open and laparoscopic approaches. *Langenbecks Arch. Surg.* 2005 Sep;390(5):442-7.
[57] Nunobe S, Hiki N, Fukunaga T, et al. Laparoscopy-assisted pylorus-preserving gastrectomy: preservation of vagus nerve and infrapyloric blood flow induces less stasis. *World J. Surg.* 2007 Dec;31(12):2335-40.
[58] Hiki N, Nunobe S, Kubota T, Jiang X. Function-preserving gastrectomy for early gastric cancer. *Ann. Surg. Oncol.* 2013 Aug;20(8):2683-92.
[59] Nakajima K, Nishida T, Takahashi T, et al. Partial gastrectomy using natural orifice translumenal endoscopic surgery (NOTES) for gastric submucosal tumors: early experience in humans. *Surg. Endosc.* 2009 Dec;23(12):2650-5.
[60] Morita S, Katai H, Saka M, Fukagawa T, Sano T, Sasako M. Outcome of pylorus-preserving gastrectomy for early gastric cancer. *Br. J. Surg.* 2008 Sep;95(9):1131-5.
[61] Hiki N, Sano T, Fukunaga T, Ohyama S, Tokunaga M, Yamaguchi T. Survival benefit of pylorus-preserving gastrectomy in early gastric cancer. *J. Am. Coll. Surg.* 2009 Sep;209(3):297-301.
[62] Jiang X, Hiki N, Nunobe S, et al. Long-term outcome and survival with laparoscopy-assisted pylorus-preserving gastrectomy for early gastric cancer. *Surg. Endosc.* 2011 Apr;25(4):1182-6.
[63] Kumagai K, Hiki N, Nunobe S, et al. Totally laparoscopic pylorus-preserving gastrectomy for early gastric cancer in the middle stomach: technical report and surgical outcomes. *Gastric. Cancer.* 2014 Jan 31.

[64] Maruyama K, Sasako M, Kinoshita T, Sano T, Katai H. Surgical treatment for gastric cancer: the Japanese approach. *Semin. Oncol.* 1996 Jun;23(3):360-8.
[65] Jeong GA, Cho GS, Kim HH, Lee HJ, Ryu SW, Song KY. Laparoscopy-assisted total gastrectomy for gastric cancer: a multicenter retrospective analysis. *Surgery.* 2009 Sep;146(3):469-74.
[66] Lee SE, Ryu KW, Nam BH, et al. Technical feasibility and safety of laparoscopy-assisted total gastrectomy in gastric cancer: a comparative study with laparoscopy-assisted distal gastrectomy. *J. Surg. Oncol.* 2009 Oct 1;100(5):392-5.
[67] An JY, Youn HG, Choi MG, Noh JH, Sohn TS, Kim S. The difficult choice between total and proximal gastrectomy in proximal early gastric cancer. *Am. J. Surg.* 2008 Oct;196(4):587-91.
[68] Bo T, Zhihong P, Peiwu Y, et al. General complications following laparoscopic-assisted gastrectomy and analysis of techniques to manage them. *Surg. Endosc.* 2009 Aug;23(8):1860-5.
[69] Jiang X, Hiki N, Nunobe S, et al. Laparoscopy-assisted subtotal gastrectomy with very small remnant stomach: a novel surgical procedure for selected early gastric cancer in the upper stomach. *Gastric. Cancer.* 2011 Jun;14(2):194-9.
[70] Hiki N, Yamamoto Y, Fukunaga T, et al. Laparoscopic and endoscopic cooperative surgery for gastrointestinal stromal tumor dissection. *Surg. Endosc.* 2008 Jul;22(7):1729-35.
[71] Nunobe S, Hiki N, Gotoda T, et al. Successful application of laparoscopic and endoscopic cooperative surgery (LECS) for a lateral-spreading mucosal gastric cancer. *Gastric. Cancer.* 2012 Jul;15(3):338-42.
[72] Abe N, Mori T, Takeuchi H, et al. Laparoscopic lymph node dissection after endoscopic submucosal dissection: a novel and minimally invasive approach to treating early-stage gastric cancer. *Am. J. Surg.* 2005 Sep;190(3):496-503.
[73] Abe N, Takeuchi H, Ohki A, et al. Long-term outcomes of combination of endoscopic submucosal dissection and laparoscopic lymph node dissection without gastrectomy for early gastric cancer patients who have a potential risk of lymph node metastasis. *Gastrointest. Endosc.* 2011 Oct;74(4):792-7.
[74] Ahn SH, Park DJ, Son SY, Lee CM, Kim HH. Single-incision laparoscopic total gastrectomy with D1+beta lymph node dissection for proximal early gastric cancer. *Gastric. Cancer.* 2013 May 17.
[75] Asakuma M, Cahill RA, Lee SW, Nomura E, Tanigawa N. NOTES: The question for minimal resection and sentinel node in early gastric cancer. *World J. Gastrointest Surg.* 2010 Jun 27;2(6):203-6.
[76] Cho WY, Kim YJ, Cho JY, et al. Hybrid natural orifice transluminal endoscopic surgery: endoscopic full-thickness resection of early gastric cancer and laparoscopic regional lymph node dissection--14 human cases. *Endoscopy.* 2010 Feb;43(2):134-9.
[77] Omori T, Oyama T, Akamatsu H, Tori M, Ueshima S, Nishida T. Transumbilical single-incision laparoscopic distal gastrectomy for early gastric cancer. *Surg. Endosc.* 2011 Jul;25(7):2400-4.

In: Laparoscopy
Editor: Christos Iavazzo

ISBN: 978-1-63321-404-0

Chapter 9

Laparoscopic Ventral Hernia Repair: Techniques and Complications

Zachary Williams, M.D.[1], Helene Seita, M.A.[2] and William W. Hope, M.D.[3*]

[1]Department of Surgery, New Hanover Regional Medical Center, South East Area Health Education Center, Wilmington, North Carolina

[2]Clinical Research Assistant, South East Area Health Education Center, Wilmington, North Carolina

[3]Assistant Professor, University of North Carolina-Chapel Hill, Department of Surgery, New Hanover Regional Medical Center, South East Area Health Education Center, Wilmington, North Carolina

Abstract

Laparoscopy has revolutionized the field of surgery allowing for faster recovery times and smaller incisions. Laparoscopic incisional hernia repair has become well-accepted due to a low probability of conversion to an open procedure, shorter hospital stays, acceptable complication rates, and low recurrence rates.

In this chapter, the technical aspects of the laparoscopic repair are discussed. The laparoscopic approach is based on the Rives-Stoppa retromuscular, sublay repair. This requires adequate mesh fixation and wide overlap of the defect. While typically well tolerated, surgeons must be aware of the potential complications. Recognition of these complications and strategies to minimize them are discussed in this review.

Laparoscopic ventral hernia repair should be in the armamentarium of all hernia surgeons. Long-term follow-up data support the durability of the laparoscopic repair. The procedure is an invaluable tool in difficult patient populations, such as the morbidly obese, smokers, and patients with prior failed attempts at repair.

* Corresponding Author: Department of Surgery, New Hanover Regional Medical Center, 2131 South 17th Street, PO Box 9025, Wilmington, NC 28401; Email: William.Hope@seahec.net,

Keywords: Hernia, Laparoscopy, Ventral, Incisional

Introduction

Ventral hernia repairs are among the most common surgeries performed by general surgeons. Of the 2 million abdominal operations performed in the United States each year, incisional hernias occur at a rate of 3% to 20% [1]. As a result, approximately 90,000 ventral hernia repairs occur annually. Many factors, both technical and patient related, contribute to incisional hernia formation [2]. These hernias contribute greatly to patients' long-term morbidity; therefore, repair of incisional hernias will remain an important and common component of general surgery. There have been numerous techniques described for the repair of ventral hernias. Tissue-based repairs involve suture approximation of healthy fascia on either side of the defect. While sometimes appropriate, primary tissue based repairs result in high recurrence rates ranging from 31% to 54% [3, 4]. The introduction of prosthetic mesh revolutionized hernia surgery with the concept of a tension-free repair. Compared with suture repairs, hernias repaired with mesh significantly decreased recurrence rates in a prospective randomized trial with long-term follow-up [5, 6]. Since their introduction, there has been an explosion of available mesh products. These meshes range from permanent synthetic meshes such as polypropylene, polyester, and polytetrafluoroethyelene meshes, to biologic meshes made from human and animals, and now synthetic absorbable materials [7]. Placement of appropriately sized mesh often requires large incisions with extensive tissue dissections. This contributes to the higher rate of wound and mesh infections.

The laparoscopic technique for repair of ventral hernias (LVHR) was developed with the hope of incurring the benefits of other laparoscopic surgeries, such as improved cosmesis, shorter recovery times, less pain, and decreased hospital stays. The technique is based on the open, preperitoneal repair described by Stoppa and Rives [8, 9]. In this technique, a large piece of mesh is placed in the preperitoneal location, facilitating an even distribution of forces along the surface area of the mesh. One notable difference is that in the laparoscopic approach the mesh is placed intra-abdominally just posterior to an intact peritoneum. The technique requires wide mesh overlap of the defect, and the mesh is made secure with transfascial sutures and tacks. One potential drawback of the repair is that the hernia defect is traditionally not closed. Recently, authors have reported on laparoscopic repairs with closure of the hernia defect [10]. Further study is needed to determine if closing the defect will have clinical benefit related to improvement of seromas, recurrence rates, or in abdominal wall physiology.

Laparoscopic ventral hernia repair has been clearly established as safe and effective in studies with large series of patients and good long-term follow-up [11-13]. This method had been demonstrated to have fewer complications, reduced surgical site infections, faster recovery, and similarly low recurrence rates when compared with open repair [14, 15].

Technique

Once general anesthesia has been induced, the patient is placed supine with both arms tucked. The bladder and stomach are typically decompressed with a Foley catheter and oral gastric tube. Prophylactic antibiotics are administered. The abdomen is then prepped and draped. An Ioban drape is used to minimize mesh contact with skin flora. Instruments used include a 30-degree angled laparoscope, 5-mm bowel graspers, scissors, clip appliers, a 5-mm spiral tacker, and an energy device if needed.

The abdomen is accessed in the left upper quadrant using either a cut-down technique, a Veress needle and optical trocar technique, or optical trocar alone. Laparoscopic access can be quite challenging in patients with incisional hernias or patients who have multiple abdominal operations and should be chosen based on the individual patient and surgeon preference [17]. The 5-mm optical trocar is placed at the left mid-clavicular line just below the costal margin. Two additional 5-mm ports are placed under direct visualization along the left anterior axillary line. One of the 5-mm ports on the left lateral abdomen can be upsized to a 10-mm port for optimal visualization using a 10-mm camera, as well as for placement of larger sized meshes. A fourth and sometimes a fifth port can be placed in the right lateral abdomen to expedite mesh fixation using tacking devices. A typical laparoscopic ventral hernia setup is shown in Figure 1. These port locations are adjusted as needed based on the location of the hernia.

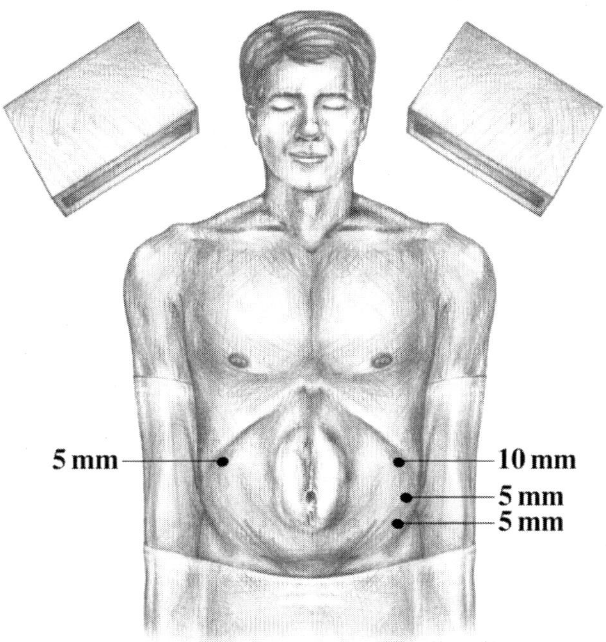

Figure 1. Typical trocar placement and setup for laparoscopic ventral hernia repair. (Used with permission from Elsevier Publishers)

The abdominal cavity is visually inspected and adhesions taken down sharply with scissors. Extreme caution is taken and the use of electrocautery minimized to avoid inadvertent bowel injury. Once adhesiolysis is completed, the facial defect is inspected and hernia contents reduced. This can be done with a combination of external manual compression and gentle traction with traumatic graspers. With the hernia contents reduced, the defect can be accurately measured. Spinal needles are placed perpendicularly through the abdominal wall at the superior, inferior, and lateral edges of the hernia defect. The defect is then measured intracorporeally using either a ruler or a suture that can then be measured extracorporeally (Figure 2).

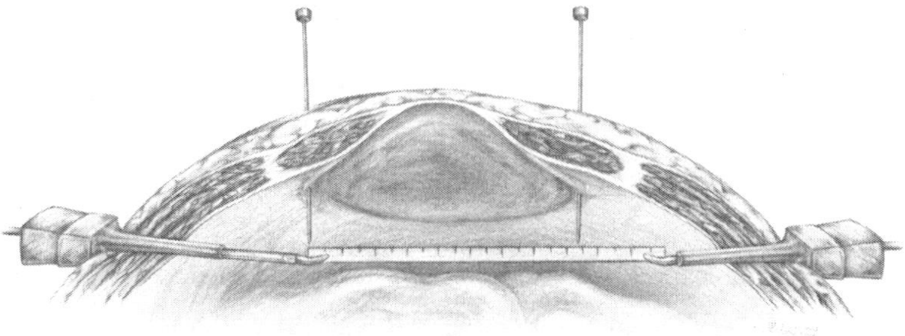

Figure 2. Intracorporeal measurement of hernia defect spinal needles and a ruler. (Used with permission from Elsevier Publishers)

Based on the defect measurements, a mesh is chosen which allows for at least 4 cm of overlap on all sides of the hernia defect. Mesh choice should be the surgeon's preference but typically includes Gore-tex based meshes or polyester and polypropylene-based meshes that have been coated with an anti-adhesion barrier. Four size zero permanent monofilament or polytetrafluoroethylene (PTFE) sutures are then placed in the superior, inferior, and lateral positions of the mesh. The Ioban drape is marked at the planned externalization sites of the four transfascial sutures. The mesh is then rolled up as a scroll on its long axis and inserted into the 10-mm trocar (Figure 3).

Once in the abdomen, the mesh is unfurled and oriented. The sutures are then pulled through the abdominal wall with a suture passer (Figure 4). The sutures should be pulled taut to evaluate for overlap and tension prior to tying. The abdomen is then desufflated and all four transfascial sutures tied. The skin is released with a hemostat to avoid dimpling. A 5-mm spiral tacker is then used to further fix the mesh. We typically place the tacks at 1 cm intervals circumferentially at the border of the mesh.

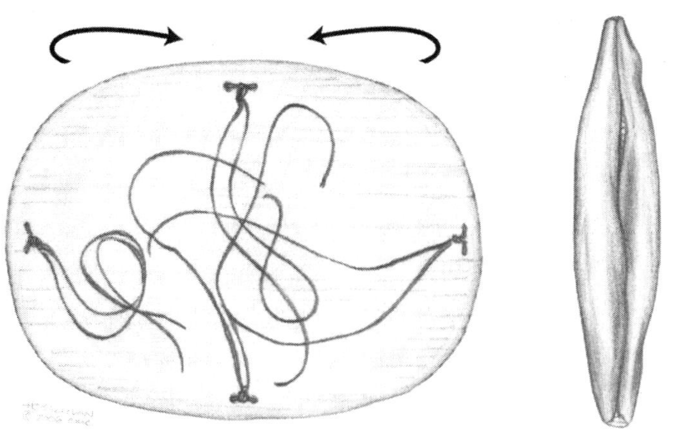

Figure 3. Sutures are placed at the four middle portions of the mesh, and then it is rolled as a scroll to allow for placement down the 12-mm trocar. (Used with permission from Elsevier Publishers)

Adequate tack placement is ensured with external compression against the tacker's tip prior to each placement (Figure 5). The mesh should be taut with wide overlap of the hernia defect. Additional transfascial sutures can be placed depending on the size of the hernia defect and the amount of mesh overlap. The abdomen is inspected for hemostasis, and the bowel inspected for potential occult bowel injuries. The 10-mm trocar is removed and fascia closed with the suture passer or under direct visualization. Local anesthetic is administered to the four transfascial suture sites and port sites. Skin defects are then closed with absorbable suture.

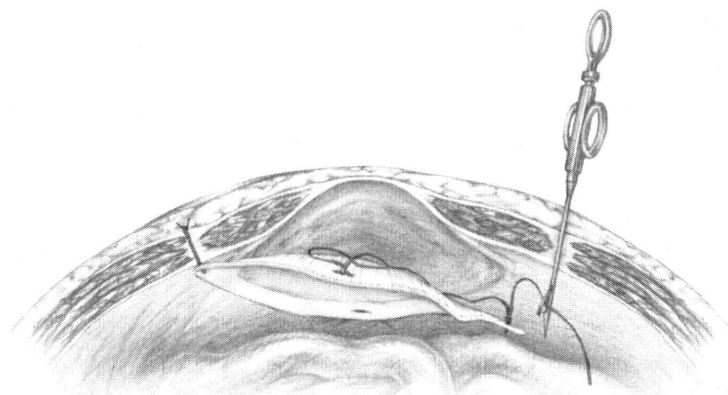

Figure 4. A suture passer is used to pull the transfascial suture up to the abdominal wall with a small stab incision made on the abdomen. (Used with permission from Elsevier Publishers)

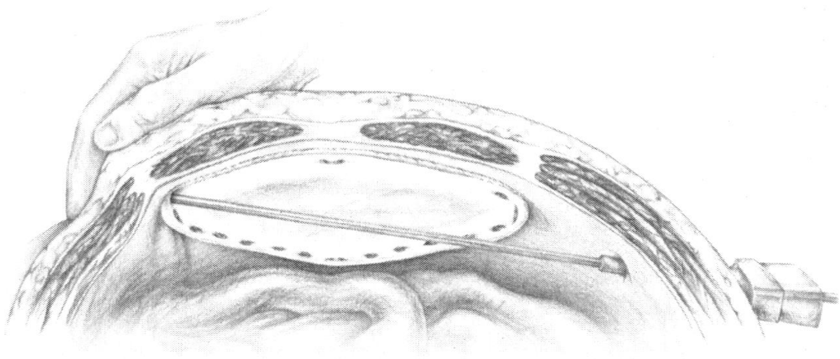

Figure 5. A tacking device is used to fix the mesh circumferentially approximately 1 cm apart and 0.5-1 cm from the edge of the mesh. Absorbable and permanent fixation devices are currently available. (Used with permission from Elsevier Publishers)

Outcomes

Recurrence

In a recent large series with mean follow-up of over a year, the overall rate of recurrence for LVHR was 4.3% [16]. An important technical point that can significantly impact recurrence is the method of mesh fixation. The majority of surgeons performing LVHR use both transfascial sutures and tacks to fix the mesh. However, some surgeons have eliminated or decreased the use of transfascial sutures, relying on the laparoscopic tacker for fixation to potentially decrease operative times and postoperative pain [13, 17]. A large series of 270 repairs, performed without suture fixation used both an inner and outer layer of tacks, had an average follow-up of 44 months and a recurrence rate of 4.4% [13]. Thus, the use of transfascial sutures and fixation methods continues to be debated [18-20].

Another potential cause of recurrence is a hernia that was not identified and repaired intraoperatively. Complete visualization of the fascia via laparoscopy allows for identification of small "Swiss-cheese" defects that would likely be missed in an open repair [21].

Mesh Infection

In open ventral hernia repairs, a large amount of soft-tissue dissection is required for placement of large pieces of mesh. Consequently, mesh infections remain an uncommon but serious complication with severe consequences. Infections of polypropylene mesh can often be managed by surgical drainage and excision of exposed, unincorporated segments. However, meshes containing PTFE typically require removal of the entire mesh prosthetic. There has been a case report of successful management with local drainage of PTFE mesh and placement of a vacuum-assisted wound device [22]. When evaluating wound and mesh infectious complications from series with at least 50 patients, LVHR had a rate of 1.7% [16] which compares favorably with 12% to 18% after open hernia repair [8, 23-25].

Seroma

Seroma formation commonly occurs in both the open and laparoscopic approach. In LVHR, the hernia sac is typically not excised, and the seromas develop above the mesh and within the retained hernia sac. Several large case series have observed the incidence of seroma formation at 4 to 8 weeks to be 11% [16]. Seromas can be sterilely aspirated or allowed to resolve and only rarely result in long-term problems. Large seromas are rare but can place tension on the skin causing necrosis and placing the patient at risk of mesh infection. Seromas that enlarge or persist should be aspirated to avoid this complication [11]. Given their common occurrence, the surgeons must inform their patients preoperatively about the likelihood of seroma formation.

Persistent Pain

Pain at the trans-abdominal suture site after LVHR occurs at a rate of 1% to 3% of patients in several reported series [11, 12, 26, 27]. This pain typically resolves within 6 to 8 weeks [28]. The exact etiology of this pain is unknown, but possible explanations include entrapment of intercostal nerves or local muscle ischemia. The first line of treatment should be nonsteroidal anti-inflammatory therapy. If the pain persists, local anesthesia can be injected at the painful suture sites. In one study, 92% of patients undergoing injection at transfascial suture sites had complete relief of their symptoms [29].

Morbid Obesity

Many patients that present for ventral herniorrhaphy are morbidly obese. Obesity has been clearly established as a risk factor for development of incisional hernias and is associated with increased intra-abdominal pressure [30]. Higher pressure creates more strain on the mesh placed during herniorrhaphy and likely causes increased recurrence following repair. The laparoscopic approach is ideal in the obese patient due to the smaller wounds and consequently decreased wound complications [31].

Complications of open ventral herniorrhaphy such as wound infection and recurrence are elevated in the obese population. Laparoscopic ventral hernia repair is ideally suited for the morbidly obese patient. One case series of 278 obese patients revealed a low rate of conversion to laparotomy, a 12% rate of minor complications, mean hospital stay of 2.6 days, and a recurrence rate of 5.5% at 25 months [32].

Previous Failed Repairs

LVHR is an excellent choice for hernias that have failed a prior attempt at open repair. This technique is ideal for patients with failed preperitoneal or onlay repairs using prosthetics, because the laparoscopic mesh placement avoids disrupting these meshes and risking infection. However, the "hostile abdomen" with numerous failed repairs and several pieces of mesh are likely best served by an open repair due to the difficulty of laparoscopic adhesiolysis. The "Swiss cheese" abdomens with multiple small defects are well suited for LVRH. Complete visualization of the fascia via laparoscopy facilitates wide mesh coverage and identification of all defects.

In one large series, patients with failed prior open attempts at repair had a higher rate of complications (17.8% versus 10.4%), longer operative times (134 minutes versus 111 minutes), increased risk of subsequent hernia recurrence (7.1% versus 2.3%), with no difference found in the rate of conversion to open surgery [11]. These patients are more technically challenging but they can be safely treated with LVHR.

Quality of life

With improvement in traditional outcomes such as wound infections and recurrence rates, more emphasis is being placed on functional outcomes such as quality of life. One study revealed that at six months follow-up, LVHR afforded a significantly better quality of life than open hernia repair using both a generic and hernia-specific quality of life survey [36]. Quality of life information will continue to be an important outcome measure in hernia repair when evaluating novel techniques and mesh products.

Conclusion

Laparoscopic ventral hernia repair results in short hospital stays, low rates of conversion to open surgery, low risk of wound infections, low recurrence rates at long-term follow-up, and an acceptable overall complication rate. The laparoscopic approach continues to be a vital tool in the treatment of complex patients, especially those who are obese and who have had failed prior open repairs. Laparoscopic ventral hernia repair should be considered the standard of care for these difficult patient populations.

References

[1] Read RC, Yoder G. Recent trends in the management of incisional herniation. *Arch. Surg*. 1989 Apr;124(4):485-8.

[2] Hope W. Prevention of incisional hernia development. *Minerva. Chir*. 2011 Apr;66(2):145-52. Epub 2011/05/20.

[3] Anthony T, Bergen PC, Kim LT, Henderson M, Fahey T, Rege RV, et al. Factors affecting recurrence following incisional herniorrhaphy. *World J. Surg*. 2000 Jan;24(1):95-100;discussion 1.

[4] Luijendijk RW, Lemmen MH, Hop WC, Wereldsma JC. Incisional hernia recurrence following "vest-over-pants" or vertical Mayo repair of primary hernias of the midline. *World J. Surg*. 1997 Jan;21(1):62-5; discussion 6.

[5] Burger JW, Luijendijk RW, Hop WC, Halm JA, Verdaasdonk EG, Jeekel J. Long-term follow-up of a randomized controlled trial of suture versus mesh repair of incisional hernia. *Ann. Surg*. 2004 Oct;240(4):578-83; discussion 83-5. Epub 2004/09/24.

[6] Luijendijk RW, Hop WC, van den Tol MP, de Lange DC, Braaksma MM, JN IJ, et al. A comparison of suture repair with mesh repair for incisional hernia. *N. Engl. J. Med*. 2000 Aug 10;343(6):392-8. Epub 2000/08/10.

[7] Novitsky YW, Harrell AG, Hope WW, Kercher KW, Heniford BT. Meshes in hernia repair. *Surg. Technol. Int*. 2007;16:123-7. Epub 2007/04/13.

[8] Stoppa RE. The treatment of complicated groin and incisional hernias. *World J. Surg*. 1989 Sep-Oct;13(5):545-54.

[9] Rives J, Pire JC, Flament JB, Palot JP, Body C. [Treatment of large eventrations. New therapeutic indications apropos of 322 cases]. *Chirurgie*. 1985;111(3):215-25.

[10] Orenstein SB, Dumeer JL, Monteagudo J, Poi MJ, Novitsky YW. Outcomes of laparoscopic ventral hernia repair with routine defect closure using "shoelacing" technique. *Surg. Endosc. 2011* May; 25(5):1452-7. Epub 2010/11/06.

[11] Heniford BT, Park A, Ramshaw BJ, Voeller G. Laparoscopic repair of ventral hernias: nine years' experience with 850 consecutive hernias. *Ann .Surg*. 2003 Sep;238(3):391-9; discussion 9-400. Epub 2003/09/23.

[12] Franklin ME, Jr., Gonzalez JJ, Jr., Glass JL, Manjarrez A. Laparoscopic ventral and incisional hernia repair: an 11-year experience. *Hernia*. 2004 Feb;8(1):23-7.

[13] Carbajo MA, Martp del Olmo JC, Blanco JI, Toledano M, de la Cuesta C, Ferreras C, et al. Laparoscopic approach to incisional hernia. *Surg. Endosc*. 2003 Jan;17(1):118-22. Epub 2002/10/26.

[14] Forbes SS, Eskicioglu C, McLeod RS, Okrainec A. Meta-analysis of randomized controlled trials comparing open and laparoscopic ventral and incisional hernia repair with mesh. *Br. J. Surg*. 2009 Aug;96(8):851-8. Epub 2009/07/11.

[15] Sajid MS, Bokhari SA, Mallick AS, Cheek E, Baig MK. Laparoscopic versus open repair of incisional/ventral hernia: a meta-analysis. *Am. J. Surg*. 2009 Jan;197(1):64-72. Epub 2008/07/11.

[16] Cobb WS, Kercher KW, Heniford BT. Laparoscopic repair of incisional hernias. *Surg. Clin. North Am*. 2005 Feb;85(1):91-103, ix.

[17] Morales-Conde S, Cadet H, Cano A, Bustos M, Martin J, Morales-Mendez S. Laparoscopic ventral hernia repair without sutures--double crown technique: our experience after 140 cases with a mean follow-up of 40 months. *Int. Surg*. 2005 Jul-Aug;90(3 Suppl):S56-62. Epub 2006/02/09.

[18] LeBlanc KA. Laparoscopic incisional hernia repair: are transfascial sutures necessary? A review of the literature. Surg Endosc. 2007 Apr;21(4):508-13. Epub 2007/02/09.

[19] Reynvoet E, Deschepper E, Rogiers X, Troisi R, Berrevoet F. Laparoscopic ventral hernia repair: is there an optimal mesh fixation technique? A systematic review. *Langenbecks Arch. Surg*. 2013 Oct 13. Epub 2013/10/15.

[20] Wassenaar E, Schoenmaeckers E, Raymakers J, van der Palen J, Rakic S. Mesh-fixation method and pain and quality of life after laparoscopic ventral or incisional hernia repair: a randomized trial of three fixation techniques. *Surg. Endosc*. 2010 Jun;24(6):1296-302. Epub 2009/12/25.

[21] Park A, Birch DW, Lovrics P. Laparoscopic and open incisional hernia repair: a comparison study. *Surgery*. 1998 Oct;124(4):816-21; discussion 21-2.

[22] Kercher KW, Sing RF, Matthews BD, Heniford BT. Successful salvage of infected PTFE mesh after ventral hernia repair. *Ostomy Wound Manage*. 2002 Oct;48(10):40-2, 4-5.

[23] McLanahan D, King LT, Weems C, Novotney M, Gibson K. Retrorectus prosthetic mesh repair of midline abdominal hernia. *Am. J. Surg*. 1997 May;173(5):445-9. Epub 1997/05/01.

[24] Rios A, Rodriguez JM, Munitiz V, Alcaraz P, Perez D, Parrilla P. Factors that affect recurrence after incisional herniorrhaphy with prosthetic material. *Eur. J. Surg*. 2001 Nov;167(11):855-9.

[25] White TJ, Santos MC, Thompson JS. Factors affecting wound complications in repair of ventral hernias. *Am. Surg*. 1998 Mar;64(3):276-80.

[26] LeBlanc KA, Whitaker JM, Bellanger DE, Rhynes VK. Laparoscopic incisional and ventral hernioplasty: lessons learned from 200 patients. *Hernia*. 2003 Sep;7(3):118-24.

[27] Bower CE, Reade CC, Kirby LW, Roth JS. Complications of laparoscopic incisional-ventral hernia repair: the experience of a single institution. *Surg. Endosc*. 2004 Apr;18(4):672-5.

[28] Heniford BT, Park A, Ramshaw BJ, Voeller G. Laparoscopic ventral and incisional hernia repair in 407 patients. *J. Am. Coll. Surg*. 2000 Jun;190(6):645-50.

[29] Carbonell AM, Harold KL, Mahmutovic AJ, Hassan R, Matthews BD, Kercher KW, et al. Local injection for the treatment of suture site pain after laparoscopic ventral hernia repair. *Am. Surg*. 2003 Aug;69(8):688-91; discussion 91-2.

[30] Sugerman HJ, Kellum JM, Jr., Reines HD, DeMaria EJ, Newsome HH, Lowry JW. Greater risk of incisional hernia with morbidly obese than steroid-dependent patients

and low recurrence with prefascial polypropylene mesh. *Am. J. Surg*. 1996 Jan;171(1):80-4. Epub 1996/01/01.

[31] Ramshaw BJ, Esartia P, Schwab J, Mason EM, Wilson RA, Duncan TD, et al. Comparison of laparoscopic and open ventral herniorrhaphy. *Am. Surg*. 1999 Sep;65(9):827-31; discussion 31-2.

[32] Birgisson G, Park AE, Mastrangelo MJ, Jr., Witzke DB, Chu UB. Obesity and laparoscopic repair of ventral hernias. *Surg. Endosc*. 2001 Dec;15(12):1419-22.

In: Laparoscopy
Editor: Christos Iavazzo

ISBN: 978-1-63321-404-0

Chapter 10

Analgesia in Robotic and Laparoscopic Urological Procedures

Sian E. Batley[1], Nikhil Vasdev*[2], Timothy Lane[1], Gregory Boustead[2], James M. Adshead[2] and Shanmugasundaram Gowrie-Mohan

[1]Department of Anesthetics, Lister Hospital, Stevenage, UK
[2]Hertfordshire and South Bedfordshire Robotic Urological Cancer Centre, Department of Urology, Lister Hospital, Stevenage, UK

Abstract

With the increased use of robotic and laparoscopic and techniques in Urological surgery there has been a concomitant increase in the interest in the use of optimum analgesic techniques to prevent and treat pain specifically caused by urological robotic and laparoscopic surgery. With the introduction of laparoscopic and robotic urological procedures, the aim of the techniques is to optimize patient care but post operative analgesia is crucial to enhance patient recovery. We present a detailed book chapter that explains the mechanism of pain pathways involved in robotic and robotic urological procedures. We also review current evidence pertaining to systemic and regional analgesia methods.

Introduction

Robotic and Laparoscopic surgery reduces post operative pain; the benefits of this reduces morbidity, enables a shorter hospital stay, costs less and increases patient satisfaction

* Correspondence: Mr Nikhil Vasdev, Robotic Urological Fellow, Hertfordshire and South Bedfordshire Robotic Urological Cancer Centre, Department of Urology, Lister Hospital, Stevenage, UK, Email – nikhilvasdev@doctors.

[1,2]. Although robotic and laparoscopic surgery reduce postoperative pain due to a reduction in tissue handling and a reduced incision size[3], no procedure is pain free and there are different challenges in treating this specific type of pain.

Pain relief is crucial but risks and side effects from the analgesic technique must also be taken into consideration and not cause increased morbidity such as nausea, ileus, reduction in consciousness and autonomic dysfunction[1] thus preventing the early discharge that the minimally invasive surgery has facilitated in the first place.

There are multiple analgesic techniques available to prevent and treat pain specifically caused by urological laparoscopic and robotic surgery; this article will explain the mechanism of pain pathways involved in laparoscopic procedures and review current evidence pertaining to systemic and regional analgesia methods.

Causes and Mechanisms of Pain

There are several types of pain associated with robotic and laparoscopic surgery; incisional port site pain, pain from the peritoneum being distended with carbon dioxide, visceral pain, and shoulder tip pain. Rapid insufflation of the peritoneum with carbon dioxide causes tearing of blood vessels, traumatic traction of nerves and release of inflammatory mediators [1].

Residual gas post procedure causes shoulder tip pain, back pain and upper abdominal pain by diaphragmatic stretching and phrenic nerve irritation [4, 5]. The fact that there are different mechanisms of pain involved in laparoscopy makes it challenging to treat.

The most severe pain is immediately post operative period [1, 6] and decreases with time; however there are often further peaks of pain up to three days later which must be effectively and safely managed in an outpatient setting. If pain is not treated effectively re-admission for pain makes the previous benefit of laparoscopic surgery for a shorter hospital stay redundant; conversely if strong analgesics are used inappropriately in the outpatient setting this may too be problematic.

Literature searches specifically for analgesia for robotic and laparoscopic urological surgery were carried out and yielded few results, there is lacking evidence for techniques used specifically in urological robotic and laparoscopic procedures and further studies are needed in this area. However, searches for robotic and laparoscopic procedures not specific to urological surgery can be extrapolated and used to mount evidence for best practice and therefore have been included for discussion.

Method

Literature searches were carried out using Medline (PubMed), Cochrane, and Tripdata. Search words specifically for urological procedures included urology + analgesia +pain + robtotics+laparoscopy. This yielded 98 results of which studies were excluded for not having a type/method of analgesia for laparoscopic surgery as a primary reason for the study. This resulted in only five studies comparing different analgesic methods which have been reviewed first in this study.

The urological laparoscopic studies based their research on laparoscopic general surgery and gynecological procedures, therefore, due to lack of evidence from the preliminary search a second search was carried out. Search words included the analgesia/technique+ robotics+laparoscopy+ surgery + analgesia.

Review of Analgesia for Laparoscopic Urological Procedures

The first literature review was specific to analgesia for urological procedures. Four of the five were retrospective studies and only one was a prospective double-blind study. All had very small numbers of participants with a total of 494 participants and 300 of those coming from one trial, the remainder were split amongst four very small trials. Two of the studies looked at the use of the local anesthetic bupivacaine, two looked at ketorolac as an adjunct to analgesia, and one looked at multimodal analgesia using NSAIDs and pregabalin. Various urological procedures were included in the study including prostatectomy, nephrectomy and pyeloplasty however all were laparoscopic. End points were reduction in pain scores, reduction in analgesic requirements-especially opioid based, reduction in length of stay, incidence of nausea and vomiting, and serum creatinine levels.

The first small retrospective trial by Trabulsi et al. [7] looked at multimodal analgesia in 60 patients who were undergoing robotic-assisted laparoscopic radical prostatectomy. In group one thirty patients received pre-emptive pregabalin, calecoxib and 975mg paracetamol two hours prior to surgery. In group 2, 30 patients received post operative intravenous ketorolac, oxycodone and 325mg paracetamol.

Mean morphine administration was measure intra- and post-operatively. The study showed a reduction of mean total morphine administration in group one ($P<0.001$) but no changes to length of stay, antiemetic use or post-operative serum creatinine levels. There are multiple variables and confounding factors with this study (different timings of medications, different paracetamol doses, different NSAIDs used, no mention of regional anesthesia or local infiltration).

Yoost et al., [8] investigated how continuous infiltration of bupivacaine into the incision site via an elastomeric pump reduced pain post operatively of patients undergoing laparoscopic nephrectomy and compared it with intravenous and oral analgesia. 38 patients were included in the study of which 18 had local anaesthetic infiltration and 20 had systemic analgesia.

They stated that initial experience suggested a reduction in opioid use and a reduction in length of stay compared to those not receiving local anaesthetic infiltration. However, this again is a very small retrospective study which did not give statistically significant results.

Another study involving bupivacaine looked at the effectiveness of aerosolized intraperitoneal bupivacaine to reduce post operative pain [9]. This study was done in the pediatric population undergoing laparoscopic pyeloplasty. 41 cases were reviewed in this retrospective trial, all received 'standard' peri-operative analgesia (ketorolac at the end of surgery, plus codeine/morphine/hydrocodone or oxycodone prn). 5 cases also received intraperitoneal aerosolized bupivacaine just prior to trochar removal and 17 had aerosolized bupivacaine earlier in the procedure (prior to incising peri-renal fascia). 19 children had no bupivacaine intervention.

The study showed a reduction in post-operative opioid use in the group that had bupivacaine at the beginning of surgery but not in those who received it at the end of the procedure. All 22 patients receiving some form of bupivacaine had shorter length of stay (P<0.01). This is a small retrospective study in just a pediatric population however it demonstrates some benefit of pre-emptive multimodal analgesia in laparoscopic urological procedures.

The largest retrospective study by Breda et al. [10] found involved 300 patients undergoing laparoscopic donor nephrectomy. In non-urological studies ketorolac has been proven to reduce opioid requirement by 50% and owing to opioids propensity to cause nausea and vomiting and constipation the authors were keen to promote its use to improve patient experience and to shorten length of stay, however, they were concerned about the effect ketorolac may have on renal function. All subjects received ketorolac (1st does given on removal of the kidney, then every 6 hours for a maximum of 48 hours) as well as a strict bowel preparation regime pre-operatively.

The results showed mean hospital stay of 1.1 days (96.7% discharged on day 1), 97% ate post-operatively with no nausea/vomiting and 97% of patients received only oral analgesia. Only 6 patients required additional post-operative intravenous opioid analgesia. It is not clear how much bowel preparation and ketorolac contributed individually to the results and so it would be useful to investigate this separately, there also seems to be significant bias in this study. It does however give strength to the analgesic effect of ketorolac as adjunct analgesia and in the selected patients did not cause renal impairment.

The only prospective trial by Chow et al. [11] was a double blind study looking at the effect of ketorolac administration after laparoscopic urological surgery. Fifty five subjects completed the study and all received patient controlled analgesia post operatively. Half the subjects also received ketorolac whilst half received a placebo and underwent a variety of urological procedures. Analogue pain scores were used to measure pain; average pain score was lower in those receiving ketorolac (P<0.005) and mean morphine use was less in the ketorolac group P=0.077. There was no demonstrated change in the length of stay, blood loss, time to resume oral intake, or creatinine levels between the two groups. It was noted that patients undergoing laparoscopic pyeloplasty needed more opioid analgesia than other procedures. In this small study ketorolac was found to decrease subjective perception of pain and decrease opioid use.

Robotic urological laparoscopic procedures are relatively new and for this reason there is a paucity in data in the most suitable analgesia for these procedures. The above studies are too few in number and lack power, they are also too heterogeneous to enable statistical analysis. There is a need for good quality highly powered randomized controlled trials. Due to this, we have to base our preliminary research on laparoscopic studies in colorectal and gynecological surgery.

Taking the above into consideration a second literature search was carried out looking at specific techniques which are already used for analgesia in other laparoscopic procedures and could prove efficacious for urological procedures and provide a basis for future investigation.

Practical Solutions

There is correlation of amount of residual intra-peritoneal gas and pain scores post operatively. Therefore, using lower abdominal pressures when insufflating and aspirating residual gas at the end of the procedure reduces post operative pain [4]. A Cochrane database systematic review of 15 trials (690 patients) also demonstrated less shoulder tip pain and reduced analgesic requirement with lower pressure pneumoperitoneum. A randomized controlled trial by Yasir et al., [13] compared low pressure (8mmHg) and high pressure (14mmHg) for abdominal insufflation for laparoscopic cholecystectomy; this study demonstrated reduced reporting of shoulder tip pain (reduced frequency and intensity) 4 hours post operatively though did not show statistical significance at 8 and 24 hours. Analgesic requirement and shorter hospital stay were also shown amongst the lower pressure group.

Another study by Sandhu T et al., [14] showed a tendency for less pain but in this trial of 140 patients this reduction was not statistically significant.

Mechanical ventilation tidal volumes did not have any effect on shoulder tip pain post laparoscopic surgery in one prospective trial containing 64 patients [15].

Multimodal

Multimodal analgesia involves the use of different classes of analgesics and different sites of analgesic administration to provide superior dynamic pain relief with reduced opioid analgesia-related side effects [16]; this can be particularly challenging in laparoscopic procedures due to the different types of pain produced by the procedure [1].

Those undergoing multimodal analgesia have shown improved recovery, less nausea and vomiting, and less opiate side effects; these can culminate into shorter hospital stays, less morbidity and increased patient satisfaction.

Multi-modal analgesia should utilize non-opiate systemic analgesics plus regional techniques, these should be administered/performed pre-emptively [17].

Pre-Emptive

The initial concept of preemptive analgesia was formulated by Crile [18] in 1913 when he described the use of regional techniques to prevent post operative pain; it is thought to prevent central sensitization and hyper-excitability which decreases post operative pain by preventing wind-up and is thought to decrease the incidence of chronic pain [19]. Pre-emptive analgesia is defined as any treatment that prevents establishment of central sensitization caused by incisional and inflammatory injuries and should start before incision, cover the surgical period and the initial post operative period [10, 19, 20].

There remains controversy over the effectiveness and timing of preemptive analgesia, there is only one study which looks at preemptive analgesia in a urological laparoscopic procedures[7] and one systematic review and meta-analysis from non-urological studies that looks at the impact of local analgesia timing and postoperative pain [21]. Coughlin et al.

analyzed 26 studies and showed that surgeons should use local analgesia in laparoscopic surgery to decrease postoperative pain (infiltration at port sites or intraperitoneally), but the timing of administration is significant only for intraperitoneal infiltration but not for port infiltration with local anesthetic. Pre-incisional use of bupivacaine has been recommended (Grade A evidence) in another systematic review of interventions in laparoscopic cholecystectomy [22].

Systemic Analgesia

There were no reviews of preemptive systemic analgesia although a review of 8 prospective, double blind, randomized controlled trials (RCT) [7, 23-29] mostly showed benefit in using adjunct systemic analgesia in laparoscopy prior to incision. Ketamine showed a reduction in pain in one trial but made no difference in pain relief in another, however, the overall conclusion in 8 of the trials (746 participants) showed statistically significant results in the reduction of pain. Drugs used involved NSAIDs (diclofenac, paracoxib, etorcoxib, calecoxib), ketamine, gabapentin and intravenous lignocaine. NSAIDs and cox-2 inhibitors showed promising results and showed benefit from their administration and demonstrated a good side effect profile.

Paracetamol has been shown to be effective and should be used in combination with other analgesics but can not be used in isolation [30].

Although these RCTs are promising, there is a need for more good quality randomized controlled trials in laparoscopic procedures plus systematic review and meta-analysis of these studies and then application to urological procedures.

Intravenous lidocaine infusion has shown benefit in analgesia in patients undergoing laparoscopic and open procedures. Although no data regarding urological procedures, it has been described in laparoscopic cholecystectomy and colorectal surgery. In a systematic review [31] of 764 patients, 369 patients received intravenous lidocaine and underwent an open or laparoscopic procedure. The results showed in both the open and laparoscopic groups a reduction in pain, reduced opioid consumption, earlier return of bowel function and shorter hospital stays. The study also states that there was no toxicity, nor any clinically significant adverse effects. Lidocaine seems to be a safe, effective, and economical [32] and therefore warrants further investigation as an intravenous analgesic.

Magnesium has also been used and compared to lidocaine as an analgesic in laparoscopic cholecystectomy. In a small (120 subject 40 in each group) double blinded study magnesium and lidocaine both reduced intra operative and post operative opioid requirements and pain scores [33]. Magnesium showed a reduction in pain scores and opioid sparing effects in another randomized controlled trial [34] though further research is required. The use of magnesium gives us another potential target for non-opioid analgesia in laparoscopic surgery.

Clonidine has been used intrathecally in spinal anesthesia pain and orally as a premedication prior to laparoscopic cholecystectomy [35]. No statistical difference was found in the oral clonidine premedication group but this was an extremely small study that would need to be done on a larger scale to increase its power. In a meta-analysis intrathecal clonidine extends the time to first analgesia and decreases the amount of morphine used.

However, there was also an increase in hypotension which must be considered [36] as well as the high risk:benefit of spinal anesthesia in laparoscopic procedures.

Steroids (dexamethasone and methyl prednisolone) have been shown to reduce post operative nausea and vomiting and post operative pain relief, both of which will improve patient well being and aid earlier discharge. In a systematic review of 1801 women [37] undergoing laparoscopic gynecological procedures prophylactic dexamethasone decreased nausea and vomiting but did not show a difference in analgesic requirements. Conversely in another met-analysis on colorectal laparoscopic procedures by Joshi et al. [38] showed that preemptive dexamethasone improved post operative pain relief as well as nausea and vomiting. They also recommended infiltration of surgical incisions with local anesthetic, NSAIDs, paracetamol and rescue opioids. Intravenous lignocaine was recommended as a second line treatment and neuroaxial blocks were discouraged.

Regional Analgesia

Neuro Axial Blockade

Epidural anesthesia lacked superiority over other multimodal analgesic techniques in one evidence based review of laparoscopic colorectal surgery undertaken by the procedure-specific postoperative pain management (PROSPECT) working group [38]. Minimally invasive procedures are less painful and there are more adverse effects associated with epidural analgesia (hypotension, pruritis, from motor blockade [39]).They concluded that neuroaxial blocks are not necessary in colorectal laparoscopic surgery based on a high risk:benefit ratio. The same review also looked at spinal morphine versus intravenous patient controlled analgesia and concluded that although there are reduced pain scores with intrathecal opiates there is a higher incidence of pruritis and respiratory depression. The risk:benefit ratios need to be carefully considered taking into account using neuroaxial blockade for urological laparoscopic procedures although there may be benefit if there is a high probability of converting to an open procedure.

Intercostal Block

The somatic supply of the skin, muscles and parietal peritoneum of the anterior abdominal wall are from the anterior divisions of T7-L1. T7 to T11 are intercostal nerves so intercostal blocks may be of benefit in pain relief caused by laparoscopic surgery in the upper abdomen; intercostal nerves 9, 10 and 11 are likely to be blocked from a transversus abdominis (TAP) block therefore extending this block by use of bilateral intercostal blocks may be of benefit in laparoscopic procedures.

One prospective, double-blinded randomized controlled trial involving 61 patients undergoing laparoscopic cholecystectomy reported that patients who had received intercostal block had a significantly lower pain score ($p<0.001$) than those who did not receive an intercostal block [40].

TAP Block

A Cochrane review looked at the benefit of transversus abdominis plane (TAP) blocks for non-laparoscopic procedures; 8 studies with 358 participants showed limited evidence of their benefit (analgesia and reduction in opioid use) however further studies were awaited and will be reviewed again in the future [41].

Another review and meta-analysis of the clinical effectiveness of TAP blocks was published by Johns et al. [42]; the authors concluded that the block could be used as part of multimodal analgesia and enhanced recovery, it was safe and reduced opioid requirements. A review of TAP blocks for laparoscopic procedures and the methods used to carry out TAP blocks (blind, ultrasound guided or laparoscopic guided) is required; there is also a need for comparison with other regional techniques.

Paravertebral Block *(PVB)*

The use of this block was used in an expanded case report of 30 patients undergoing hand-assisted laparoscopic nephrectomy and compared with conventional opioid therapy [43]. They found that utilizing a PVB as part of multi-modal analgesia improved dynamic pain scores and decreased opioid requirements. A prospective randomized controlled trial was carried out in patients who had a PVB (level T5-T6) undergoing laparoscopic cholecystectomy [44]; the small study group failed to show a statistically significant decrease in post operative pain. Larger randomized controlled trials are lacking and due to a skill shortage in Anesthetists trained to carry out this block this will be difficult to accomplish. Autonomic nervous system may be involved in the pathogenesis of acute as well as chronic pain [45] and Stellate ganglion blockade may contribute to post operative pain relief [46].

Airseal® Integrated Access System for Laparoscopic and Robotic Surgery

AirSeal® is an integrated access system for laparoscopic and robotic surgery, representing a revolutionary transformation of conventional insufflation, trocar, and filtered tubing systems. The system provides a stable pneumoperitoneum, continuous smoke evacuation, and valve-free access to the abdominal cavity.

The AirSeal® System (Milford, CT, USA) which consists of the 3 mode IFS Control Unit, Valve-less Trocar and Smoke Evacuation Filter Tube component has been reported to provide Stable Pneumoperitoneum even under constant aspiration, Automatic smoke evacuation, less patient CO_2 absorption [47], less operative time [48] along with other improved operating efficiencies[1] during laparoscopic and robotic surgery. Further, when compared to conventional insufflator this device has been shown to maintain stable pneumoperitoneum [49] with unimpeded visualization. Recently an abstract was presented at the recent AAGL3 congress in which a pilot study describes how in comparison to conventional insufflation the AirSeal® System significantly reduced pain, pain medication.

Conclusion

In our experience caudal analgesia (with bupivacaine 0.25% 40 ml, clonidine 150 microgram and fentanyl 100 microgram) provides very good intraoperative and post operative pain relief after robotic assisted laparoscopic prostatectomy (ongoing observational study).

Although limited data there seems to be benefit from pre-emptive, multi-modal analgesia, use of systemic analgesic adjuncts and regional anesthesia. There is less benefit and also undesirable side effects from large quantities of systemic opioids including those delivered by patient controlled analgesia systems and neuroaxial blockade.

Robotic urological procedures are relatively new but offer great benefit to patients-reduction in morbidity, shorter hospital stay, economical benefit and increased patient satisfaction. However, pain from laparoscopic procedures can prove difficult to treat and will have a negative impact if not dealt with effectively and with minimal side effects.

The current urological laparoscopic studies are limited by lack of good quality randomized controlled prospective trials and small participant number. There is huge scope for further study and research in this area, especially since more urological robotic laparoscopic surgery is being successfully carried out.

References

[1] Alexander JI. Pain after laparoscopy. *British Journal of Anesthesia* 1997;79:369-378

[2] Efficacy and safety of fast-track recovery strategy for patients undergoing laparoscopic nephrectomy. Recart A, Duchene D, White PF, Thomas T, Johnson DB, Cadeddu JA SO *J Endourol.* 2005;19(10):1165.

[3] Midley S, Tolley DA. *Anaesthesia for Laparoscopic Surgery in Urology* 2006 EAU-EBU Update Series 4;241-245

[4] Fredman B, Jedeikin R, Olfsanger D. Residual pneumoperitoneum: a cause of postoperative pain after laparoscopic cholecystectomy. *Anesth Analg* 1994;79:152.

[5] Jackson SA, Laurence AS, Hill JC. Does post-laparoscopy pain relate to residual carbon dioxide? *Anaesthesia* 1996;51:485-487

[6] Perla Ekstein, Amir Szold, Boaz Sagie, Nachum Werbin, Joseph M. Klausner, Avi A. Weinbroum. Laparoscopic Surgery May Be Associated With Severe Pain and High Analgesia Requirements in the Immediate Postoperative Period. *Ann Surg.* 2006 January; 243(1): 41–46.

[7] Trabulsi EJ, Patel J, Viscusi ER, Gomella LG, Lallas CD. Preemptive multimodal pain regimen reduces opioid analgesia for patients undergoing robotic-assisted laparoscopic radical prostatectomy. *Urology.* 2010. Nov;76(5):1122-4.

[8] Yoost TR, McIntyre M, Savage SJ. *J Endourol. Continous Infusion of local anesthetic decreases narcotic use and length of hospitalisation after laparoscopic renal surgery.* 2009 Apr;23(4):632-6.

[9] Freilich DA, Houck CS, Meier PM, Passerotti CC, Retik AB, Nguyen HT. The effectiveness of aerosolized intraperitoneal bupivacaine in reducing postoperative pain in children undergoing robotic-assisted laparoscopic pyeloplasty. *J Pediatr Urol.* 2008 Oct;4(5):337-40. doi: 10.1016/j.jpurol.2008.04.006. Epub 2008 Jun 16.

[10] Breda A, Bui MH, Liao JC, Schulam PG. Association of bowel rest and ketorolac analgesia with short hospital stay after laparoscopic donor nephrectomy. *Urology*. 2007 May;69(5):828-31

[11] Chow GK, Fabrizio MD, Steer T, Potter SR, Jarrett TW, Gelman S, Kavoussi LR. Prospective double blind study of effect of ketorolac administration after laparoscopic urological surgery. *J endourol.* 2001 March;15(2):171-4.

[12] Gurusamy KS, Samraj K, Davidson BR. Low pressure versus standard pressure pneumoperitoneum in laparoscopic cholecystectomy. *Cochrane Database of Systematic Reviews 2009,* Issue 2. Art. No.: CD006930. DOI: 10.1002/14651858.CD006930.pub2.

[13] Yasir M, Mehta KS, Hussain V, Banday, Aiman A, Masood I, Iqbal B. Evaluation of post operative shoulder tip pain in low pressure versus standard pressure pneumoperitoneum during laparoscopic cholecystectomy. *The Surgeon - April 2012* (Vol. 10, Issue 2, Pages 71-74, DOI: 10.1016/j.surge.2011.02.003)

[14] Sandhu T, Paiboonworachat S, Ko-iam W.Effects of preemptive analgesia in laparoscopic cholecystectomy: a double-blind randomized controlled trial.*Surg Endosc.* 2011 Jan;25(1):23-7. doi: 10.1007/s00464-010-1122-y. Epub 2010 Jun 30.

[15] Shin HY, Kim SH, Lee YJ, Kim DK. The effect of mechanical ventilation tidal volume during pneumoperitoneum on shoulder pain after a laparoscopic appendectomy. *Surg Endosc.* 2010 Aug;24(8):2002-7. doi: 10.1007/s00464-010-0895-3. Epub 2010 Feb 5.

[16] Joshi GP. Multimodal analgesic techniques and postoperative rehabilitation. *Anesthesiol Clin North America*. 2005 Mar;23(1):185-202.

[17] Ahn Y, Woods J, Connor S. *A systematic review of interventions to facilitate ambulatory laparoscopic cholecystectomy*. HPB (Oxford). 2011 Oct;13(10):677-86.

[18] Crile GW: The kinetic theory of shock and its prevention through anoci-association. *Lancet* 1913; 185: 7–16.

[19] Kissin I, Preemptive Analgesia. *Anesthesiology*. 1993 October;93(4) 1138-1143.

[20] Jorgen D, Moiniche S. Pre-emptive analgesia. *Br Med Bull* (2004) 71 (1): 13-27.doi: 10.1093/bmb/ldh030.

[21] Coughlin SM, Karanicolas PJ, Emmerton-Coughlin HM, Kanbur B, Kanbur S, Colquoun PH. Better late than never? Impact of local analgesia timing on postoperative pain in laparoscopic surgery: a systematic review and metaanalysis. *Surg Endosc*. 2010 Dec;24(12):3167-76. doi: 10.1007/s00464-010-1111-1. Epub 2010 May 20.

[22] Pourseidi B, Khorram-Manesh A. Effect of intercostals neural blockade with bupivacaine on postoperatove pain post laparoscopic cholecystectomy. *Surg Endosc.* 2007 Sep;21(9):1557-9.

[23] Kim TH, Kang H, Choi YS, Park JM, Chi KC, Shin HY, Hong JH. Pre- and intraoperative lidocaine injection for preemptive analgesics in laparoscopic gastrectomy: a prospective, randomized, double-blind, placebo-controlled study.*J Laparoendosc Adv Surg Tech A*. 2013 Aug;23(8):663-8. doi: 10.1089/lap.2012.0542. Epub 2013 Apr 24.

[24] Singh H, Kundra S, Singh RM, Grewal A, Kaul TK, Sood D.Preemptive analgesia with Ketamine for Laparoscopic cholecystectomy.*J Anaesthesiol Clin Pharmacol.* 2013 Oct;29(4):478-84. doi: 10.4103/0970-9185.119141.

[25] Bunyavejchevin S, Prayoonwech C, Sriprajittichai P.Preemptive analgesic efficacy of parecoxib vs placebo in infertile women undergoing diagnostic laparoscopy:

randomized controlled trial.*J Minim Invasive Gynecol.* 2012 Sep-Oct;19(5):585-8. doi: 10.1016/j.jmig.2012.05.002. Epub 2012 Jul 3.

[26] Ratchanon S, Phaloprakarn C, Traipak K. Pain control in laparoscopic gynecologic surgery with/without preoperative (preemptive) parecoxib sodium injection: a randomized study.*J Med Assoc Thai.* 2011 Oct;94(10):1164-8.

[27] Wang Q, Li Z, Wang ZP, Cui C. *Preemptive analgesic effect of parecoxib sodium in patients undergoing laparoscopic colorectal surgery.* Nan Fang Yi Ke Da Xue Xue Bao. 2010 Nov;30(11):2556-7.

[28] Nesek-Adam V, Grizelj-Stojčić E, Mršić V, Rašić Z, Schwarz D.Preemptive use of diclofenac in combination with ketamine in patients undergoing laparoscopic cholecystectomy: a randomized, double-blind, placebo-controlled study.*Surg Laparosc Endosc Percutan Tech.* 2012 Jun;22(3):232-8. doi: 10.1097/SLE.0b013e31824f8ae4.

[29] Phinchantra P, Bunyavehchevin S, Suwajanakorn S, Wisawasukmongchol W.The preemptive analgesic effect of celecoxib for day-case diagnostic laparoscopy.*J Med Assoc Thai.* 2004 Mar;87(3):283-8.

[30] Gousheh SM, Nesioonpour S, Javaher Foroosh F, Akhondzadeh R, Sahafi SA, Alizadeh Z.Intravenous paracetamol for postoperative analgesia in laparoscopic cholecystectomy. *Anesth Pain Med.* 2013 Summer;3(1):214-8. doi: 10.5812/aapm.9880. Epub 2013 Jul 1.

[31] McCarthy GC, Megalla SA, Habib AS. Impact of lidocaine infusion on postoperative analgesia and recovery from surgery: a systematic review of randomised controlled trials. *Drugs* 2010 Jun 18;70(9):1149-63.

[32] De Oliveira GS Jr, Fitzgerald P, Streicher LF, Marcus RJ, McCarthy RJ. Systemic lidocaine to improve postoperative quality of recovery after ambulatory laparoscopic surgery. *Anesth Analg.* 2012 Aug;115(2):262-7.

[33] Saadawy IM, Kaki AM, Abd El Latif AA, Abd-Elmaksoud AM, Tolba OM. Lidocaine vs magnesium: effect on analgesia after laparoscopic cholecystectomy. *Acta Anaesthesiol Scand.* 2010 May;53(5):549-56.

[34] Mentes O, Harlak A, Yigit T, Balkan A, Balkan M, Cosar A, Savaser A, Kozak O, Tufan T. Effect of intraoperative magnesium sulphate infusion on pain relief after laparoscopic cholecystectomy. *Acta Anaesthesiol Scand.* 2008 Nov;52(10):1353-9.

[35] Sung CS, Lin SH, Chan KH, Chang WK, Chow LH, Lee TY. Effect of oral clonidine on perioperative hemodynamic response and postoperative analgesic requirments for patients undergoing laparoscopic cholecystectmy. *Acta Anaesthesiol Sin.* 2000 Mar;38(1):23-9.

[36] Engelman E, Marsala C. Efficacy of adding clonidine to intrathecal morphine in acute postoperative pain: metanalysis. *Br J Anaes.* 2013 Jan;110(1):21-7.

[37] Wang B, He KH, Jiang MB, Liu C, Min S. Effect of prophylatic dexamethasone on nausea and vomiting after laparoscopic gynacological operation: meta-analysis. *Middle East J Anesthesiol.* 2011 Oct;21(3)397-402.

[38] Joshi GP, Bonnet F, Kehlet H, on behalf of the PRSOPECT collaboration. Evidence-based postoperative pain management after laparoscopic colorectal surgery. *Colorectal Disease.* 2013 Feb;15:2 146-155.

[39] Wheatley RG, Schug SA, Watson D. Safety and efficacy of postoperative epidural analgesia. *Br.J.Anaesth.* 2001 Feb; 87(1):47-61.

[40] Pourseidi B, Khorram-Manesh A. Effect of intercostals neural blockade with Marcaine (bupivacaine) on postoperative pain after laparoscopic cholecystectomy. *Surg Endosc.* 2007 Sep;21(9):1557-9. Epub 2007 Mar 7.

[41] Charlton S, Cyna AM, Middleton P, Griffiths JD. TAP blocks (nerve blocks) for analgesia after abdominal surgery - See more at: *http://summaries.cochrane.org/CD007705/tap-blocks-nerve-blocks-for-analgesia-after-abdominal-surgery#sthash.2m4MkcaH.dpuf*

[42] Johns N, O'Neill S, Ventham NT, Barron F, Brady RR, Daniel T Clinical effectiveness of transversus abdominis plane (TAP) block in abdominal surgery: a systematic review and meta-analysis. *Colorectal Disease October* 2012 14(10);635-642.

[43] Clendenen SR, Wehle MJ, Rodriguez GA, Greengrass RA. Paravertebral block provides signiificant opioid sparing after hand held laparoscopic nephrectomy: An expanded case report of 30 patients. *J Endourol.* 2009 Dec;23(12):1979-83.

[44] Naja MZ, Ziade MF, Lonnqvist PA. General Anaesthesia combined with bilateral paravertebral blockade (T5-T6) vs general anaesthesia for laparoscopic cholecystectomy: a prospective randomised clinical trial. *Eur J Anaesthesiol.* 2004 Jun;21(6):489-95.

[45] Bantel C, Trapp S. The role of the autonomic nervous system in acute surgical pain processing – what do we do? *Anaesthesia* 2011; 66: 539-544.

[46] McDonnell JG, Finnerty O, Laffey JG. Stellate ganglion blockade for analgesia following upper limb surgery. *Anaesthesia* 2011; 66: 611-614.

[47] Herati AS, Andonian S, Rais-Bahrami S, Atalla MA, Srinivasan AK, Richstone L, Kavoussi LR., Use of the valveless trocar system reduces carbon dioxide absorption during laparoscopy when compared with standard trocars. *Urology*, 2011. 77(5): p. 1126-32.

[48] Nepple, K.G., D. Kallogjeri, and S.B. Bhayani, Benchtop evaluation of pressure barrier insufflator and standard insufflator systems. *Surg Endosc*, 2013. 27(1): p. 333-8.

[49] Jérémy Sroussi, Agnès Rigouzzo, Antoine Elies, Nicolas Louvet, Anne Sophie Chevalier, Mathilde Piketty, Matthieu Mezzadri, Jean-Louis Benifla *Laparoscopic surgery at low (7mm Hg) pressure with AirSeal® System; A comparative prospective pilot study with a standard insufflation (15mm Hg) in 60 patients.*

In: Laparoscopy
Editor: Christos Iavazzo
ISBN: 978-1-63321-404-0

Chapter 11

Single-Site Port Laparoscopic Hysterectomy

Christos Iavazzo,[1] M.D., Ph.D. and Ioannis D. Gkegkes,[2] M.D.
[1]Gynaecological Oncology Department, Christie Hospital, Manchester, UK
[2]First Department of Surgery, General Hospital of Attica "KAT", Athens, Greece

Abstract

Minimally invasive surgical techniques as standard care of treatment in gynecological oncology have made laparoscopic hysterectomy a common practice. Recently, the application of single-site port laparoscopic technique represents an innovative, scarless option in the field of hysterectomy. The reduced number of surgical ports may have a reduction in port-associated complications, faster hospital recovery and better cosmetic outcome. The presence of a single entry point, normally situated at the umbilical region, implies co-axial entry of the laparoscopic instruments. The lack of triangulation and the absence of flexibility between the instruments represent the most important technical issues that should be overcome in order to make single-site port hysterectomy a therapeutical option of everyday practice.

Minimally invasive surgical techniques represent the standard of everyday treatment options in gynecology. [1] The utilization of a single-site port in the field of gynecologic surgery is not considered a novelty. Forty years ago, Wheeless et al. was the first to report the surgical sterilization of 3,600 women with the application of single trocar laparoscopy. [2] In 1991, Pelosi et al. has carried out the first hysterectomy by using single-trocar technique. [3] Nevertheless, the single-site port did not become a standard of care in gynecologic surgery due to technical issues, such as the absence of specific port devices, the lack of specific optical systems and the absence of laparoscopic articulating instruments, that have prevented the widespread use of this technique. Langebrekke et al., in 2009, performed the first single-port access laparoscopic hysterectomy. [4]

The available published data on minimally invasive surgery have revealed that single-port access laparoscopic hysterectomy can be applied even in patients with cervical cancer with the need of more radical treatment. The decreased number of surgical ports, which represents an attempt to reduce port-associated complications and improvement of cosmetic outcomes, the accuracy in surgical steps, the reduced blood loss and the shorter recovery time are the principal advantages of single-port access technique (Table). [5]

Table. Principal advantages and disadvantages of the single-site port hysterectomy

Advantages	Disadvantages
• Decrease number of ports. • Good physical status of the patient. • Better cosmetic outcome. • Reduced blood loss. • Shorter recovery time.	• Central obesity. • Uterus of large dimension. • Metastatic disease / peritoneal carcinomatosis. • Poor pulmonary function. • Prior umbilical surgery. • Triangulation effect. • Instrument crowding.

The commercially available port systems present several different properties. Some of these single use multichannel single-port systems usually consist of a wound retractor with a flexible inner ring joined to an outer ring with an also flexible cover. The necessary length of the incision required for the retractor may range from 15 to 70 mm. Moreover, the diameter of the outer ring can reduce the instrument crowding, allowing more liberty at the movement of the instruments. [1] Multichannel devices with fixed ports accesses permit the placement and the removal of laparoscopic instruments without the loss of pneumoperitoneum, in contrary to the surgical glove made ports. Also, the variability of the angle entrance of the different ports permits the decrease of instrument crowding. The ideal port device may have the necessary depth so as to assist at the application of the device in obese patients. In addition, the restricted dimensions of the port require the port removal in order to pass through the fascial incision when it is obligatory the retrieval of organ specimens. Last but not least, the application of surgical gloves with conventional wound retractors does not present any limitation regarding the diameter of the utilized ports and the length of the necessary fascial incision.

In conventional laparoscopy, the effect of triangulation represents a fundamental condition in order to provide the minimal, necessary flexibility for instruments and ports. However, the existence of a single site port for both the camera and the laparoscopic instruments eliminate the effect of triangulation. An easy and cheap solution at this problem is that the surgeon can simply cross the instruments. Nonetheless, this act may possibly cause counterintuitive movements as the surgeon maneuvers the instruments on the reverse side of the surgical field, causing confusion. Furthermore, the creation of curved coaxial instruments with double bending (S-Portal curved instruments, Karl Storz GmbH & Co. KG) allows the crossing over, by passing the problem of triangulation. Lastly, the development of flexible endoscopes can also represent an alternative to rigid instruments increasing their practicality and the range of their use as well. [6].

Regarding the learning curve of the single-port technique, the published evidences are not sufficient. According to Paek et al. study, the single-port accessed hysterectomy appears to be a relative safe technique that can be learned by surgeons after the realization of at least 40 cases. [7]

Surgical Technique

The low lithotomy position with the legs in stirrups is the preferred position for the candidate patients. The arms are placed at the sides of the patient. After the intubation, a Foley catheter and a uterine manipulator are positioned. A laparoscopic motorized endoscope holder such as ViKY® (Endocontrol Medica, La Tronche, France) can also be placed in order to be utilized as surgeon's third hand. A vertical incision (up to 30 mm) is typically made at the inferior of the umbilicus via an open Hasson approach. A single-port multiple channel device, which allows the position of a high-definition camera, two curve robotic cannulae and an insufflator port, is placed through the incision with the use of either a Mayo-Guyon clamp or a pair of Farabeuf elevators. With the insufflation of CO_2 (up to 12 mmHg) into the abdomen, pneumoperitoneum is created. The patient then is placed in a Trendelenburg position (in 30–35°). The high-definition camera is positioned at the upward port with the intention to reduce collisions between the other instruments and to provide a great range of movements to laparoscopic instruments. A surgeon's assistant can place an endoscopic suction device and a standard atraumatic grasper through the assistant port. The organs of the pelvis can be exposed by holding back both the small bowel and the rectosigmoid colon out of the pelvis with the use of atraumatic laparoscopic graspers.

Simple Hysterectomy Technique

The uterus and the ovaries are inspected. Both the round ligament and the infundibulopelvic ligament are coagulated and ligated, while the retroperitoneal space is opened to identify the ureter. The uterine arteries are also coagulated and ligated. The bladder is dissected below the level of the colpotomy cup and then a colpotomy is performed. When the colpotomy is completed, the uterus and adnexae are removed through the vaginal canal. The vaginal cuff is closed with interrupted sutures, in preference with barbed sutures. The ovaries could be preserved, in younger patients with benign diagnosis, with the aim to avoid menopausal symptomatology.

Pelvic Lymphadenectomy Technique

The peritoneum is incised along to the external iliac artery. Moreover, the external iliac vessels are successively cauterized and moved anterior and laterally, away from the muscle psoas, in order to avoid any injury to the genitofemoral nerve, which is situated anteriorly along the muscle. Using the Cadiere grasper, paravesical and pararectal spaces are created by gentle dissection. Lymph nodes from the mid portion of the common iliac artery superiorly, to the circumflex iliac vein inferiorly and from the mid-portion of the psoas muscles laterally, to the ureters and the hypogastric artery and vein medially. In addition, lymph nodes within the obturator fossa are also dissected. The excised lymph nodes are placed in endoscopic bags and through the assistant channel port within the single-port device. In the same mode is performed the dissection of the left pelvic lymph nodes, remaining always within the same anatomic boundaries as the right pelvic lymph nodes. The round and infundibulo pelvic ligaments are then skeletonized and dissected bilaterally with the use of Cadiere grasper. A bladder flap is created with the use of curved scissors and electrocautery, while uterine vessels are cauterized and dissected with the Maryland bipolar forceps. Furthermore, when the bladder is finally dissected below the cervico-vaginal junction, then a colpotomy is completed. The formed vaginal cuff is closed with interrupted sutures. In the case that radical hysterectomy is necessary, ureters are both mobilized, upper vaginectomy is carried out while the reflection of the bladder should be further extended. Also, the removal of the parametria and paracervical tissues is obligatory.

Single-site port surgery is currently applied in everyday practice in various surgical specialties. In gynecologic surgery, the existing evidence seems to be promising. Nevertheless, the adoption of the robotic-assisted technology as standard surgical treatment as well as the development of new port and laparoscopic instrumentation may open new prospectives on gynecological oncology.

References

[1] Uppal S, Frumovitz M, Escobar P, Ramirez PT. Laparoendoscopic single-site surgery in gynecology: review of literature and available technology. *J Minim Invasive Gynecol* 2011; 18:12–23.

[2] Wheeless CR Jr, Thompson BH. Laparoscopic sterilization. Review of 3600 cases. *Obstet Gynecol* 1973; 42:751–758.

[3] Pelosi MA, Pelosi MA 3rd. Laparoscopic hysterectomy with bilateral salpingo-oophorectomy using a single umbilical puncture. *N J Med* 1991; 88:721–726.

[4] Langebrekke A, Qvigstad E. Total laparoscopic hysterectomy with single-port access without vaginal surgery. *J Minim Invasive Gynecol* 2009; 16:609–611.

[5] Iavazzo C, Gkegkes ID. Single-site port robotic-assisted hysterectomy: a systematic review. *Arch Gynecol Obstet.* 2014; 289, 725-731.

[6] Escobar PF, Starks D, Fader AN, Catenacci M, Falcone T. Laparoendoscopic single-site and natural orifice surgery in gynecology. *Fertil Steril* 2010; 94:2497–2502.

[7] Paek J, Kim SW, Lee SH et al. Learning curve and surgical outcome for single-port access total laparoscopic hysterectomy in 100 consecutive cases. *Gynecol Obstet Invest* 2011; 72:227–233.

In: Laparoscopy
Editor: Christos Iavazzo

ISBN: 978-1-63321-404-0

Chapter 12

Laparoscopy in Pediatric Surgery

Mario Lima, Francesca Destro, Noemi Cantone, Dora Persichetti Proietti, Michela Maffi, Stefania Pavia and Andrea Gentili
S. Orsola Hospital
Department of Pediatric Surgery, University of Bologna, Italy
Department of Anesthesiology and Intensive Care Unit

Abstract

Laparoscopy carries with it the advantages of being minimally invasive procedures that have less postoperative pain, excellent cosmetic results and reduced hospitalization with decreased socio-economic costs. This is particularly true in pediatrics. In the last two decades technologic and instrumental improvements have led to the widespread application of laparoscopy also in children. We report some general considerations about pediatric anesthesiological management required during laparoscopic procedures, techniques used and available instrumentation. We take into consideration the main pediatric pathologies (congenital and aquired) that can be managed through laparoscopic surgery. Anatomical districts group these diseases. For each of them we provide a short definition, epidemiology, clinical presentation and treatment focusing on technical details and postoperative complications.

The Chapter will be divided into the following paragraphs:

1. Anesthesiological management
2. Instrument and techniques
3. Laparoscopy in pediatric surgery:
    a) Diaphragmatic and esophageal pathologies: hernias, gastro-esophageal reflux and achalasia, gastrostomy
    b) Acute abdomen: acute appendicitis and its complications, Meckel diverticulitis, intussusception
    c) Intestinal malformations: intestinal atresia and stenosis, intestinal duplications, lymphangiomas

d) Abdominal masses
e) Hepato-biliary and splenic pathologies
f) Ano-rectal malformations and Hirshprung disease
g) Inguinal hernia, cryptorchidism and varicocele
h) Gynecologic affections
i) Urologic pathologies

Introduction

Surgery has developed considerably over the years and modern surgery tries not only to treat the illnesses but also to *minimize the patient's discomfort and to optimize the therapeutic success.* Surgical procedures are evolving into minimally invasive procedures that tend to limit the trauma of the intervention.

Minimally invasive surgery (MIS) has the same goals as classical "open" surgery and takes advantage of access sites that reduces surgical trauma. However, minimally invasive surgery is not free from risks: intraoperative complications may develop, especially with inexperienced operators. The biggest difference is that MIS is characterized by the loss of tactile sensation and by the bi-dimensional field of view with loss of depth perception.

Pediatric minimally invasive surgery was born from the need to reduce tissue damage during surgery. Modern laparoscopy was introduced in the seventies and it was used in pediatric age for diagnostic purposes until 1990 when it became operative.

MIS therapeutic and diagnostic potentialities were soon clear and there has been great development over the last decades. This was possible thanks to the experience acquired by surgeons and the introduction of new instruments fitted for children. All this led to the spread of endosurgery also for cancer treatment. Benign and malignant pathologies are now dealt with through MIS with good results, as in traditional surgery.

Laparoscopy was initially based on the introduction of the Veress needle in the peritoneal cavity through the inferior umbilical margin. The needle was used to inflate CO2 creating the pneumoperitoneum. A trocar for the camera was then inserted and the surgical image was transmitted to a monitor. The open technique was introduced in children to limit organ damage. It consisted of blunt spindle insertion through a small laparotomy (2 cm) below the umbilicus. The pneumoperitoneum is then created and the trocars are inserted. All the instruments are placed under direct vision reducing the risk of damage. Gas inflation is performed with 0.5 L/min of flow in infants. It is completed in 30 – 60 seconds in small children (2-4 years) with 300 ml of gas. A 12-14 year-old boy requires 5 L to obtain full abdominal distension.

Advantages of minimally invasive surgery

A fundamental advantage is to limit surgical aggression not only in terms of aesthetic results but also to limit general impairment of the patient. This is demonstrated by reduced hospitalization, reduced complication rate and reduced postoperative pain.

Complications and disadvantages

Unfortunately there are some disadvantages related to CO2 inflation. Pneumoperitoneum changes the features of the abdominal circulation affecting vital organs as heart (reduced flow in inferior vena cava and reduced cardiac output) and liver.

Minimally invasive surgery complications:

- Lesions during instruments introduction: bowel perforation, solid organs lesions, vascular lesions
- Trocar site related complications: infection, hematoma, seroma, hernia
- Insufflation related complications: nerve stimulation (vagus), gas embolism
- Bleeding: vascular lesions
- Electric lesions: electric arc lesions, thermal lesions

Lesions during instrument movements: wrong instrument choice, wrong technique or force.

Laparoscopic Instruments

Endosurgical pediatric instruments have evolved rapidly in recent years. At first pediatric endosurgery was performed with instruments designated for adults that were too big for small children.

The equipment is classified according to its use: support and conduction.

The support equipment includes insufflators, scopes and video camera systems, coagulation devices and instruments for irrigation and aspiration (Fig. 13). All these tools are housed on endoscopic surgery towers.

Operative devices represent the conduction equipment.

Inflation Instruments

Trocars

The way to look inside the peritoneum requires a space in which the light enters and the instruments move. This space is obtained creating an artificial pneumoperitoneum. Tubular sleeve-like devices called ports allow the introduction of gas and instruments through the abdominal wall. Every port has a valve mechanism that allows instruments to be inserted without gas losses. They are disposable or non-disposable with dimensions between 1.5 and 12 mm. Disposable trocars are made of metal and they are heavier, without security systems during introduction and are subjected to valve deterioration. Ports are positioned through the abdominal wall with trocars that are spike-like devices placed inside the port sleeve. Trocars can have a conical tip, a pyramidal tip or a blunt tip. The blunt tip leaves a smaller incision in the abdominal wall and allows a stronger adhesion between tissues when the trocar is removed avoiding gas looses. It is used in the open technique. Some ports have fixation devices that prevent them from moving (pneumatic anchorage, cannula with external thread).

It is possible to use 5 mm instruments through bigger trocars thanks to reducers that allow movements without losing gas.

Insufflator

The insufflator is an instrument that delivers a gas monitoring flow rate, pressure of delivery and internal pressure. It also automatically regulates small internal pressure losses.

- The most common gasses used are carbon dioxide, nitrogen dioxide and air. They are easy to manage, cheap and slightly soluble in blood reducing the risk of embolism.
- Carbon dioxide is used the most because of its minimal collateral effects. It may irritate the peritoneum in longer procedures (> 2 hours) causing acid-base balance alterations. It is thus important to monitor CO2 and 02 blood pressures in order to detect alterations of the acid-base balance.
- Nitrogen dioxide is preferred in case of diagnostic laparoscopy because it is quickly disposed of. Unfortunately it is inflammable (it is not possible to use coagulation devices).
- Air has minimal collateral effects but it is less indicated because it is slowly eliminated.
- At the beginning gases are inflated slowly (0.5 – 1 L/min depending on the patient's size). Later the flow can be increased (2 – 3 L/min) until the internal pressure is between 6 and 12 mmHg.
- Gas temperature should be 37°C to reduce the effects on thermoregulation. In small children and infants the wall is suspended with instruments in order to avoid long gas exposure.

Instruments for Endoscopic Vision and its Reproduction

Optics

The vision system consists of the telescope (or laparoscope). The telescope is an inoxidizable tube containing a lens system designed by Hopkins-Rod that has various dimensions (1.5 – 12 mm). The system consists of a series of glass rod lenses separated by air. The light passes through the air; it is refracted until it reaches the ocular lens that is a magnifier lens. Transferred images are bright and clear, without peripheral distortion ("fisheye effect").

Scope size ranges from 5 to 10 mm in diameter; 3 mm scopes are available but they offer a limited view. Scopes are also sorted by angle of lenses: 0°, 25°, 30°, 45° and even 120°. The majority of the procedures are performed using 0°, 30° and 45° angles.

Different angles of the lens allow the inspection of organs otherwise difficult to explore.

A 20 cm scope is used in neonates and infants whereas a 30 cm scope is preferred in older children.

Beside the optical component, operating scopes (10 mm in diameter) have a work channel that allows the introduction of 5 mm instruments.

Scopes are connected with cameras, video recording systems and light sources (alogen or xenon) through fiberoptic cables.

The light heats the tip of the scopes even if we are using “cold lights”, with potential inflammation of drapes and gowns after prolonged contacts and potential damage of internal organs during surgical maneuvers.

Camera

The camera is an optic-electronic conversion unit at the end of the laparoscope. A cable connects the camera with an electronic processor that modifies the image and transmits it to the video recorder.

White balancing is necessary to obtain an accurate spectrum of colors every time the camera is turned on. Keeping a white object in front of the scope and pressing the appropriate button achieves white balancing.

In the majority of cases cameras can automatically adjust the lens opening according to light variations during their use.

Presently, cameras give high-resolution images through digital systems.

It is also possible to obtain 3D images using specific personal lenses.

The most recent cameras are based on a digital system with high definition capacity, allowing the use of 1-2 mm optics (ideal for diagnostic procedures).

The camera is connected with a computer through specific software that can obtain real time Bitmap or Jpeg images. This is an important tool for storage and transmission of data.

Irrigation / Aspiration Devices

The irrigation and aspiration system permits the introduction and aspiration of sterile fluid in intracorporeal cavities in order to wash them. It also permits the aspiration of pre-existent fluids.

Modern instruments have just one channel for both aspiration and irrigation, which may be associated with the smoke aspirator during surgical dissection. The most efficient irrigation devices are those that use pressured CO_2 to deliver saline solution. A delivery pressure of 300 mmHg is adequate to mobilize clots and to identify bleedings. Some instruments have a valve that regulates the delivery pressure.

This property is also used to dissect tissues. Probes are made of one or two channels for an overall diameter of 5 mm. In case of two channels each canal has a diameter of 2 mm that is the limitation to remove big clots.

Electrosurgery Devices

They use the heat produced by short electric waves that divides and coagulates tissues. The heat is conducted through the electric monopolar scalpel or modified laparoscopic instruments (isolation of handles and stem). The electrocoagulation should be used with caution, since sparks released by the instrument can damage the intestine. This risk can be avoided if the tip of the instrument is in contact with the tissue prior to starting. The tip must not be in contact with the laparoscopic cannula, because other tissues, including the skin, may be affected by electrical conduction. There is a conduction system, called bipolar, which cauterizes only the tissue between the claws, ensuring greater safety against accidental injury. The laser has been recently inserted between laparoscopic instruments as an alternative to electrocautery. It uses photons to cut and coagulate, avoiding damage to adjacent tissue.

The Ultracision (ultrasonic dissector) is both a dissector and coagulator. It is very expensive and it uses the energy of the piezoelectric element placed on the claw of the handpiccc to coagulate. If it is kept closed for a longer time it dissects the tissue itself. This type of cauterization decreases the risk of accidental damage and does not cause the "fog effect" which decreases the endoscopic vision.

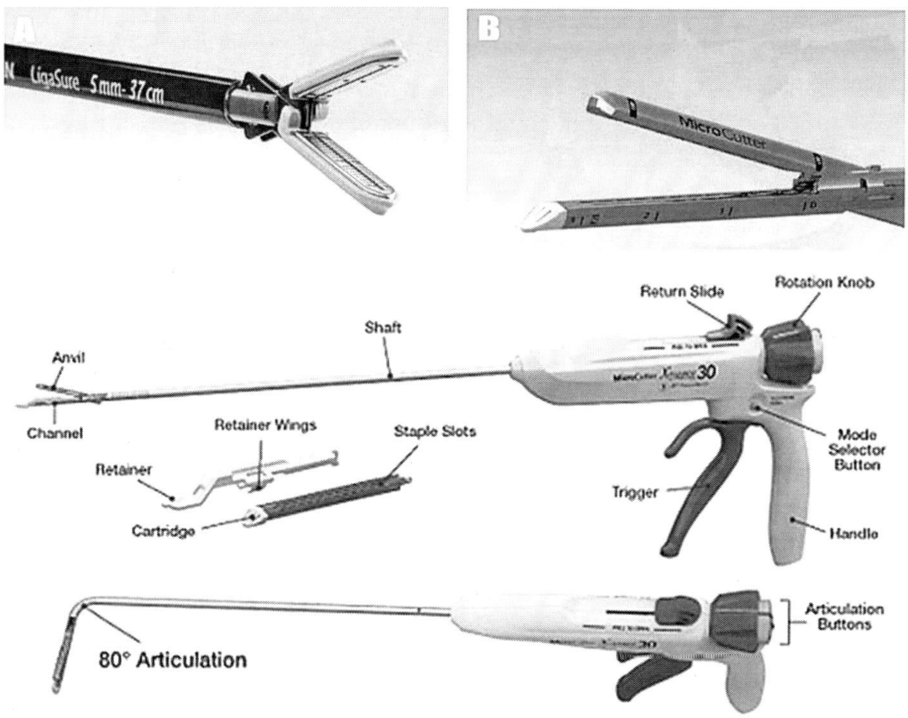

Figure 1. Five millimetres Ligasure^{TM} (a) and stapler (b). The stapler is a cartridge-based instrument with 80 degree articulation (figure below) that eliminates the need to upsize trocars to 12 mm just to fire the stapler.

Conduction Equipment

The conduction equipment includes a series of complex operative instruments. The function of these instruments is similar to those for traditional surgery but the handle and the movements are different. The instruments are divided as disposable or non-disposable.

They all have conductor tips and isolated stems. In the majority of cases they can rotate around their axes. For children, the diameter of the instruments usually varies from 2 to 5 mm. The ideal position of the instrument during surgical procedures uses one-third outside and two-thirds inside the body in order to obtain precise movements inside with minimal efforts outside.

Forceps

They are instruments used to catch or retract tissues. They are divided into blunt grasping and biopsy forceps. They can have single or double action jaws. Their diameter can vary from 2 to 10 mm (the most common in pediatric surgery is between 2 and 5 mm). Forceps are similar to a small Klemmer. They may be straight or curved, but they may also have the characteristic duckbill appearance with 3 or 5 blunt prongs. Long and penetrating teeth may form their terminal part, by rings or by structures similar to the Duval of traditional surgery.

Dissectors

They are the most important tools in laparoscopic surgery. The terminal part is similar to the "mosquito", with an atraumatic bite. They separate and divide the tissue with minimal trauma.

Scissors

The scissors can be disposable or non-disposable, as in traditional surgery, straight or curved, blunt or pointed, but also with one or two mobile branches. They can move around their own axis and can be angled up to 80°. Hooked scissors have tips that can be closed before the branches, in order to traction the tissue and to highlight the underlying or adjacent structures such as vessels, before cutting. This possibility is very important as the sense of depth is lacking and the two-dimensional perspective can deceive the surgeon.

The biggest inconvenience of disposable scissors is the deterioration of the blades over time.

Retractors

They are used for manually maneuvering tissue that would otherwise obstruct the view of the operative site. They are straight or curved and they may have a 3 mm or 5 mm diameter.

They are sized for insertion through ports and they open into the cavity (abdomen or thorax). They have a wide range of action, a flat surface and a cylindrical handle.

Monopolar hook

Every laparoscopic instrument can act as a laparoscopic electrocoagulator if an insulating material coats it with a clamp on the handle for a monopolar electrical connection.

Some concerns have been expressed regarding the use of electrocautery devices in the closed abdominal cavity. Many authors have shown that complications are related to inexperience of the operator.

Needle Holders, Sutures and Knot Pushers

The suture is performed with classical sutures and needles or staplers. The needle is handled with the needle holder that has a diameter of 3-5 mm and it is supplied with spring grip or rack. The spring grip needle holders (Castro - Viejo) require a certain force on the handle to open. The shape of the grip is variable: simple U-shape, angled handle or with a handle that is parallel to the major axis. If the node is prepared outside, a special instrument called a "knot pusher" is used to transfer the node inside the abdomen and to close it. Knot pushers allow a prepared knot to be pushed down through the length of the suture.

The diameter can be 3 or 5 mm. The tip of the knot pusher has a groove for the thread and a notch to lock the node.

Suture threads can be absorbable or non-absorbable, monofilament or twisted. They have three lengths: 70 – 120 cm for extracorporeal stitches, 20 cm for linear sutures, 7 cm for interrupted sutures. Some sutures are prepared (pre-tied) in order to simplify extracorporeal passages of the knotting procedure. Endoloops are used for peduncolated structures.

Needles are usually curved but they can also be straight or they can have particular shapes ("sky needle" or "canoe needle"). Straight needles give major penetration in tissues because they don't rotate on the needle holder but they don't allow delicate maneuvers. Curved needles are gentler but they don't pass through ports. The optimal design is that of the sky needle (curved tip and straight stem). Laparoscopic needles are burnished to avoid bright reflexes from the optic light.

Clip appliers are the simpler way to obliterate cave structures as vessels and ducts. Their diameter varies from 5 to 10 mm and the grip has differentiated branches. They can be disposable or non-disposable and clips can be absorbable or non-absorbable (titanium). Clips are placed in the distal tip (double jaws with a central channel). The structure to close is placed between the clips. Closing the grip you close the clip. Endoscopic staplers accost tissues with metallic "U-shaped" staples that are closed in a "B-shape". When the instrument is closed the legs of the staples are driven through tissues and they are folded. The B-shape allows the passage of little capillary vessels that vascularize the margins of the resection.

Staplers are divided as linear or circular (depending on the suture line) or transecant (with a blade that permits the simultaneous resection of tissue between the suture lines).

Linear staplers produce a double layer of stitches that allows a rapid and safe closure. Circular staplers produce a circular double-staggered row of staples. When the instrument is closed a circular blade sections the excess tissue. Care should be taken in port selection: most staplers can only be used with 10 mm ports.

Creation of the Pneumoperitoneum

This is the most dangerous maneuver in small children. There are two techniques: percutaneous (Verres needle) or open (Hasson technique or variants). At our Institution we use the Hasson technique or open technique. The procedure is based on the opening of the peritoneal cavity and the trocar insertion under direct vision. For the peri-umbilical insertion of the cannula, a proper skin incision is performed up to the linea alba. The latter and the peritoneum are dissected and a purse-string absorbable suture is performed to optimize trocar placement. We use a disposable trocar with pneumatic anchorage and external block so there is no need for suturing.

Once the pneumoperitoneum has been created the abdominal cavity is explored in order to choose the sites to introduce the remaining trocars. The location and number of trocars depend on the type of surgical procedure, the size of the patient and the presence or absence of abdominal scars or other abdominal pathologies.

Congenital Diaphragmatic Hernia

Introduction

Congenital diaphragmatic hernia (CDH) is a malformation characterized by abnormal diaphragmatic patency that allows the passage of abdominal organs into the thorax. The failure to close the pleuro-peritoneal canal leads to a postero-lateral defect, more frequently on the left side (80% of all postero-lateral defects): this type of hernia is the most common (plus 90% of all CDH) and it is termed Bochdalek hernia (through the foramen of Bochdalek). Developmental abnormalities of the sternocostal bundles result in anterior defect (1 to 6% of all cases): Larrey hernia on the left sternocostal hiatus and Morgagni hernia on the right one. Frequently both hiatus are involved and the defect is called Morgagni-Larrey hernia.

CDH is a common birth anomaly (1:3000-5000) with important health consequences according to the size, the location of defect and the association with others malformations (neural tube defects, heart malformations, gastrointestinal malformations, etc.) or syndromes (Down syndrome, Fryns syndrome, Denys-Drash syndrome, etc.).

Diagnosis

The presumptive diagnosis can be made prenatally (after the second trimester) and it is based on the demonstration of polyhydramnios, on the absence of an intrabdominal stomach (no gastric bubble) and on the presence of abdominal viscera in the thorax causing mediastinal shift and pulmonary hypoplasia.

At birth the baby may present with respiratory distress or respiratory symptoms (cyanosis, gasping, etc.) according to the grade of pulmonary hypoplasia and hypertension (severe in cases of large postero-lateral defects). The distress may also be related to pneumothorax.

In cases of small defects (e.g. Morgagni-Larrey hernia), the baby can be asymptomatic in the neonatal period and in first infancy. Late onset is characterized by recurrent bronchopneumonia or gastrointestinal symptoms (vomiting or intestinal (sub)occlusion). In these cases the diagnosis is frequently made during thorax X-ray performed for other reasons (incidental finding).

The differential diagnosis includes pulmonary cystic lesions, congenital hiatal hernia, congenital eventration of the diaphragm (abnormal elevation of all or a part of the hemidiaphram). In doubtful cases a contrast upper X ray is useful.

Treatment

Surgical treatment is mandatory even in the asymptomatic diaphragmatic hernia and it should be planned according to the patients' general condition and hemodynamic stability. The treatment provides for the repair of the defect by direct suture or by patch interposition in cases of large defects or recurrence. Different techniques have been described and include open or endoscopic procedure through a transthoracic or transabdominal approach. The laparoscopic technique is indicated in children with a delayed presentation, a symptom-free interval and none or mild respiratory symptoms. Moreover, laparoscopic treatment is the gold standard for anterior hernia.

The first trocar is placed with open technique through a classical subumbilical or supraumbilical incision (midline incision); we use a 0° and rarely 30° 10mm optic. The pressure and the flow of insufflation varies according to age and weight (pressure of 8-10 mmHg and flow of 0.5-1 L/min).

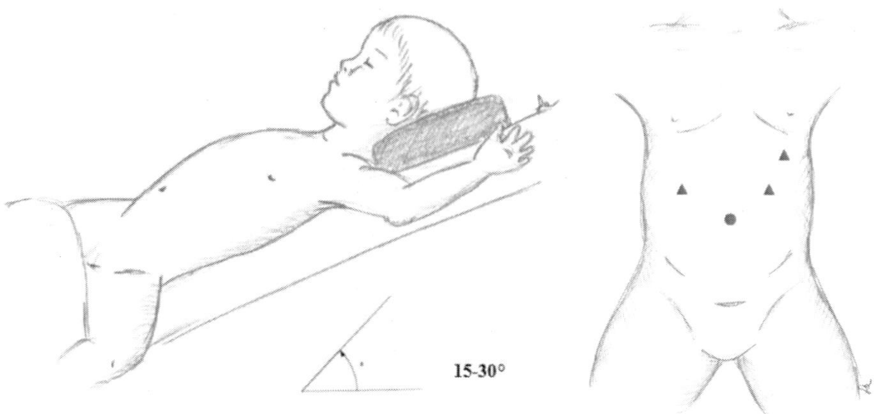

Figure 2. The patient lies in the supine, anti-trendelenburg position (image on the left). Lens (circle) is placed in the umbilicus and operative trocars in the right and left hypocondrium and on the left subcostal margin (triangles).

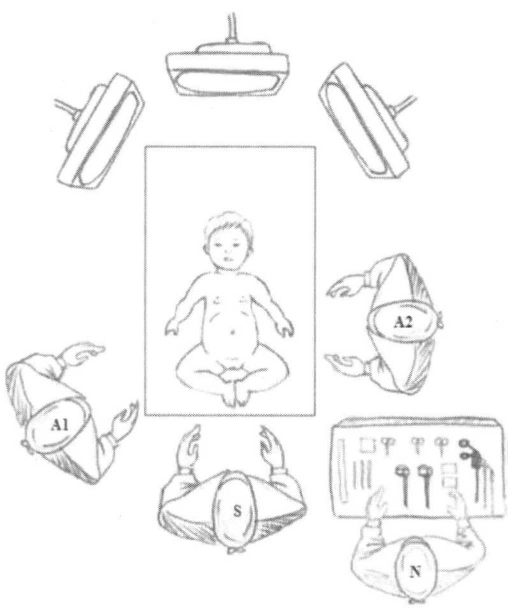

Figure 3. Operative set-up. S = surgeon; A1 = assistant 1; A2 = assistant 2; N = scrub nurse.

The other trocars are placed under direct vision. After a careful exploration of the abdominal cavity, we gently reduce the herniated organs in the abdomen and examine the size of the defect. We try to remove the hernia sac, when present. If this maneuver is difficult, we freshen the edges of a diaphragmatic rib to allow healing of tissue. When primary repair is possible, we close the defect with an interrupted non-absorbable 3-4/0 suture: to facilitate the repair and reduce the tension over the margins, we put in one or more transparietal stitches that can be removed at the end of the procedure. Knots can be performed intra or extracorporeally. If the defect is too large, a synthetic or biologic patch is used: the aim is to perform a floppy, tension free closure.

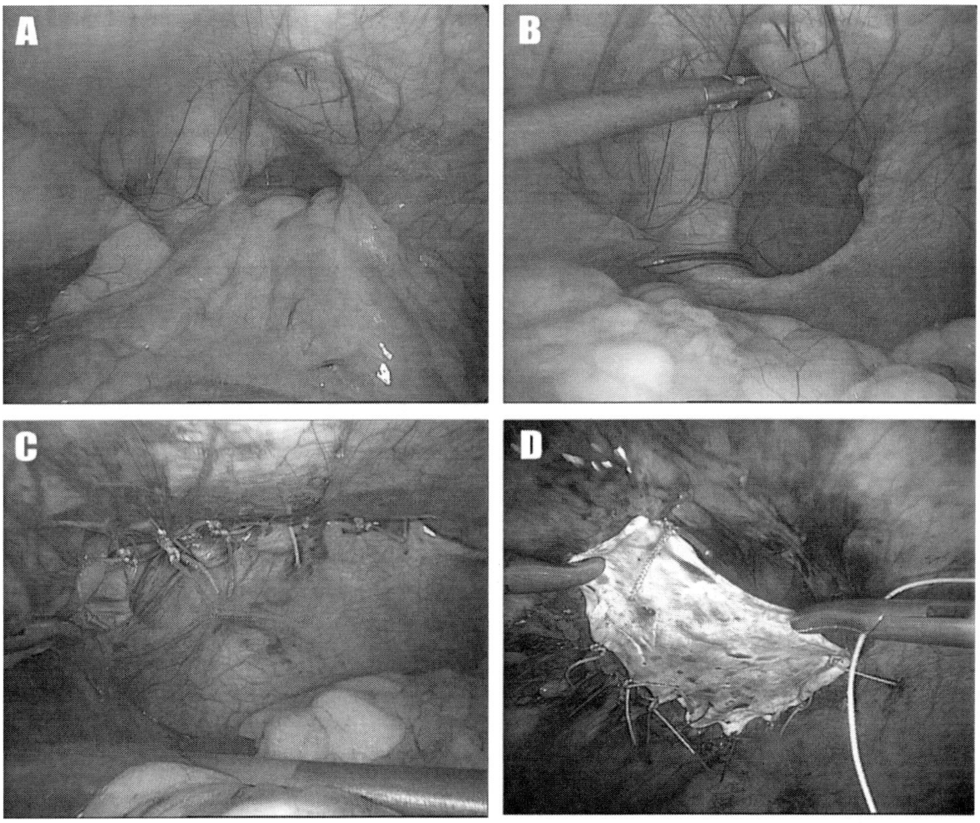

Figure 4. The colon herniates through the diaphragmatic defect (A). The colon is reduced in the abdomen and the defect is clearly visible (B). The defect is closed by direct interrupted suture (C) or by patch interposition (D).

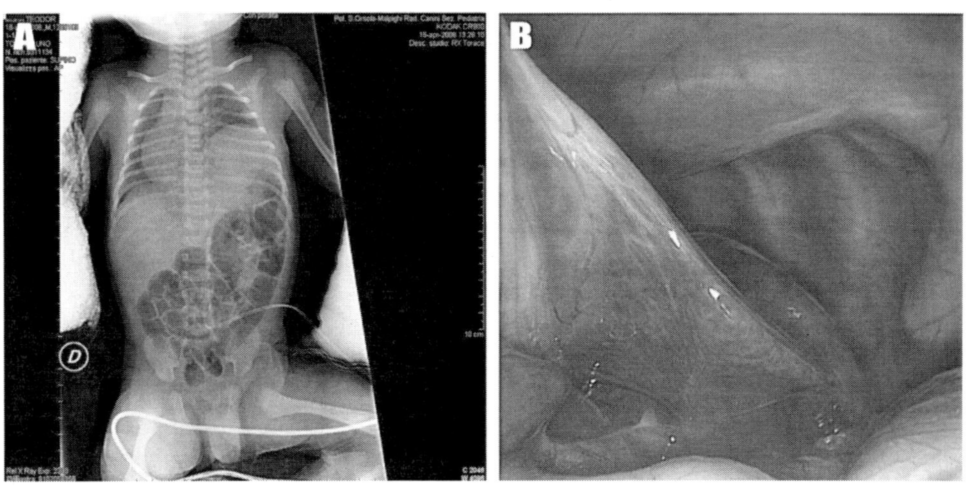

Figure 5. Bochdalek hernia: preoperative x-ray and laparoscopic view of the diaphragmatic defect.

Complications

Complications are the same as the open technique: abdominal compartment syndrome due to an increase of abdominal pressure, abdominal organ injuries (especially splenic injuries) during the reduction, infection or dislodgment of prosthetic patch. Recurrence rates vary widely in various reports from 5% to 60%; recognized risk factors are the use of extracorporeal membrane oxygenation (ECMO), the need of a patch and the size of the defect (large).

References

Arca M, Barnhart D, Lelli J et al. Early experience with minimally invasive repair of congenital diaphragmatic hernias: results and lessons learned. (2003) *J Pediatr Surg,* 11: 1563–1568ù

De Kort LM, Bax KM. Prosthetic patches used to close congenital diaphragmatic defects behave well: a long-term follow-up study. (1996) *Eur J Pediatr Surg.* 6(3): 136-8.

Keijzer R, Puri P. Congenital diaphragmatic hernia. *Semin Pediatr Surg.* 2010. Aug;19(3):180-5. Review.

Marhuenda C, Guillén G, Sanchez B et al. Endoscopic repair of late-presenting Morgagni and Bochdalek hernia in children: case report and review of the literature. (2009) *J Laparoendosc Adv Surg Tech.* 19: S95–S101

Rowe DH, Stolar CJ. Recurrent diaphragmatic hernia. (2003) *Semin Pediatr Surg.*12(2):107-9.

Shah SR, Wishnew J, Barsness K, Gaines BA, Potoka DA, Gittes GK, Kane TD. Minimally invasive congenital diaphragmatic hernia repair: a 7-year review of one institution's experience. *Surg Endosc.* 2009 Jun;23(6):1265-71.

Gastro-Esophageal Reflux

Introduction

The definition of gastro-esophageal reflux (GER) refers to the involuntary passage of the gastric content in the esophagus. It is caused by the incomplete maturation of anti-reflux mechanisms in children thus being very frequent in infants and small children. It is estimated that 7 out of 10 infants have symptomatic GER. Only 5% of them will develop a disease related to the reflux (GERD) that is characterized by esophageal damage and/or symptoms that interfere with the quality of life.

The pathophysiological alteration responsible for the GER is the incompetence of the antireflux barrier at the level of the gastro-esophageal junction (GEJ). The GEJ separates a negative pressure zone (the esophagus) from a positive pressure zone (the stomach). The antireflux barrier prevents the passage of the gastric acid content in the esophagus. It includes a high-pressure zone (2-5 mm) that is similar to the adult zone and it consists of: intra-abdominal esophagus, angle of His, pinchcock action of the right diaphragmatic crus, phreno-esophageal membrane.

Other factors that influence the GER damage are: esophageal clearance and peristalsis, gastric volume and emptying, gastric acidity, Helicobacter infection and jatal hernia.

Diagnosis

The clinical picture varies with age (Table 1). Beside the classical presentation that affects older patients (regurgitation, vomiting, pirosis), there are atypical symptoms (respiratory and neuro-behavior involvement).

Table 1. GER symptoms

First year of age	Older children
Regurgitation, vomiting, irritability, crying, coughing, failure to thrive, bronchospasm, esophagitis, sleep disorders, Sandifer's syndrome, pneumonia, laryngospasm, cyanosis, sudden death apnea syndrome.	Regurgitation, vomiting, heartburn, chest / epigastric pain, dysphagia, irritability, esophagitis, tachycardia, cough / respiratory diseases, recurrent abdominal pain, sleep disorders, anemia, hematemesis / melena.

The diagnosis is clinical; history and physical examination are sufficient to make diagnosis.

Diagnostic procedures are performed in selected cases. Distal esophagus ultrasound is useful in infants as screening. An upper gastrointestinal contrast series is neither specific nor sensitive but it is not invasive and may detect malformations (pyloric stenosis, malrotation, duodenal obstructions). The endoscopic evaluation is required in the case of suspected esophagitis. The gold standard for the diagnosis of GERD remains the esophageal pH-monitoring that should be performed in case of complicated GER (non responsive cases or atypical symptoms).

Differential diagnosis includes: hyperalimentation, allergy to cow's milk proteins, hypertrophic pyloric stenosis, anatomical causes (e.g. duodenal stenosis or atresia below Vater papilla), and metabolic alterations.

Treatment

The treatment of uncomplicated GER includes changes in lifestyle (smaller and frequent feeding, thickened feeding, hypoallergenic milk, positioning therapy). In case of failure or when there are symptoms and signs of GERD, drugs can be useful: procinetics and acid suppressants are the main types of pharmacotherapies.

Surgical treatment of GERD in children is indicated in the following cases:

- Medical therapy failure (at least 8 weeks of PPI treatment) or strong dependence with medical therapy;
- Onset of GERD complications such as esophageal peptic stenosis, severe esophagitis or gastric esophageal metaplasia;
- Respiratory symptoms with potentially lethal events such as apnea and / or ab ingestis;
- Presence of jatal hernia, esophageal atresia, diaphragmatic hernia;
- Neurological impairment.

There are different surgical techniques that greatly vary with surgical preference. The most common procedure in children is the Nissen complete fundoplication. Partial fundoplication is indicated in patients with esophageal motility disorders. (e.g. Dor, Thal and Toupet). All the techniques respect the three cardinal principles of GERD surgery: distal esophagus isolation (with increment of its abdominal part), esophageal jatus reduction and fixation of the gastric fundus to the diaphragm. Over the last decade all of these procedures are performed laparoscopically.

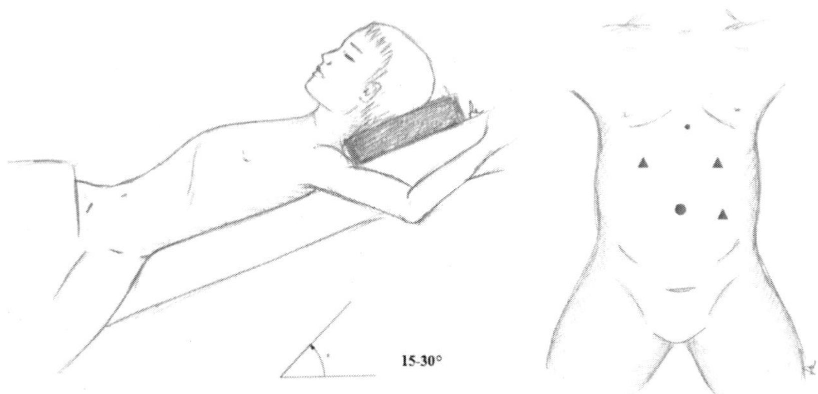

Figure 6. The patient lies in the supine, anti-trendelenburg position. Lens is inserted in the umbilicus (circle on the right figure); operative trocars are inserted in the right and left hypocondrium and on the left paraumbilical line (triangles). Hepatic retractor is generally placed in the epigastrium (small circle).

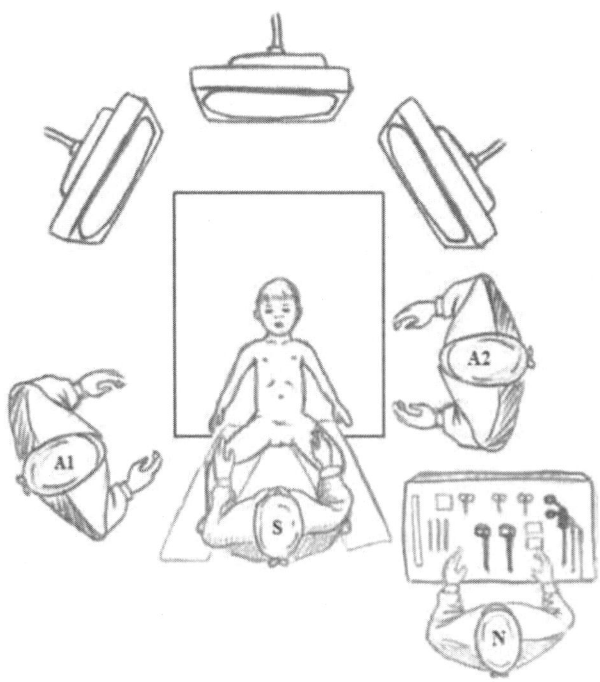

Figure 7. Operative set-up. S = surgeon; A1 = assistant 1; A2 = assistant 2; N = scrub nurse.

The 5 mm optic is inserted through an umbilical incision with the open technique. The abdomen is insufflated with 8-10 mmHg and 0.5-1 L/min. The remaining trocars are inserted under direct vision (see Fig.). The anterior abdominal wall is lifted up through a wall hanger or a big stitch placed in the xiphoid region encircling the falciform ligament. At the same time the stomach is pulled to the right. The esophageal jatus is then exposed with the hepatic retractor. The distal end of the esophagus is mobilized circumferentially: the ephato-gastric ligament and phreno-esophageal membrane are cut with a monopolar hook until the right pillar is exposed and the peritoneum is dissected on the anterior esophageal wall up to the left diaphragmatic pillar. It is important to spare the anterior branch of the vagus nerve during this maneuver. The esophageal isolation ends with the creation of a retro-esophageal window that is used to loop a silicon tape around the esophagus. At this time the fundus of the stomach is mobilized. Short gastric vessels do not usually require ligation to reach a sufficient gastric mobilization. In some cases it is important to do a plastic of the jatus with one or two non-absorbable stitches that approximate the two pillars. The fundus is then fitted 360° around the esophagus (a reticular may be useful). The gastric fundus is sutured to the opposite stomach and to the anterior esophageal wall with 2/0 non-absorbable three stitches and a sky-needle (extracorporeal knotting). The fundoplication should be 3-4 cm long. Sutures need to be performed over a rigid probe to avoid stenosis. Fundoplication can be secured to the right diaphragmatic pillar in order to avoid its slip toward the thorax.

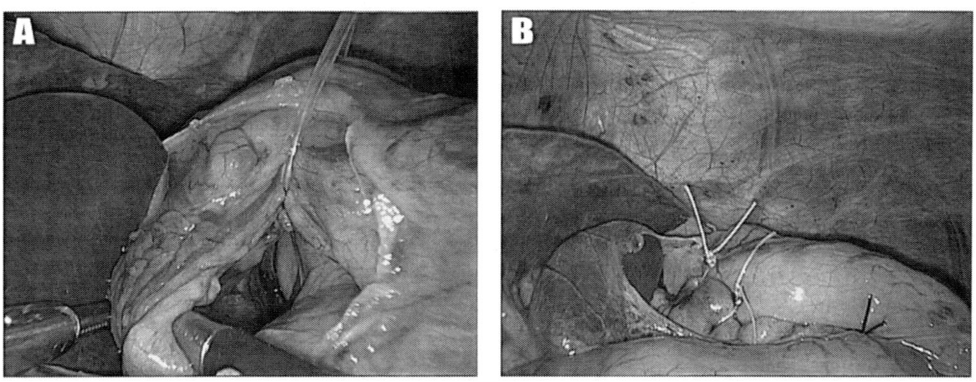

Figure 8. The retro-esophageal window is created by blunt dissection (A) to perform Nissen fundoplication (B).

In the Toupet technique the esophagus is dissected in the same manner as for a Nissen fundoplication. The gastric fundus is pulled behind the abdominal esophagus as a wrap. The anterior wall of the fundus on the left side is sutured on the right part of the esophagus secured to the right crus. The opposite side of the wrap is sutured to the right edge of the esophagus. A 270° wrap is thus created. As for the other anterior techniques, the creation of the retro-esophageal window is not necessary. In our center we often use the Dor fundoplication that includes the same ligament dissection of the Nissen techniques. The anterior 180° fundoplication is obtained using 4 stitches. The first two stitches are placed between the gastric fundus and the left lateral part of the esophagus. The other two are used to unite the gastric fundus to the anterior esophageal wall, involving the right pillar.

The naso gastric tube is removed after 12-24 hours when the feeding starts.

Complications

Intraoperative (2-5%)

- Gastric perforation;
- Esophageal perforation;
- Pneumothorax (due to strong jatal dissections)

Postoperative

- Long-term dysphagia (2%), which should be differentiated from the immediate postoperative dysphagia (40% for the Nissen, rare for the Dor), is related to wrong convalescence feeding. Rarely (<1%) a strong plastic of the jatus can led to recurrent vomiting and severe dysphagia, which requires surgical revision.
- Recurrent GER (2-5% two years after surgery for the Nissen; 7% for the Dor) is due to sleeve intrathorax slip and fundoplication dehiscence.

References

Czinn SJ, Blanchard S. Gastroesophageal reflux disease in neonates and infants: when and how to treat. *Paediatr Drugs.* 2013 Feb;15(1):19-27. Review

Esposito C, Montupet Ph, Rothemberg S. The Gastroesophageal Reflux in Infants and Children. Diagnosis, Medical therapy, Surgical management. *Springer* 2004

Lima M, Bertozzi M, Ruggeri G, Dòmini M, Libri M, Parigi GB, De Biagi L, Franzoni E, Bernardi F. Laparoscopic antireflux surgery in neurologically impaired children. *Pediatr Surg Int* 2004; 20: 114-117

Lima M, Esposito C, Papparella A, Mattioli G. Malattia da Reflusso Gastro-Esofageo. In Laparoscopia, *Toracoscopia e Retroperitoneoscopia pediatrica.* 2004; cap 3.2: 89-94

Montupet P Toupet's fundoplication in children. *Semin Laparosc Surg* 2002; 9: 163-167

Rossetti M. Antireflux surgery: from Nissen to mini-invasive technics. *Minerva Chirurgica* 1995; 50: 104-108

Van der Zee DC, Rvekamp MH, Pull ter Gunne AJ, Bax NMA. Surgical treatment for Reflux esophagitis: Nissen versus Thal procedure. *Pediatr Surg Int* 1994; 9: 334-337

Achalasia

Introduction

The term achalasia refers to a motor acquired disorder of the lower end of the esophagus. It is characterized by an uncoordinated peristaltic wave activity of the esophageal body and by an incomplete and delayed or absent relaxation of the lower esophageal sphincter (LES).

This condition is relatively rare in young children and it mainly affects adolescents and adults.

There are two types of achalasia: primary (low intrinsic inhibitory activity of the esophageal innervation due to inflammation) and secondary (vagus damage, infections such as the Tripanosoma cruzi, other causes). The primary form probably has a congenital origin as shown by the association with syndromes (familiar glucocorticoid deficit, Razycki syndrome). The result is the esophageal dilatation with muscular hypertrophy.

Diagnosis

Symptoms include dysphagia (a typical feature is the paradox dysphagia for liquids), regurgitation of undigested food, scialorrhea, cough, retrosternal pain and loss of weight. At first the dysphagia does not affect the patients' general conditions and it can also disappear (thanks to the esophageal hypertrophy). Eventually the esophagus loses its function and symptoms become severe.

The barium meal is often diagnostic because the esophagus is large (megaesophagus) and it contains stagnant fluids. The peristalsis is reduced and the esophago-gastric junction has a characteristic "beard's beak shape". The endoscopic evaluation rules out the presence of anatomical strictures and esophagitis. The gold standard for the diagnosis is the manometry that records high pressures on the LES (hypertonic LES) and the absence of proper peristalsis.

Treatment

Many therapeutic options have been proposed in the last decade with unsatisfactory results (pharmacological therapy with calcium antagonists, endoscopic cardial pneumatic dilatations, cardial injection of botulin toxin). Therefore the treatment of the esophageal achalasia remains the surgical correction with the extramucosal longitudinal modified Heller cardiomiotomy (the double myotomy proposed by Heller was modified into a procedure that provides for the anterior cut alone). We always perform an anterior fundoplication along with the Heller myotomy in order to avoid the onset of gastro-esophageal reflux and to protect the esophageal mucosa. The myotomy can be performed laparoscopically or thoracoscopically. Laparoscopy is associated with lower recurrence rate because the myotomy can be easily extended also on the gastric side (complete distal myotomy) and it allows the execution of antireflux procedures. A liquid diet is administrated 72 hours before surgery in order to avoid the presence of food in the esophagus and blood should be available for transfusions during surgery.

At the beginning the procedure is similar to that used for the fundoplication alone (umbilical trocar inserted with open technique, creation of pneumoperitoneum and placement of the trocars under direct vision).

The esophago-gastric junction is exposed after the retraction of the left hepatic lobe and the phreno-esophageal ligament opening. At this point the anterior and lateral walls of the esophagus are isolated after the identification of the anterior vagal nerve branch. The posterior wall is not included because of the high risk of damaging the vagal nerve and the jatal region. A monopolar hook is used to mark the zone for the myotomy in the muscular esophago-gastric wall. The miotomy extends proximally until the point of the mediastinum where the anterior vagal branch crosses the anterior esophageal wall from the left to the right side (that is the point where the esophagus dilates).

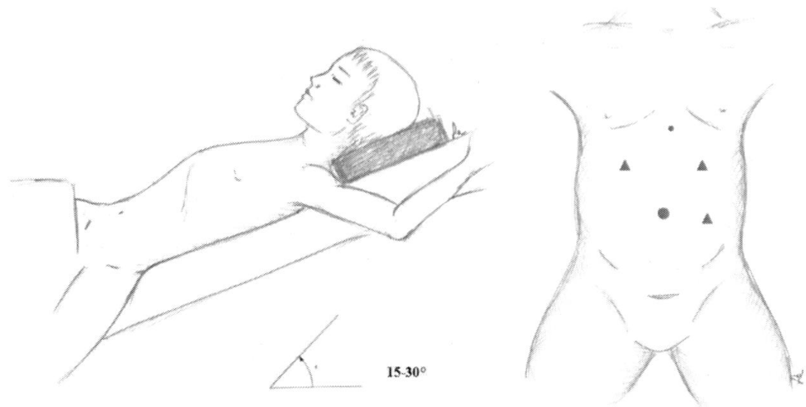

Figure 9. The patient lies in the lithotomic anti-trendelenburg supine position. The optic is inserted in the umbilicus (circle on the right figure); operative trocars are placed in right and left hypocondrium and on the left paraumbilical line (triangles on the right figure); hepatic retractor is in the epigastrium (small circle).

Distally the miotomy ends on the stomach where transversal muscular fibers become vertical (2 cm from the esophago-gastric junction). The overall length of the miotomy is almost 6-8 cm. Both longitudinal and circular esophageal muscles are cut letting the mucosa herniate. Muscular bleedings at the margins of the miotomy are usually self-limited and therefore should not be treated with electrocautery. At the end of the procedure the insufflations of air through the naso-gastric tube is used to check the tightness of the mucosa prior to the execution of the Dor fundoplication. After surgery antibiotics are administrated for 24 hours. The nasogastric tube is removed when the patient awakes. On the 1st – 2nd postoperative day a contrast x-ray is performed and feeding follows it. The patient is discharged after 2-3 days.

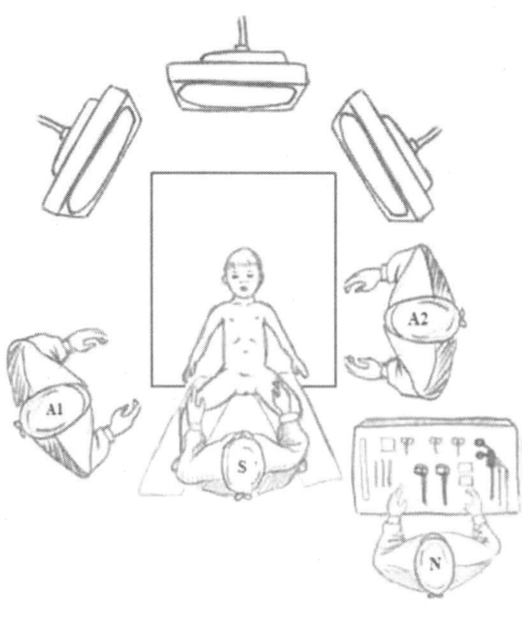

Figure 10. Operative set-up (S = surgeon; A1 = assistant 1; A2 = assistant 2; N = scrub nurse).

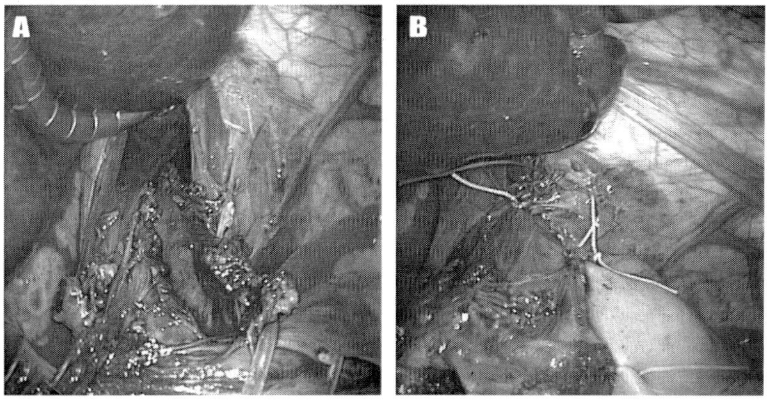

Figure 11. Gastric muscular wall has been opened preserving the integrity of nerves and inner mucosa (A). Dor fundoplication is performed at the end (B).

Complications

Described complications are:

- Esophageal perforation (10%): the most frequent localization of perforations is the esophago-gastric junction where muscular layer becomes thinner. The perforation is usually detected and treated during surgery without future consequences or need for conversion;
- Dysphagia recurrence (14%): it is usually related to incomplete myotomy on the gastric side. The treatment with endoscopic dilatations has great results.

References

Boeckxstaens GE, Zaninotto G, Richter JE. Achalasia. *Lancet.* 2014 Jan 4;383(9911):83-93. Review.

O'Neill OM, Johnston BT, Coleman HG. Achalasia: a review of clinical diagnosis, epidemiology, treatment and outcomes. *World J Gastroenterol.* 2013 Sep 21;19(35):5806-12. doi: 10.3748/wjg.v19.i35.5806. Review.

Torres-Villalobos G, Martin-Del-Campo LA. Surgical Treatment for Achalasia of the Esophagus: Laparoscopic Heller Myotomy. *Gastroenterol Res Pract.* 2013;2013:708327. Epub 2013 Nov 18. Review.

Gastrostomy

Introduction

In children gastrostomy is mostly indicated in cases of swallowing disorders (often secondary to neuropathies), food refusal and all the conditions that require long-term enteral nutrition. In some cases it is useful for decompression purposes.

Surgery

In our Unit the gastrostomy is performed by video-assisted procedure. In case of neurological patients frequently affected by GERD gastrostomy is often associated with anterior fundoplication. The need to routinely perform a fundoplication is still debated because the alteration of the standard gastric anatomy leads to the risk of developing GER. The video-assisted gastrostomy follows the Stamm procedure principles.

The definitive site of the gastrostomy is marked over the anterior abdominal wall before the beginning of the laparoscopic step. In fact the abdominal distension due to the pneumoperitoneum may alter the anatomical relationships. Gastrostomy is usually placed between the superior third and the lower two-thirds of an ideal line that joins the umbilicus with the middle left inferior rib margin.

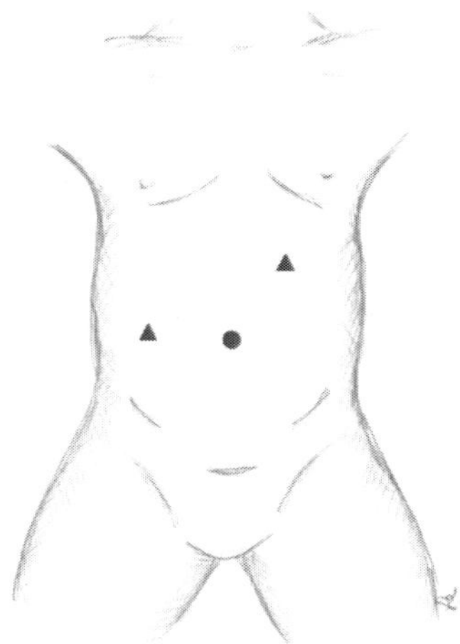

Figure 12. Trocars' position (circle = lens; triangles = operative trocars).

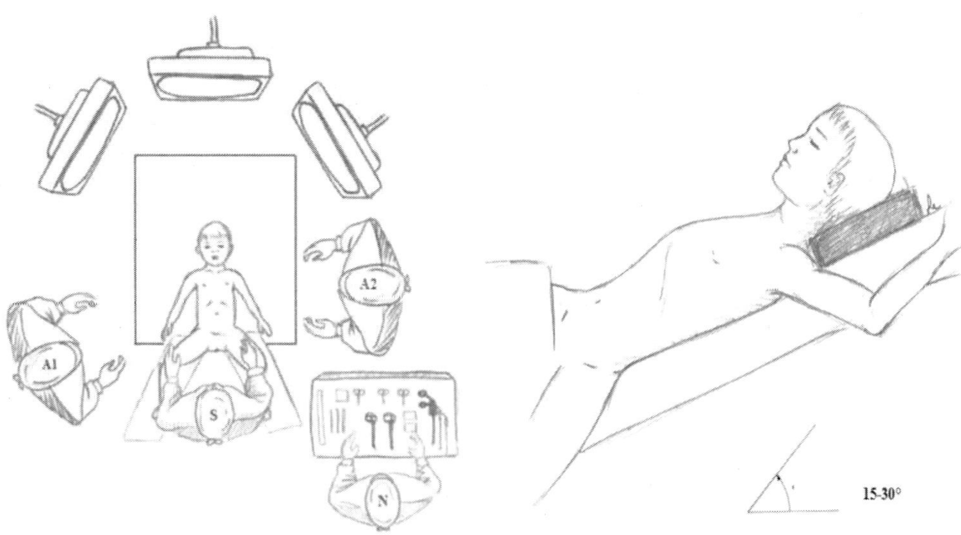

Figure 13. The patient lies in the lithotomic anti-trendelenburg supine position (S = surgeon; A1 = assistant 1; A2 = assistant 2; N = scrub nurse).

The first trocar is the umbilical one for the 5 mm / 0° optic. The pneumoperitoneum is created (8-10 mmHg of pressure and 1 L/min) and an operative trocar is inserted at the point chosen for the gastrostomy. The proper site for the gastrostomy is identified on the great curve. The stomach is grasped at this site and pulled up through the abdominal wall after the enlargement of the trocar site. The chosen point should neither be too close to the pylorus, which may be obstructed by the anchoring balloon, nor too close to the fundus, acting as an obstacle for fundoplication. Two concentric purse string sutures are performed outside the abdomen. The stomach is opened in the center of the purse string sutures in order to insert the gastrostomy probe. At this point four stabilizing angular stitches are placed on the margins of the gastric hole and anchored to the abdominal muscular fascia. Purse string sutures are tied and the skin around the gastostomy is closed with non-absorbable interrupted suture. At the end of the procedure we always perform a laparoscopic check.

The advantages of this technique are the precise placement of the gastrostomy at the chosen site and the safety of a direct vision procedure without the risk of intestinal perforation.

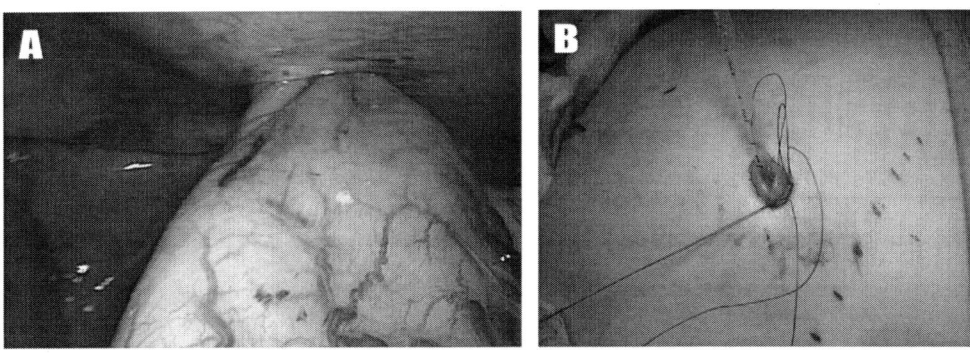

Figure 14. The stomach is approximated to the anterior abdominal wall and it is exteriorized (A). Gastrostomy is then performed outside the abdomen (B).

Feeding is gradually reintroduced after 3-4 days, meanwhile the gastrostomy is kept open to empty the stomach. Neurological therapies can already be administered in the immediate postoperative period. Anti-secretive therapy is maintained to reduce acid secretion may lead to local complications. If the tube goes out it can be reinserted because the Stamm procedure guarantees high security levels.

Complications

The main complication is ostomy dehiscence with endoperitoneal aliments/gastric acid diffusion.

References

Ostlie DJ, Holcomb GW 3rd. Laparoscopic fundoplication and gastrostomy. *Semin Pediatr Surg*. 2002 Nov;11(4):196-204. Review

Wragg RC, Salminen H, Pachl M, Singh M, Lander A, Jester I, Parikh D, Jawaheer G. Gastrostomy insertion in the 21st century: PEG or laparoscopic? Report from a large single-centre series. *Pediatr Surg Int.* 2012 May;28(5):443-8.
Zamakhshary M, Jamal M, Blair GK, Murphy JJ, Webber EM, Skarsgard ED. Laparoscopic vs percutaneous endoscopic gastrostomy tube insertion: a new pediatric gold standard? *J Pediatr Surg.* 2005 May;40(5):859-62

Intestinal Atresia and Stenosis

Introduction

Intestinal atresias and stenosis are common causes of intrinsic intestinal obstruction in neonates. The most frequently involved tracts are the jejunum and the ileum. Colonic atresia is very rare, accounting for only 5% of all intestinal atresias (clinical picture is the same as distal ileal atresias and a bowel enema permits the diagnosis).

Duodenal Atresia and Stenosis

Duodenal atresia is a complete obstruction of the duodenal lumen. Duodenal stenosis is an incomplete obstruction due to extrinsic (anular pancreas, Ladd adhesion, preduodenal portal vein) or intrinsic causes (incomplete diaphragm, diverticulum). The incidence is about 1/2500 live births with male preponderance. Associated anomalies are: prematurity, growth retardation, cardiac defects, esophageal atresia, ARM, uropathies and Down syndrome. The defect is probably related to a flaw in morphogenesis early in development. There are 3 types of duodenal atresias (see table 2).

Table 2. Duodenal atresias

DUODENAL ATRESIA CLASSIFICATION	
Type I	Complete membrane across the lumen of the duodenum (windsock). Duodenal wall is intact
Type II	Blind-ending proximal and distal segments connected by a fibrous cord
Type III	Separation of the two blind-ending segments with V-shaped mesentery

Diagnosis

Maternal US scan shows polyhydramnios in up to 50% of neonates. Sometimes there is a dilated stomach and first duodenum. After birth, the baby (often premature) presents with bilious vomit (85% of cases) or clear vomit if the level of the atresia is below the Vater ampulla (15% of cases). Often there is a scaphoid abdomen (not distended because the obstruction is high) or distended epigastrium (due to the distended stomach). The meconium emission can be normal within the first 24 hours of life. Late signs are icterus, dehydration and failure to thrive. Clinical picture of duodenal stenosis may be unclear with symptoms arising only late in childhood.

A plain abdominal radiograph shows the classical "double bubble" sign, caused by the dilated stomach and first part of the duodenum. The injection of gastric gas is helpful to identify the double bubble sign. The presence of gas distal to the duodenum shows incomplete obstruction. In these cases a contrast study is performed: bowel enema to exclude malrotations (Ladd), volvulus and upper contrast x-ray to exclude stenosis. Cardiological and renal evaluations are performed.

Jejunoileal Atresia

Jejunoileal atresia is a complete obstruction of the small intestine lumen and it is the most frequent cause of congenital intestinal occlusion (1/1000 live births). It seems to be related to an intrauterine ischaemic insult (fetal intussusception, midgut volvulus, thromboembolic events, mechanical problems – gastrochisis). The result of this ischemic insult can be an abnormal function of the proximal bowel segment. This must be considered at surgery in order to perform resections of tapering that will ensure optimal postoperative function. On the other hand care should be taken in order to avoid short bowel syndrome in patients with low intestinal length. Different from duodenal atresia, the association with syndromes is rare.

There are 4 types of intestinal atresia (see Table 3).

Table 3. Intestinal atresias

INTESTINAL ATRESIA CLASSIFICATION	
Type I	Complete membrane across the lumen of the intestine. Intestinal wall is intact
Type II	Blind-ending proximal and distal segments connected by a fibrous cord
Type III	a) Separation of the two blind-ending segments with V-shaped mesentery b) High jejunal atresia with huge mesenteric gap and twisted distal intestine (apple peel)
Type IV	Multiple atresias

Diagnosis

Prenatal polyhydramnios may be observed in cases of high defects.

After birth, the baby presents bilious vomit, abdominal distension and failure to pass meconium. Low birth weight may be observed. Abdominal radiograph shows dilated loops of small bowel and air-fluid levels. A bowel enema should be performed in all cases: it identifies the caecum position, the microcolon, the meconium ileus, etc.

Treatment

After birth a nasogastric tube is placed to decompress the stomach and to prevent aspiration. Fluid ev administration is started. Surgery is then required.

Nowadays there are two minimally invasive methods to treat those defects: the laparoscopic or the laparo-assisted technique. The first laparoscopic correction of a duodenal atresia was firstly described in 2001. Laparoscopy is associated with a high conversion rate (due to associated anomalies) and a high complication rate (anastomosis dehiscence, stenosis, and colic iatrogenic perforation). The pure laparoscopic correction of jejunal-ileal atresia has never been completed because of the need for proximal intestinal stump tapering.

The laparo-assisted technique is a reasonable alternative and it can be defined as an evolution of the pure laparoscopic procedure.

Duodenal Atresia and Stenosis

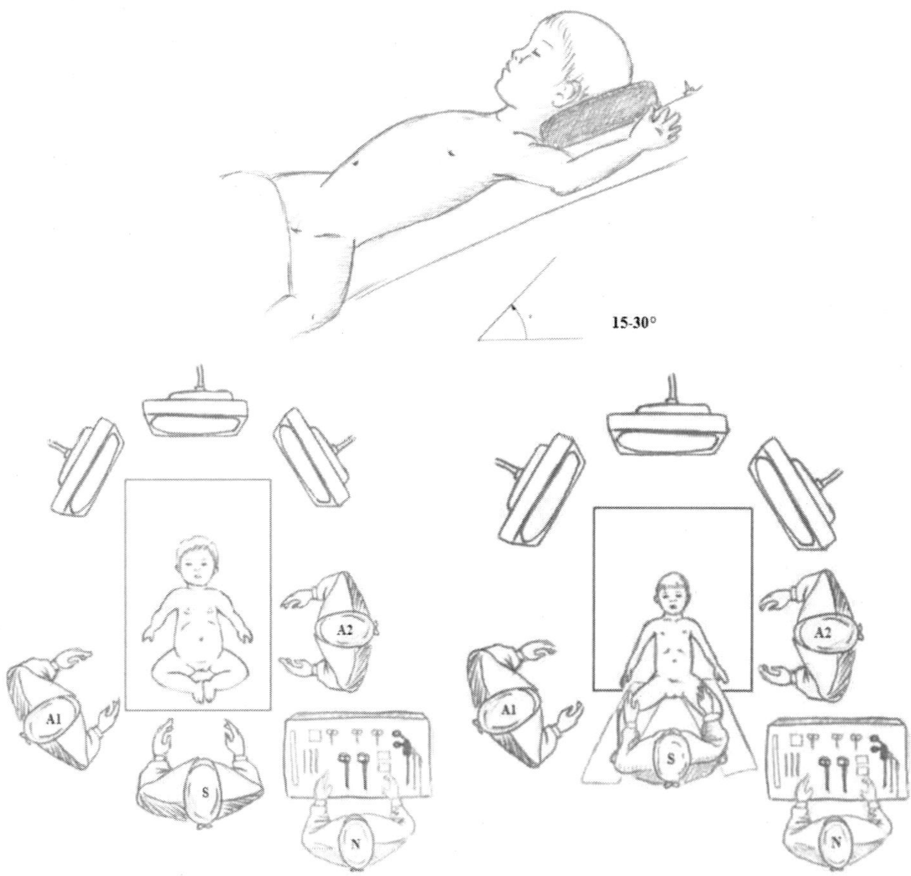

Figure 15. The patient lies in supine anti-Trendelenburg position, at the end of the operating table (S = surgeon; A1 = assistant 1; A2 = assistant 2; N = scrub nurse).

The first 10 mm trocar with pneumatic anchorage for the 0°, 5 mm optic is inserted through a supra-umbilical semicircular wound. The pneumoperitoneum is created with 6-7 mmHg of pressure and 0.5 L/min of flow and the abdominal cavity is explored. Duodenal forms require duodenum mobilization (because it is behind the peritoneum). Two 3 mm operative trocars are therefore inserted in the right flank and in the left hypochondrium under direct vision.

Once the atretic segment has been identified, it is mobilized and exteriorized through the umbilical wound. The umbilical incision can be extended upward to facilitate this maneuver. The second part of the procedure is performed outside the abdomen. The whole small intestine should be explored after exteriorization to exclude the presence of multiple atresias or associated anomalies. Also, washing out the internal bowels, before completing the anastomosis, helps to identify multiple atresias. Diaphragms are resected after duodenotomy and a duodeno-duodenostomy is performed. The anastomosis is then placed in the abdomen and the last evaluation (good anastomosis location, no bleeding) is performed laparoscopically. A trans-anastomotic tube is placed through the nose and no drains are left in place.

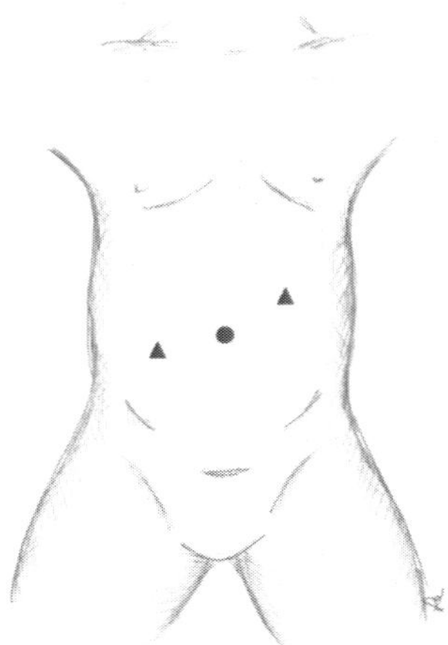

Figure 16. Trocars' position (circle = lens; triangles = operative trocars).

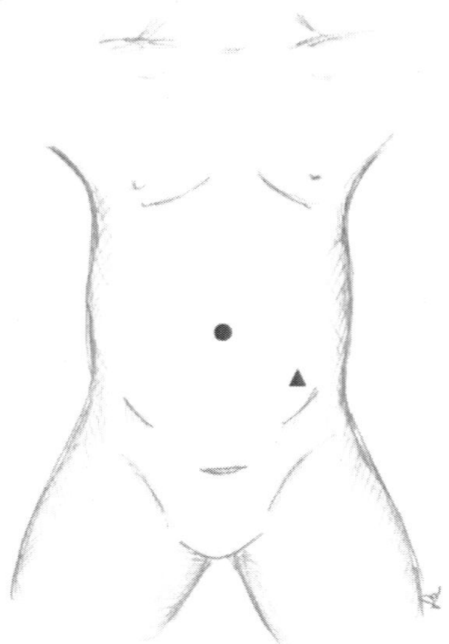

Figure 17. Trocars' position (circle = lens; triangle = operative trocars).

Jejunoileal Atresia

The jejunoileal atresia correction is performed with the same umbilical incision and 0°, 5 mm optic (through 10 mm operative trocar). Only an additional operative trocar (3 mm in the left flank) is inserted after the creation of the pneumoperitoneum.

The abdominal cavity is explored and the atretic segment is identified thanks to the difference of caliber between the proximal and distal intestinal tracts. The pathological segment is then exteriorized and resected outside the abdomen. Also in this case the whole intestine is inspected to exclude multiple forms. The anastomosis is performed after the tapering of the proximal stump, as required in the majority of cases. At the end of the procedure, the laparoscopic control is performed and no drains are left in place.

After surgery feeding is re-introduced on the 4th-5th post-operative day.

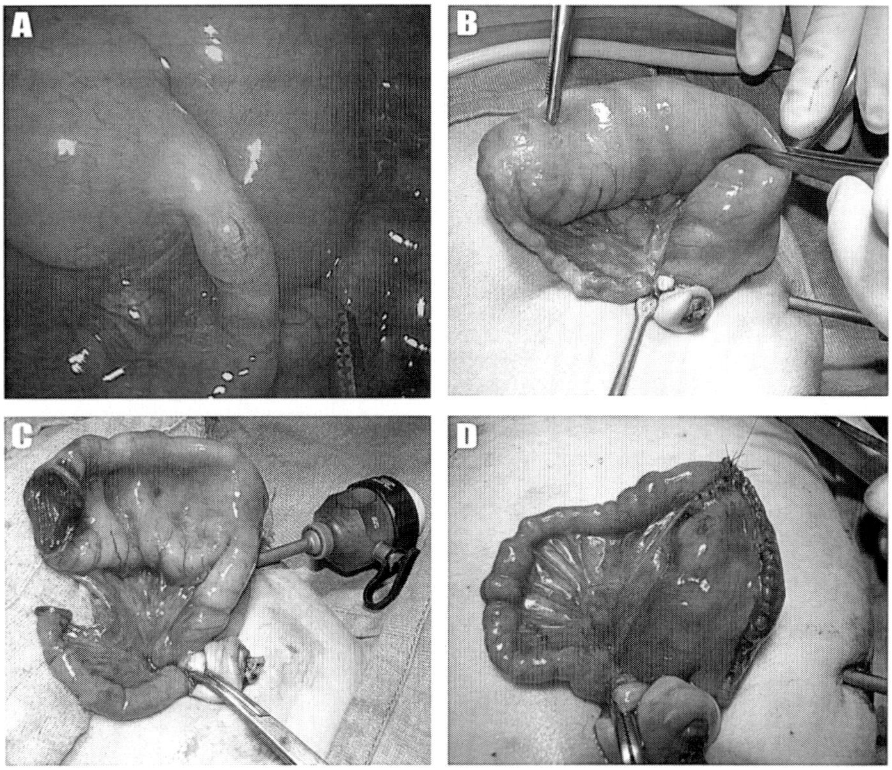

Figure 18. Identification of atresic jejunal segment (A) and its exteriorization through umbilical wound (B). Resection of the atresic segment (C). Anastomosis is performed after tapering of the dilated segment (D).

Complications

Complications are rare and they are the same as for the open approach. Described complications are anastomotic leaks, megaduodenum and short bowel syndrome. Children require intensive early and late management, often needing long-term parenteral nutrition.

References

Banieghbal B, Beale PG. Minimal access approach to jejunal atresia. *J Pediatr Surg.* 2007 Aug;42(8):1362-4.

Georgeson KE, Robertson DJ. Minimally invasive surgery in the neonate: review of current evidence. *Semin Perinatol.* 2004 Jun;28(3):212-20.

Lima M, Ruggeri G, Domini M, Gargano T, Mazzero G, Landuzzi V, Sciutti R. Evolution of the surgical management of bowel atresia in newborn: laparoscopically assisted treatment. *Pediatr Med Chir.* 2009 Sep-Oct;31(5):215-9.

Murphy FJ, Mohee A, Khalil B, Lall A, Morabito A, Bianchi A. Versatility of the circumumbilical incision in neonatal surgery. *Pediatr Surg Int.* 2009 Feb;25(2):145-7.

Yamataka A, Koga H, Shimotakahara A, Urao M, Yanai T, Kobayashi H, Lane GJ, Miyano T. Laparoscopy-assisted surgery for prenatally diagnosed small bowel atresia: simple, safe, and virtually scar free. *J Pediatr Surg.* 2004 Dec;39(12):1815-8.

Intestinal Duplications

Introduction

The term alimentary tract duplications include a wide variety of mass lesions through the gastrointestinal tract that are either tubular (25%) or cystic (75%). According to Ladd, they have three characteristics: the presence of a coat of smooth muscle, a lining epithelium representing a tract of the intestine and intimate association with the gastrointestinal tract (they are always on the mesenteric margin). They can occur anywhere in the gastrointestinal tract (from the mouth to the anus, see Table 4).

Table 4. Intestinal duplications

INTESTINAL DUPLICATIONS	
ABDOMINAL > 75%	
Jejunum-ileaum (50%)	They are cystic with mucosal lining
Colon-rectum (16%)	They can be tubular or cystic. They are often associated with other malformations
Stomach (6%)	They are cystic masses on the great curve or near the pylorus
Duodenum (5%)	They are often inside the pancreas causing obstruction or pancreatitis
THORACIC 20%	They are found in older children and they are often cystic
THORACO-ABDOMINAL 5%	They are rare diverticula that extend through the posterior mediastinum and the diaphragm in the abdomen where they end blindly

Several theories have been proposed to explain their origin but none is fully accepted: split notochord syndrome, recanalization defects and persistent diverticula.

Diagnosis

The clinical presentation varies from asymptomatic to bowel obstruction or compression over surrounding structures: dysphagia, dyspnea, etc. Sometimes they cause intussusception or volvulus. Erosions and bleedings may occur when gastric epithelium lines the mass. Gastric duplication near the pylorus may cause a clinical picture similar to that of the hypertrophic pyloric stenosis. Anal duplications may protrude or be responsible for hydro-ureteronephrosis or stipsis. There a few described cases of intestinal duplications identified in utero (prenatal US). After birth initial screening examination is abdominal US, especially for cystic forms. Radiological evaluation can be completed by contrast x-ray, CT and MR scans and ^{99m}Tc scintigraphy (in case of ectopic gastric mucosa).

Treatment

Surgery is the treatment of choice in case of intestinal duplications. Intestinal resection and subsequent anastomosis may be required in order to excise the mass entirely. During the maneuver iatrogenic perforations are not uncommon and they require surgical closure. These are the reasons for the delayed application of minimally-invasive techniques to treat these conditions. Laparoscopy was first employed for explorative purposes, in order to define the location and nature of the lesions. The resection was later performed by a focused mini-laparotomy. Laparoscopy has still the same aim (to precisely locate and to obtain information about the nature of the lesion) but it can also be therapeutic. In fact the lesion can be resected or enucleated during the same surgical procedure.

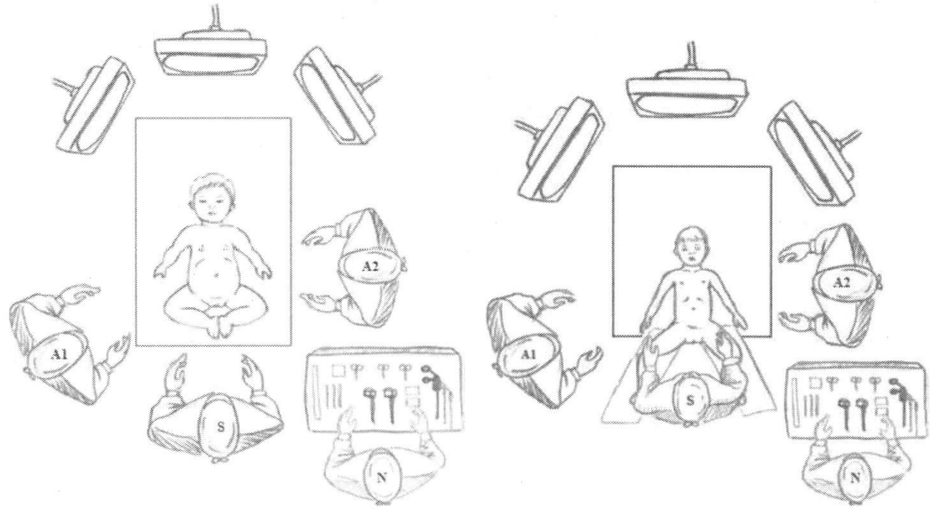

Figure 19. (Continued).

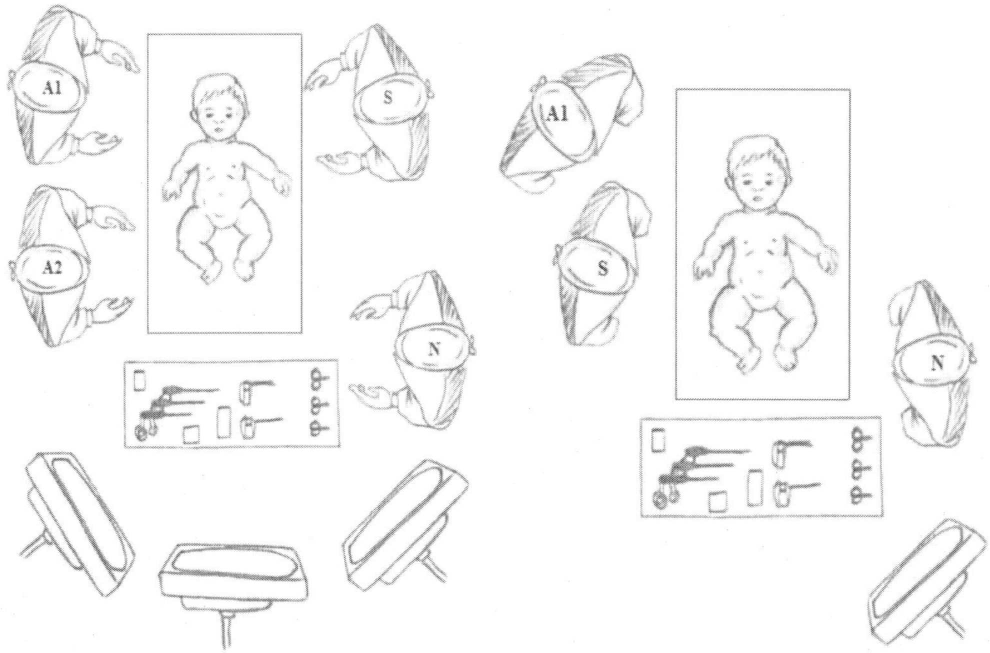

Figure 19. Operative set-up in case of gastric – duodenum – small intestine – colon duplications (up left = infant; up right = children); cecum duplications (down left); recto – sigmoid duplications (down right). (S = surgeon; A1 = assistant 1; A2 = assistant 2; N = scrub nurse).

Jejunal - ileal and cecal forms require a video-assisted approach because the bowel is easily extracted from the umbilicus; gastric, duodenal and colic duplications need a purely laparoscopic approach.

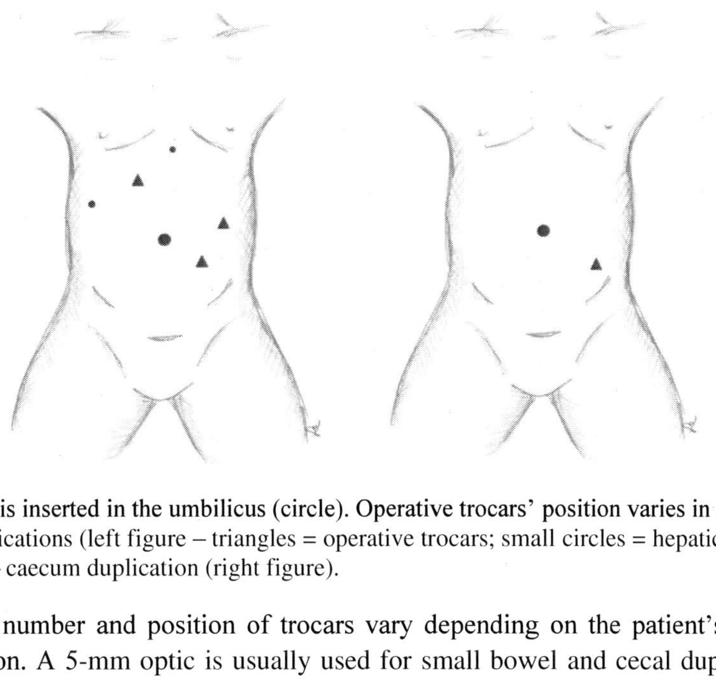

Figure 20. Lens is inserted in the umbilicus (circle). Operative trocars' position varies in case of gastric – duodenal duplications (left figure – triangles = operative trocars; small circles = hepatic retractor) or small intestine – caecum duplication (right figure).

The type, number and position of trocars vary depending on the patient's age and the lesion's location. A 5-mm optic is usually used for small bowel and cecal duplications. We recommend the use of a 10 mm pneumatic anchorage trocar for the video assisted technique. The umbilical trocar is introduced with open technique and the pneumoperitoneum is created with 8-10 mmHg of pressure and 0.5-1 L/min of flow. At the beginning of the procedure the abdominal cavity is explored in order to identify the lesion. Operative trocars are then placed under direct vision.

Gastric, Duodenal and Colic Duplications

The duplication can be removed via laparoscopic enucleation. At the end of the procedure it is important to verify the vascularization of remaining structures that could have been damaged during the procedure. The sample is extracted with an Endobag or a finger glove (the exact diagnosis is only determined by histological examination).

Jejunal, Ileal and Caecal Duplications

Also in these cases the procedure starts with the identification of the lesion. The duplicated tract is then extracted from the umbilical wound and resected (intestinal resection and subsequent anastomosis). The lesion is enucleated in case of extended duplications or caecal duplications.

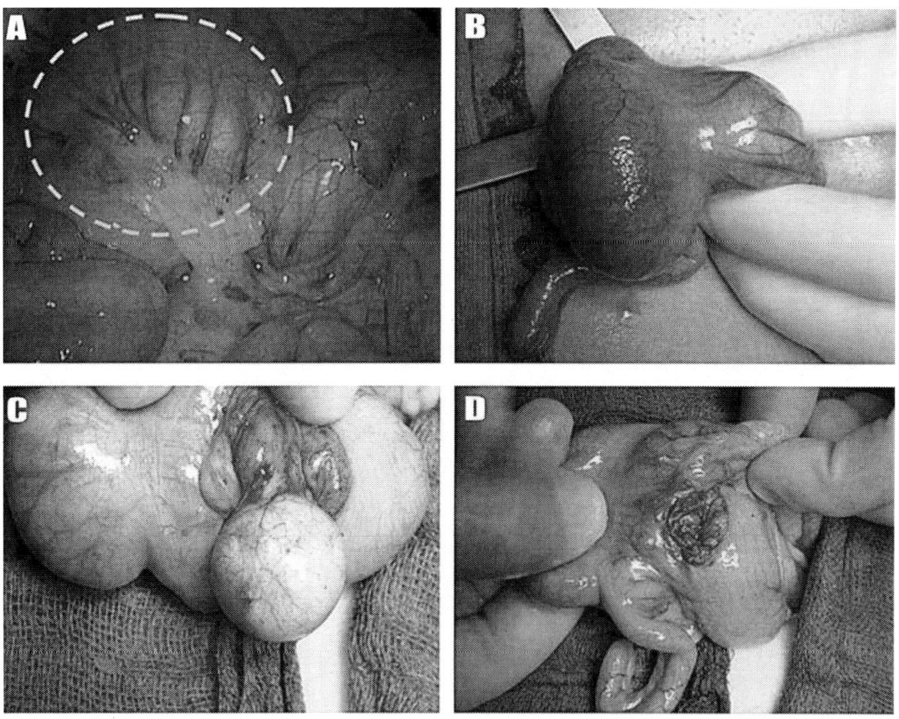

Figure 21. Laparoscopic identification of caecal duplication (Fig. A). Caecal exteriorization through the umbilical wound (Fig B). Lesion enucleation (Fig C and D).

After surgery the naso-gastric tube is maintained only in case of intestinal resection-anastomosis or in case of gastric-duodenal duplications. Fasting is kept for 24 hours in case of enucleation or for 4-5 days in case of intestinal resection. When the feeding is completely reintroduced the patient is discharged ($2^{nd} - 3^{rd}$ post operative day or $5^{th} - 6^{th}$)

Complications

Preoperative = intestinal occlusion and hemorrhage

Intraoperative = the most common complication is the intestinal perforation during enucleation. It is generally solved laparoscopically without sequelae.

Postoperative = short bowel syndrome

References

Azzie G, Beasley S. Diagnosis and treatment of foregut duplications. *Semin Pediatr Surg.* 2003 Feb;12(1):46-54.

Lima M, Molinaro F, Ruggeri G, Gargano T, Randi B. Role of mini-invasive surgery in the treatment of enteric duplications in pediatric age: a survey of 15 years. *Pediatr Med Chir.* 2012 Sep-Oct;34(5):217-22.

Merrot T, Anastasescu R, Pankevych T, Tercier S, Garcia S, Alessandrini P, Guys JM. Duodenal duplications. Clinical characteristics, embryological hypotheses, histological findings, treatment. *Eur J Pediatr Surg.* 2006 Feb;16(1):18-23.

Abdominal Lymphangiomas

Introduction

Lymphangioma is a rare benign condition characterized by proliferation of the thin-walled lymphatic spaces. It is usually found in the head and neck of children. Lymphangioma of the small-bowel mesentery is rare, having been reported for less than 1% of all lymphangiomas. Abdominal lymphangioma usually manifests in the first year of life. The etiology is unknown, although some believe that it might be associated with developmental anomalies of the lymphatic ducts. Bleedings, inflammation, abdominal trauma, abdominal surgery, radiation or lymphatic obstruction may also play a role in the genesis of lymphangioma formation.

Lymphangiomas are traditionally classified into three histologic types: 1) capillary (simple) is made of small thin-walled lymphatics, usually in the superficial dermis; 2) cavernous is made of dilated lymphatic spaces associated with lymphoid stroma. It is often connected to normal-caliber adjacent lymphatic spaces; 3) cystic that consists of dilated lymphatic spaces of various sizes associated with collagen and fibrous adventitial covering without any connection to adjacent lymphatics.

Diagnosis

There are no pathognomonic signs and symptoms of lymphangiomas. The most common symptoms in children are non-specific abdominal pain, palpable mass, vomiting, abdominal distension or acute intestinal obstruction. Complications include partial or complete intestinal obstruction, infection, perforation, torsion and hemorrhage.

The differential diagnosis should include abdominal cystic masses such as mesenteric cyst, omental cyst, enteric duplication and ovarian tumors.

Ultrasound is usually the first imaging study to be performed. CT and MRI can add important preoperative information regarding anatomical location, relations of the cyst with surrounding structure (e.g. major blood vessels), which is essential for planning the operative procedure.

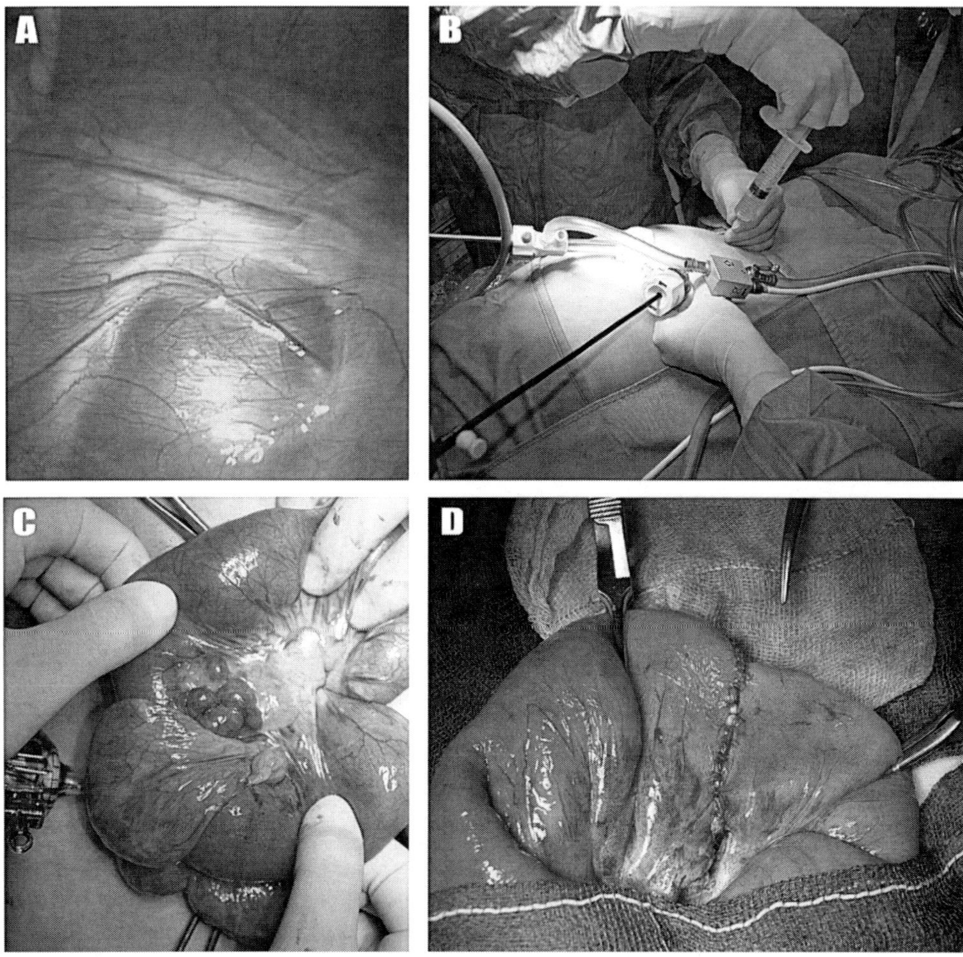

Figure 22. Abdominal cystic lymphangioma, identified during laparoscopy (A) and exteriorized after emptying (B, C). An intestinal resection was required to remove the mass and it was followed by primary anastomosis (D).

Treatment

The treatment of abdominal lymphangiomas is surgical. Laparoscopic removal has many advantages over classic laparotomy: more precise dissection, minimal trauma to abdominal structure, less pain and shorter hospital stay. At our Institution we perform video-assisted resection of abdominal lymphangiomas.

The procedure includes the insertion of a 10-mm trocar operative trocar (optic) through a sub-umbilical semi-circular or trans-umbilical incision. The lens is a 0° lens with an operative channel for 5 mm instruments. Pneumoperitoneum is created with 0,5-1 L/min of flow and 8-10 mmHg of pressure.

The abdominal cavity is explored and the mass is identified. A blunt grasper is used to approximate the mass to the anterior abdominal wall. The cyst is then emptied by transparietal puncture under laparoscopic surveillance to facilitate the extraction and creating a wider working space for the surgeon. The emptied lymphatic cyst is then grasped with blunt forceps and it is exteriorized through the umbilicus soon after the trocar's removal. Once the cyst is outside the abdomen, it is excised (with or without bowel resection) following the principles of traditional surgery.

The pure laparoscopic technique is used in presence of anatomical variants that make the exteriorization difficult. The operative trocars are placed under direct vision following the triangular principle and their position depends on the lesion's location.

In all cases, the dissection should be careful with the identification of all neurovascular structures and of all afferent lymphatic channels, which are ligated wherever possible.

Complications

Complications are uncommon when the first resection is complete. Incomplete resections often lead to recurrences.

References

De Lagausie P, Bonnard A, Berrebi D, Lepretre O, Statopoulos L, Delarue A,Guys JM. Abdominal lymphangiomas in children: interest of the laparoscopic approach. *Surg Endosc.* 2007 Jul;21(7):1153-7.

Shimura H, Ueda J, Ogawa Y, Ichimiya H, Tanaka M. Total excision of mesenteric cysts by laparoscopic surgery: report of two cases. *Surg Laparosc Endosc.* 1997 Apr;7(2):173-6.

Steyaert H, Guitard J, Moscovici J, Juricic M, Vaysse P, Juskiewenski S. Abdominal cystic lymphangioma in children: benign lesions that can have a proliferative course. *J Pediatr Surg.* 1996 May;31(5):677-80.

Tran NS, Nguyen TL. Laparoscopic management of abdominal lymphatic cysts in children. J Laparoendosc Adv Surg Tech A. 2012 Jun;22(5):505-7.

Laparoscopic Approach to Neoplastic Masses

Introduction

The use of laparoscopy in children has followed its use in adults and this also applies to the approach to cancer. As with all procedures, the target is to achieve the same therapeutic results of the open approach, adding the advantages of less invasive ones. In the case of malignancies, laparoscopy has not yet reached the acceptance that it has for the treatment of other pathologies. The purpose of this paper is to explore the possibility of MIS illustrating the indications and the concerns about its use in pediatric oncology.

Risks and Concerns

The main factors that have limited the use of the MIS are as follows:

- Loss of tactile sensation makes it difficult to individuate a little lesion in a parenchymal organ or an involved lymph node
- Intra-abdominal spillage advances grade staging of certain cancers, making the MIS not applicable. Indeed, in some cases the local recurrence significantly influences the prognosis and is difficult to treat. Obviously it is important to reduce the peritoneal contamination use an endobag or a glove finger for any sample of certain or suspected neoplastic origin.
- Margins of resection. The removal of a mass freed by laparoscopy can be performed through the umbilical wound, but this can require its morcellation. By choosing this strategy, it is much more difficult to assess the involvement of resection margins and therefore the radicality of surgery. A solution can be a service laparotomy in a more aesthetic position (Pfannenstiel incision).
- Recurrence at the trocar site. Although there are many encouraging studies, even in pediatric surgery cases are reported with this complication.

Indications

Laparoscopy in malignancies can be used in selected patients according to the protocols currently used. For this reason it is important to be familiar with oncologists' requirements and comply with it. Main abdominal neoplasms are listed in Table 1.

The surgery should be guided by clinical and radiological requirements of the patient to minimize the risks. A complete evaluation usually includes: history, physical examination, imaging (ultrasounds, X-ray, CT scan, MRI according to each case), laboratory results (blood, urine, tumoral markers, etc.).

The following are the main applications of laparoscopy

Biopsy

Masses of unknown origin or those that require a histological typing to set the most appropriate treatment protocol can be biopsied. Laparoscopy has the advantage of providing a sufficient amount of tissue (greater than radiologically percutaneous biopsy), a rapid recovery to begin therapy and reduced adhesion of further surgery. The diagnostic accuracy of laparoscopic biopsies is 85 -100%, so this approach should be considered. Among the cancers that most frequently require biopsy are neuroblastoma and lymphoma. The exception is represented by the Wilms' tumor, which should be primarily excised; in fact, the rupture of the tumor has a significant impact on treatment and prognosis.

Staging

Lymph node involvement is another important prognostic factor. Laparoscopic removal can aid correct staging of tumors. The most common site of involved lymph nodes are: celiac, portal, periaortic and pericaval, mesenteric and iliac. Obviously, the approach varies depending upon the localization.

Celiac lymph nodes and portal ones can be reached through an omental window above the lesser curvature of the stomach. Alternatively, portal nodes can be removed following the cystic duct from the gallbladder to the porta hepatis. The removal of periaortic and pericaval lymph nodes requires the mobilization of the ipsilateral colon through a peritoneal incision. It's important to be careful not to damage the mesocolon, the ureter, gonadal and iliac vessels. Mesenteric lymph nodes are easy to take, but the identification of those involved can be complex. It can require the radiological guided injection of methylene blue or India ink into the node. The iliac site can be reached with an incision of the posterior peritoneum lateral to the vessels.

Table 5. Abdominal neoplasm in pediatric age

Main abdominal neoplasm in pediatric age by location	
Liver	Hepatoblastoma Hepatocellular carcinoma Rhabdomyosarcoma Hemangiomas Mesenchymal hamartoma Adenomas Metastases
Main abdominal neoplasm in pediatric age by location	
Stomach	GIST Leiomyoma Leiomyosarcoma
Spleen	Cystic tumors Lymphomas
Pancreas	Pseudocyst Pancreatoblastoma Adenocarcinoma
Adrenal gland / sympathetic ganglia	Neuroblastoma Ganglioneuroblastoma Ganglioneuroma Pheochromocytoma
Intestine	Leiomyoma Leiomyosarcoma Lymphangioma Lymphoma
Gonads / extragonadal sites	Teratomas Endodermal sinus tumors Choriocarcinoma Sacro-coccygeal teratoma
Lymph node	Lymphoma (Hodgkin, Non Hodgkin)
Miscellaneous	Fibrosarcoma Rhabdomyosarcoma others

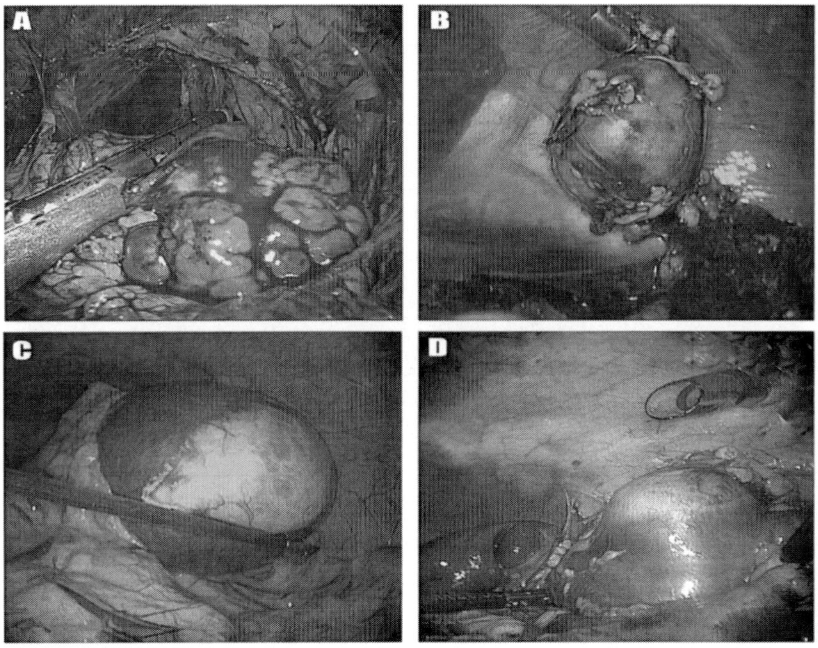

Figure 23. Laparoscopic view of abdominal masses: GIST (A), neuroblastoma (B), splenic cyst tumor (C), Wilms' tumor (D).

Evaluation of Resectability

Despite radiological images, which are becoming more technologically advanced, they are not always able to determine the actual anatomic relationship of a lesion with surrounding vital structures and thus determine the actual resectability. Laparoscopy in this case provides direct visualization of the tumor by providing more precise anatomical detail.

Removal

Laparoscopy still has limitations, however, there are now several reports that describe its use in small tumors, capsulated, mostly benign but also malignant. Examples include subcapsular liver metastases, neuroblastomas (selected cases), splenic and hepatic cysts, visceral leiomyomas, ganglioneuromas, ganglioneuroblastomi, ovarian teratomas or other tumors. In these cases a high rate of success is reported. Also, in the last few years some retrospective studies of laparoscopic nephrectomy in Wilms' tumor, with no or a low rate of complications, have been reported. Unfortunately, randomized and controlled trials have not been reported.

References

Davidoff AM, Minimally invasive surgery for pediatric cancer. In Lobe TE (ed) Pediatric laparoscopy (2003) *Landes Bioscience Georgetown,* Texas USA Ch 19 pp 157-169.

Duarte RJ, Dénes FT, Cristofani LM et al. Laparoscopic nephrectomy for Wilms' tumor. *Expert Rev Anticancer Ther.* 2009 Jun;9(6):753-61. doi: 10.1586/era.09.44.
Kumar V, Mandhani A, Srivastava A, et al. Port site metastasis after laparoscopic radical nephrectomy: a single-center experience. *Indian J Cancer.* 2012 Jan-Mar;49(1):102-6. doi: 10.4103/0019-509X.98932.
Metzelder ML, Kuebler JF, Shimotakahara A Role of Diagnostic and Ablative Minimally Invasive Surgery for Pediatric Malignancies CANCER June 1, 2007 / Volume 109 / Number 11 pp2343-2348.
Sandoval C et al. Laparoscopy in the Management of Pediatric Intraabdominal Tumors, *JSLS* (2004)8:115-118.
Zachariou Z, Otte J-B Kiely E, Godzinski J Pediatric Surgical Oncology In: Zachariou Z (ed) Pediatric Surgery Digest (2009) *Springer* Ch 28 pp541-597.

Hirschsprung's Disease

Introduction

Hirschsprung's disease (HSCR) is a common cause of neonatal intestinal obstruction. It is part of a group of congenital affections characterized by the absence of enteric ganglia in the submucosa and myenteric plexuses in the distal colo-rectum with variable proximal extension.

The disease is a congenital malformation occurring in 1/5000 live births, with the high incidence in Asian populations and the lowest in Hispanics. The male/female ratio is 4:1.

The enteric nervous system (ENS) is a division of the peripheral nervous system. It is large and complex, containing more neurons than the spinal cord.

HSCR is caused by a premature arrest of the migration of neural crest cells that will form the ENS (neurocristopathy). The effect is a motor alteration, which makes it impossible for the intestinal content to move forward (functional obstruction). The alteration is related not only to the absence of ganglia but also to the increment of colinergic Ach positive fibers and to alterations of the non-adrenergic-non-colinergic (NANC) system.

The events that led to the formation of the ENS are controlled by cellular and molecular mechanisms that are not well known.

In 1994, the causative gene HSCR was identified on the proto-oncogene RET (chromosome 10). Its alterations are responsible for autosomal dominant forms. RET mutations are found in 50% of familiar cases and in less than 30% of sporadic cases. RET is also involved in other complex neurocristopathies such as the multiple endocrine neoplasia (MEN 2A and MEN 2B). The following factors are responsible for the clinical variability:

- Colinergic fiber (Ach pos) hyperinnervation
- Adrenergic fiber increment
- NANC neuron absence
- Extension of the agangliar tract

The variable extent of aganglionosis leads to a classification of HSCR into short and long segment phenotypes.

1) Short forms (classical) include aganglionosis confined below the rectosigmoid junction (80%)
2) Long forms (20%) can extend below the splenic flexure to the whole colon (total colonic aganglionosis, TCA, 5-10%) or in the whole bowel (total intestinal)
3) The third group includes the ultra-short forms where the disease is confined to the last 2-3 cm of the distal rectum (megarectum).

Diagnosis

HSCR should be considered in any child who has a history of constipation dating back to the new-born period. The median age at which children are diagnosed with the disease has progressively decreased over time.

Clinical history can start at birth (the neonate is usually a full-term baby) with delayed meconium passage (after 24 hours), progressive constipation, distended abdomen, feeding intolerance and bilious vomiting. However several authors have found that more than 40% of neonates with HSCR pass meconium in the first 24 hours. Symptoms may be reduced by the use of water enemas. In this phase rectal examination or irrigation causes an "explosive" passage of meconium. The clinical picture can be very different in terms of severity.

Principal clinical picture:

- Neonatal persistent intestinal sub-occlusion = soon after birth the intestinal content stands in the dilated part proximal to the aganglionic tract. The clinical picture is characterized by the absence of spontaneous evacuations, progressive abdominal distension and vomit. The worse effect is the portal system embolism and intestinal perforation. It requires a colostomy / ileostomy of the normal bowel.
- Progressive constipation = initial symptoms improve spontaneously leaving a clinical picture of constipation. Recurrent sub-occlusive crisis due to fecalomas are frequent. The physical examination permits the identification of the abdominal fecal masses with an empty rectum. These patients are treated with definitive surgery without the need for a protective colostomy.
- Late sudden intestinal obstruction = patients have mild signs of the disease followed by severe constipation and chronic obstruction. They have a severe abdominal distension and general dystrophy (associated with anorexia, recurrent infections, anemia). If not treated they develop enterocolitis.
- Enterocolitis = it is characterized by the onset of diarrhea, fever and abdominal distension. It is the most feared complication. Among the proposed theories to explain the etiology there is physical dilatation of the proximal bowel, Clostridium difficile, variations in the mucin components and production, and increased prostaglandin e1 activity. Patients require urgent resuscitation and correction of electrolytes prior to the start of any treatment.

The diagnosis of HSCR is based on intestinal biopsy. Rectal manometry remains a reliable screening procedure and radiology still has an important role to suggest the presence of the disease and to detect enterocolitis.

- Supine and lateral plain films = they show gaseous distension of bowel loops with involvement of the large bowel. The level of obstruction may be identified by normal colon or rectum. Multiple air fluid levels may be shown. The presence of air in the rectum does not exclude the diagnosis.
- Bowel enema = the patient should not be prepared (no rectal wash outs and no digital examination) in order to avoid decompression of the distended proximal bowel. Plain films should exclude perforations. Oblique and lateral projections are required to identify the cone-shaped transition zone (that separates the normal colon from the aganglionic one). The principal sign is the different calibre between the pathological tract and the proximal intestine. In case of enterocolitis the enema shows mucosal edema, mucosal ulcerations, abnormal air-fluid levels, bowel wall thickening and pneumatosis.
- Rectomanometry = it allows the recording of pressure changes around hollow muscular organs of the gastrointestinal tract. It is performed after 2-3 days preparation (colon, rectum and ano-rectum should be empty). The system investigates several aspects of sphincter activity: variations of internal anorectum pressure (anorectal fluctuations), spontaneous release of the internal sphincter, inhibitory anal reflex (that is a reproduction of the defecator reflex), compliance, anorectum pressure profile.
- Histopathological diagnosis = it is the gold standard for the diagnosis and it is obtained with rectal mucosal and submucosal suction biopsies. Histochemic of HSRC has the following features: absence of nerve cells in the submucous and myenteric plexus (ganglion cells are visualized by an LDH reaction) and a typical increase in AchE activity in the parasympathetic nerve fibers of the lamina propria mucosae.

Preoperative diagnosis should be confirmed during surgery with intraoperative seromuscular biopsies sent for histological examination. This allows the identification of the exact transition area.

Treatment

Once the diagnosis has been confirmed the infant should be prepared for surgery. Until 1995 the gold standard for the treatment of HSCR was the rectosigmoidectomy with "aseptic" endorectal colon pull-through (Soave technique). After the introduction of minimally-invasive approaches, the Georgeson laparoscopic technique has become the treatment of choice. Transanal laparo-assisted endorectal pull-through (Georgeson technique) follows the steps of the Soave technique including a laparoscopic step that aims at the isolation and mobilization of the aganglionic colon and a perineal step to perform the extramucosa dissection and transanal pull-through with subsequent colo-anal anastomosis. In recent years we have modified the laparoscopic step and we have introduced a video-assisted dissection with exteriorization of the colon through the umbilical wound.

Preparation of the patient includes oral liquid intake 72 hours before surgery, rectal irrigations twice a day for 5 days before surgery until the intestines are clear, broad-spectrum antibiotics and blood available for transfusion.

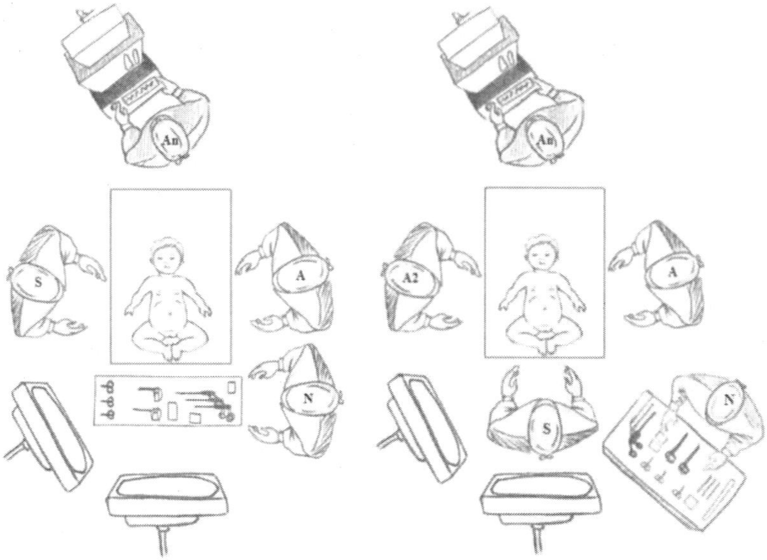

Figure 24. Operative set-up for laparoscopic (left) and perineal step (right). S = surgeon; A1 = assistant 1; A2 = assistant 2; N = scrub nurse; An = anesthesiologist.

The patient is positioned on the operating table to provide simultaneous exposure of the perineum and abdomen.

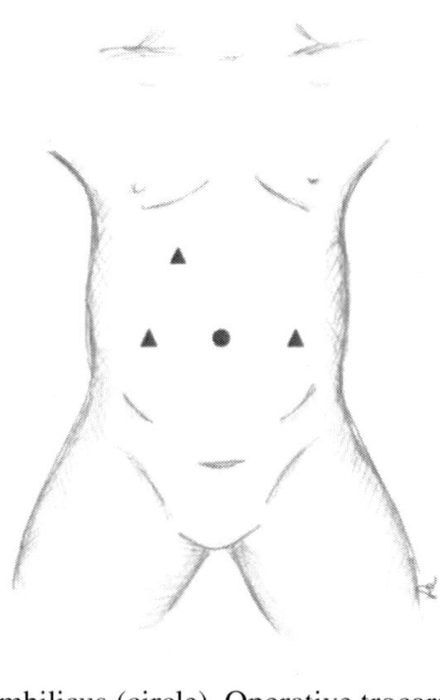

Figure 25. Lens is inserted in the umbilicus (circle). Operative trocars (triangles) are placed in the right and left flank and on the right subcostal margin.

The first step is the laparoscopic one. The first 5-10 mm umbilical trocar is inserted with open technique through the umbilicus. The trocar dimension depends on the patient's size but we usually use a 10 mm pneumatic anchorage trocar because it allows the exteriorization of the colon. Pneumoperitoneum is created with 8-10 mmHg of pressure and 0.5 L/min of flow. Remaining trocars are placed under direct vision. The procedure starts with the identification of the transition zone and of the normal colon (sero-muscular biopsies are taken along the anti-mesenteric border to determine the level of ganglionated bowel). Biopsies can be performed laparoscopically or grasping the colon and exteriorizing it through the umbilical wound (laparo-assisted). The sigma and colon are mobilized once the extension of the aganglionic tract has been identified. Mobilization length depends on the extension of the disease (it starts more proximally in long segment forms). Pure laparoscopy is used when there are difficulties in the colon exteriorization. Vascular structures can be cauterized and sectioned during laparoscopy using the harmonic scalpel or Ligasure™, recommended particularly for older patients. It is important to preserve the marginal arc (that allows the vascularization of the mobilized colon) proximally and collateral branches of the inferior mesenteric artery (that allows the vascularization of muscles) distally. When the dissection is over and the pull-through can be easily performed, the perineal step begins.

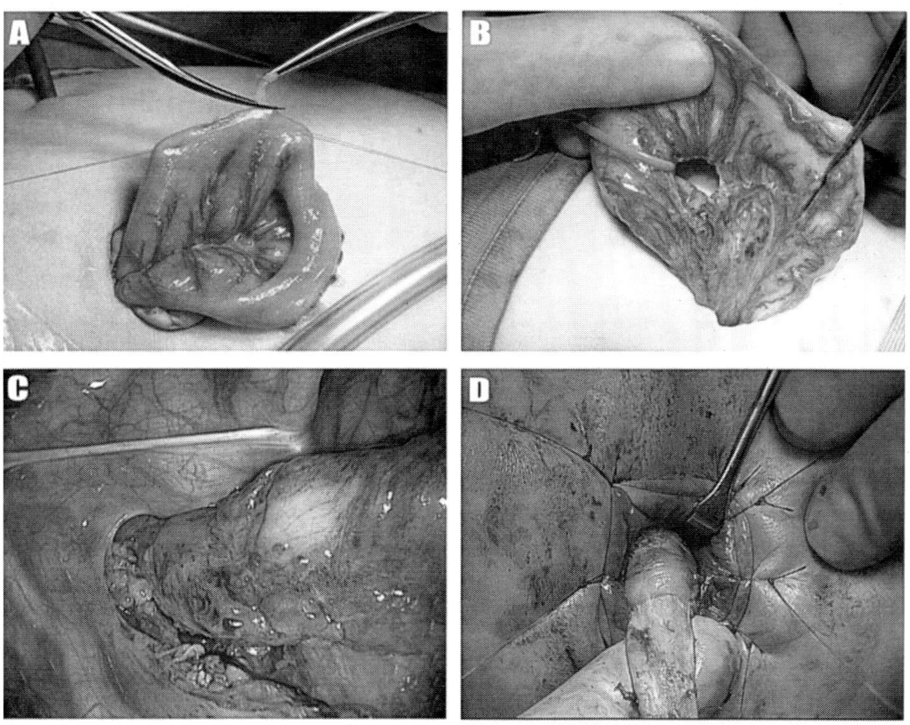

Figure 26. Sero-muscular biopsies are taken once the colon has been exteriorized through the abdominal wall (A); the colon is mobilized (B) and the pull-through is performed (C) prior to extramucous dissection (D).

The perineum is exposed and a radial traction is achieved using 6-8 stitches passing through the perineal skin and the muco-cutaneous junction. The mucous dissection starts proximally 5-10 cm below the pectineal line. The incision line is marked with the electric scalpel; traction stitches are then placed on the mucosa that is dissected following the cleavage plane with the submucosa. The maneuver can be easily performed with the use of a bipolar grasp that clots vessels. The mucosectomy continues for almost 10-15 cm until it overcomes the peritoneal reflection when the rectum prolapse is felt. Muscles are circumferentially sectioned, the colon is pulled through and the aganglionic segment is resected (the normal zone has been previously identified by the biopsy).

The muscular tract of the intussuscepted bowel is grasped with the left blunt forceps while the right blunt forceps takes the opposite part (contro-traction). The confirmation of the complete reduction can be performed outside the abdomen. The 10 mm trocar allows the exteriorization of the ileo-caecal tract or the ileo-ileal tract (even simpler). The mucosa should be opened posteriorly until the point of the future anastomosis to avoid future stenosis. Then the tract is placed in the abdomen. The purpose of that sleeve is to perform an aseptic pull-through (the bowel is never opened) and at the same time to perform a natural anastomosis between the two intussuscepted intestinal tracts (Soave's principle). The anastomosis between the neorectum and the distal anus is performed after the removal of the aganglionic tract. The procedure ends with a laparoscopic exploration to evaluate that the colic loop has good vascularization without bleeding, tractions or altered rotations of the loop itself.

Feeding is gradually re-introduced after 4-5 days and the patient is discharge on the 8th-10th post-operative day. A program of anal dilatations starts after 15 days and goes on for 6-8 weeks.

Complications

Surgical complications can develop soon after surgery or later during the follow-up. Most series report a significant incidence of early postoperative enterocolitis. Enterocolitis is more common in patients with preoperative attacks. Other serious complications are anastomotic leak, anastomotic stricture and pelvic sepsis.

- Dehiscence (1-10%): risk factors are the anastomosis tension-ischemia, poor nutritional status, steroids, residual aganglionic tracts
- Intestinal occlusion for adhesions (7-10%): many studies state that laparoscopy has drastically reduced the incidence of this complication
- Stenosis of the anastomosis (0-35%): risk factors are tension-ischemia of the anastomosis, previous dehiscence. It rarely requires surgery. Conservative therapy with dilatations is decisive in most cases.
- Stypsis (8%): it is managed with diet and behavior advice, osmotic laxatives and enemas. Severe or persistent stypsis may be the expression of a sphincteric acalasia, of the presence of an aganglionic residual segment or simply an anastomototic stenosis

References

K Hoffmann, F Schier, J Waldschmidt: J. Laparoscopic Swenson's procedure in children. *Eur J Pediatr Surg* 6: 15-7, 1996.

KE Georgeson, DJ Robertson: Laparoscopic-assisted approaches for the definitive surgery for Hirschsprung's disease. *Semin Pediatr Surg* 13:256-62, 2004.

KE Georgeson, RD Cohen, A Hebra, et al: Primary laparoscopic assisted endorectal colon pull-through for Hirschsprung's disease: a new gold standard. *Ann Surg* 229:678-683, 1999.

L De La Torre , JC Langer : Transanal endorectal pull-through for Hirschsprung's disease: techniques, controversies, pearls, pittfalls, and an organized approach to the management of postoperative obstruction symptoms. *Seminars in Pediatric Surgery* 19: 96-106, 2010.

M Lima, G Ruggeri, C Antonellini et al: Laparoscopic treatment of Hirschsprung disease. *Pediatr Med Chir* Jan-Feb 29: 19-22, 2007.

RN. Haricharan, KE Georgeson: Hirschsprung disease. *Semin Pediatr Surg* 17: 266-275, 2004.

S Turial, J Enders, V Engel: A Microlaparoscopically Assisted Pull-Through Procedure for Hirschsprung's Disease: Initial Experiences. *J Laparoendosc Surg* 21: 271-276, 2011.

Anorectal Malformations

Introduction

Anorectal malformations (ARM) include a wide spectrum of anomalies involving the urogenital and gastrointestinal tract and affecting both males and females.

The incidence of ARM is reported as 2.0-2.5/10,000 live births with significant variations in the prevalence between regions (e.g. ARM account for 15% of admissions in India). Males are affected more than females who usually have high anomalies. The only predisposing factor is familiarity, which is identified only in some syndromic forms (e.g. Currarino syndrome). There are various associations and syndromes that include ARM. It is important to define them in order to establish the risk of recurrence.

- VATER = non-random association of Vertebral defects, Anorectal malformation, esophageal atresia with or without Tracheo-esophageal fistula, Radium dysplasia and renal defects. In case of cardiac and Limbs defects the acronym becomes VACTERL. The incidence is 1/7000-10000 live births.
- Caudal regression syndrome = it is a congenital disorder in which there is abnormal fetal development of the lower spine. It is associated with ARM, vertebral agenesy, central nervous system malformations (myelomeningocele, anchored spine, etc.). The incidence is 1/7500 live births.
- Currarino syndrome = it is a singular type of caudal regression characterized by ARM, sacral agenesy and presacral mass (meningocele or presacral teratoma). It is an inherited congenital disorder.
- Townes-Brocks syndrome = it is a genetic disease with abnormalities of the external ears, ARM, hand and foot, renal and hearth abnormalities.
- FG syndrome = it is a genetic syndrome linked to the X chromosome and causing physical anomalies and developmental delays. Major clinical features include mental retardation, hyperactive behavior; severe constipation, with or without structural anomalies; macrocephaly; severe hypotonia;

Before the 5th week of fetal life the cloaca represents a single cavity in which Wolf ducts, uretra, Müller ducts and primitive intestine come out. The uro-rectal septum separates the primitive intestine and the urogenital structures. Many factors permit its caudal migration and the cloaca division into the rectum and the urogenital sinus. Then the urogenital septum descends and separates from the intestine. The rectum fuses with the anus and they both reach the perineum. An error that occurs in the urogenital migration causes the onset of altered communications between the rectum and the urogenital sinus; the sinus does not disappear and the anus becomes ectopic along the caudal septum path.

Many classifications have been proposed and multiple systems are used in different centers making comparisons difficult. In 1970 the "International" classification was proposed on the basis of normal and abnormal anatomy dividing the lesions into three groups high (supralevator), intermediate and low (translevator). The International classification was later simplified into the "Wingspread classification" that does not include rarer subtypes. In 2005 a new system was proposed (Krickenbeck classification). It does not focus on anatomical or embryological features or on imaging but on frequency of occurrence.

Table 6. ARM classification

Krickenbeck classification	
Major clinical groups	Perineal (cutaneous) fistula
	Rectourethral fistula
	Bulbar
	Prostatic
	Rectovescical fistula
	Vestibular fistula
	Cloaca
	No fistula
	Anal stenosi
Rare/Regional variants	Puch colon
	Rectal atresia/stenosis
	Rectovaginal fistula
	H type fistula
	Others

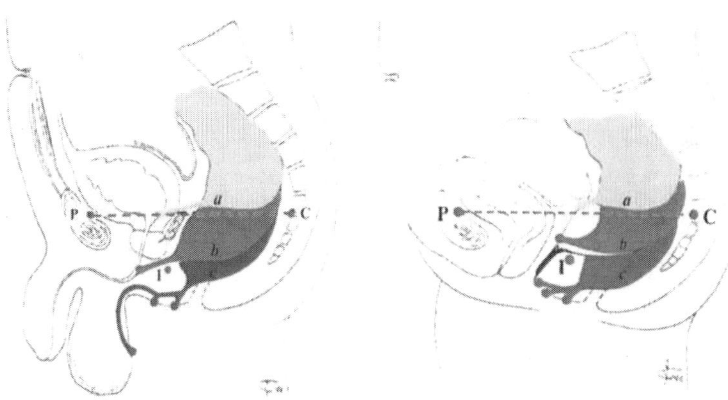

Figure 27. Types of ARM.

Diagnosis

The diagnosis should be made soon after birth (with the exception of lower forms) and it is based on accurate physical examinations. The untreated imperforated anus brings intestinal occlusion. Recto-vestibular or recto-perineal fistulas are associated with difficulties in stool passage and abdominal distension. Prenatal evaluation may detect the absence of a circular rim of hypoechogenicity in the perineum (abnormal anus), dilated colon and polyhydramnios. After birth the perineal examination should detect the presence or absence of the anus, the aspect of the perineum (flat bottom perineum is typical of male patients with rectovescical fistula), the presence of vaginal and urethral openings, the presence and the exact position of the fistula, the size of the anal dimple and midline groove and the presence of a presacral mass. The passage of meconium should be assessed as well. The management in the newborn period is shown by the following decision making algorithms (PSARP = posterior sagittal anorectoplasty). It must be remembered that radiological investigations should be performed after 24 hours of life in order to have enough intra-abdominal pressure to conquer the muscular tone of the rectal fistula making the meconium appear in urine or at the perineum. Radiological investigations are used to assess the anatomy, to plan surgery, to identify associated anomalies and to do a prognosis. It includes a first phase (diagnosis and neonate evaluation) and a second phase (study before surgery).

- Abdominal, urinary and lumbo-sacral US
- EKG, cardiological evaluation and echocardiogram
- Abdominal x-ray (after 16-24 hours of life, in two planes and with a marker on the anal dimple): it evaluates the distance between the rectum and the perineum, signs of peritonitis, associated intestinal malformations, sacral alterations
- Distal colostogram = this consists of the injection of hydrosoluble contrast material through the distal stoma. The study must be done under fluoroscopy, in the lateral position, using a Foley catheter with the balloon inflated in the distal stoma. The lower the defect, the more hydrostatic pressure the surgeon must apply to fill up the distal part of the colon. It is highly desirable to determine the precise type of anatomic defect, as it has important prognostic and therapeutic implications.
- MRI = it is important for the evaluation of the spine

Treatment

The current standard surgical management for patients with ARM is the posterior sagittal anorectoplasty (PSARP). The technique provides for excellent exposure of the anatomy and the exact placement of the rectum within the muscle complex but fecal continence is not always obtained. Since 2000 the Laparo-Assisted Anorectoplastic (Georgeson procedure - LAARP) has represented a good alternative to the PSARP. The laparoscopic procedure avoids the division and weakening of the muscular sphincter structures and it permits the correct placement of the rectum into the perineal muscle complex thanks to the use of an internal electrostimulator. LAARP includes a first laparoscopic step that aims for the isolation of the distal rectum after the ligature of the fistula and a second perineal step during which the rectum is identified and pulled down to perform the anastomosis. We prefer to perform the laparoscopic pull-through at 2-3 months of life and a distal left protective colostomy at birth. Recently some authors have proposed the surgical correction in the neonatal period without a protective colostomy with good results. The patient is prepared for surgery with a distal loop washing the night before and the same morning and antibiotic prophylaxis is administrated. Prior to surgery a nasogastric tube and a transurethral catheter are placed.

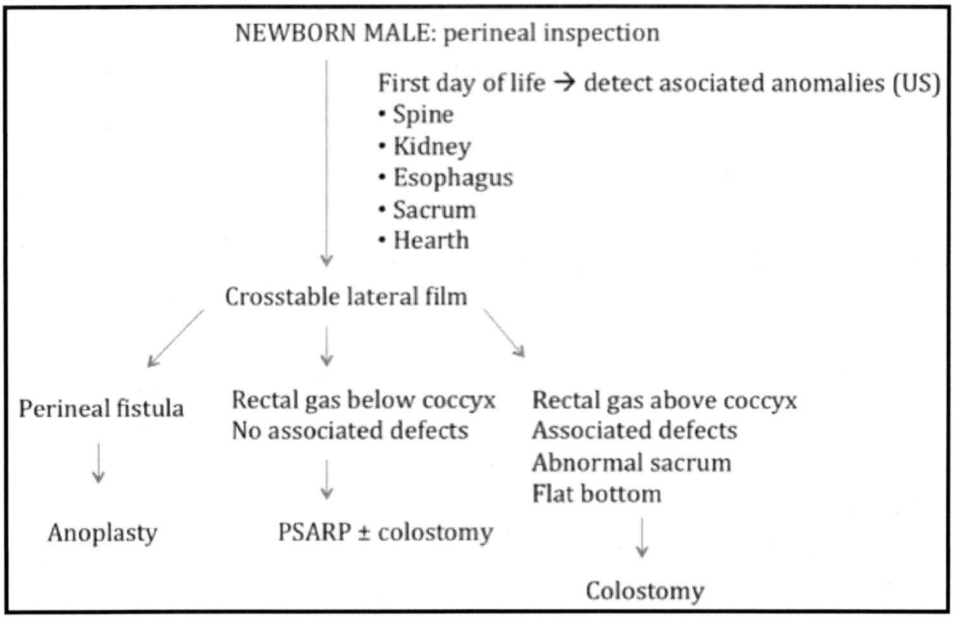

Figure 28. Management in male patients.

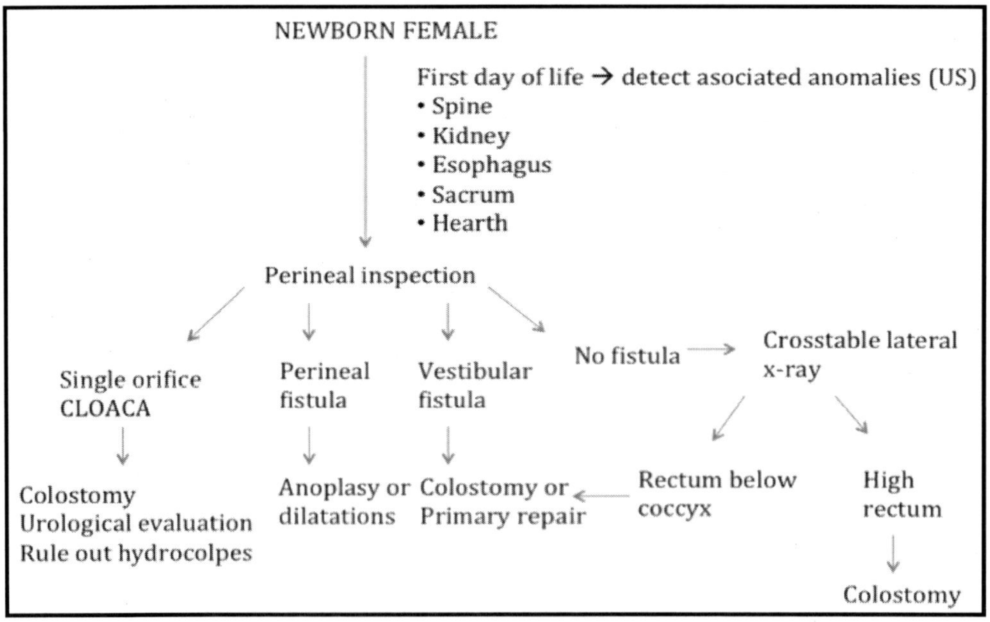

Figure 29. Management in female patients.

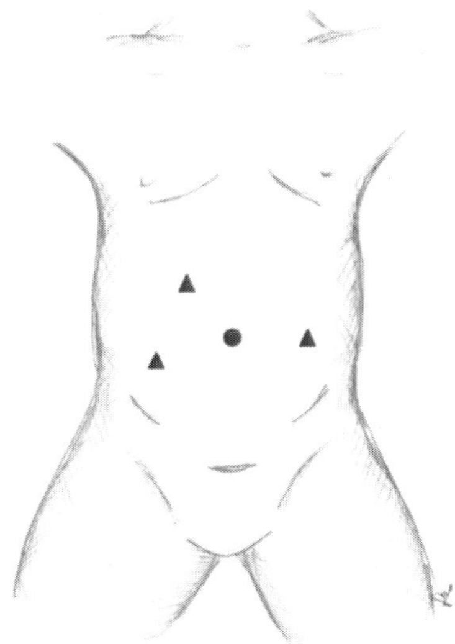

Figure 30. Trocars' position is the same as for HSCR (lens = circle; operative trocars = triangles).

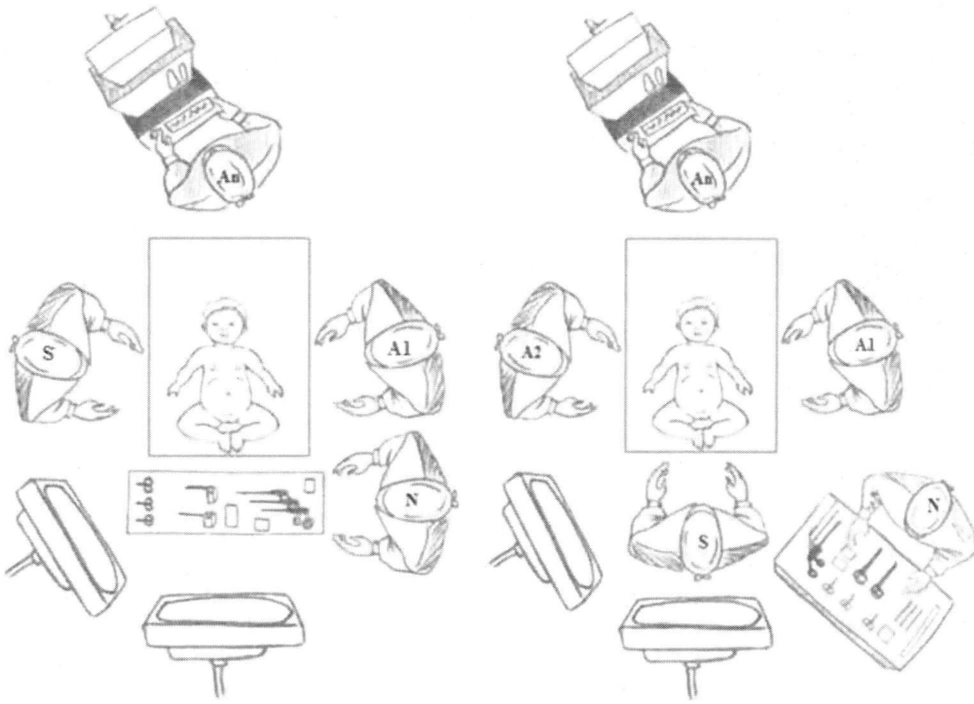

Figure 31. Operative set-up (laparoscopic step – left; perineal step – right). S = surgeon; A1 = assistant 1; A2 = assistant 2; N = scrub nurse; An = anesthesiologist.

The laparoscopic step is performed with a 5 mm trocar inserted in the umbilicus with open technique and used to create the pneumoperitoneum (8 mmHg of pressure, 0.5 L/min of flow) and two operative trocars are inserted under direct vision. Laparoscopic rectal dissection starts at the peritoneal reflection with hook cautery and it proceeds circumferentially. The recto-urinal or recto-genital fistula is identified, legated with transfixed non-absorbable stitches and dissected. The rectum is then retracted out of the pelvis in order to expose the muscles of the pelvic floor (they sometimes are poorly developed). The pubo-coccygeal muscle is identified with the use of the laparoscopic electrostimulator (intensity = 60 mA). The pull-through will be at the center of the muscle complex. The perineal step includes the precise mapping of the pelvic floor muscle with an external electrostimulator that helps to identify the area of maximum contraction. Single stitches are used to mark this area and to limit the site of the incision (1 cm, vertical midline incision). The intersphincteric plane is gently dissected until the fascial plate is reached. A trocar is then passed through this intersphincteric plane and advanced between the two bellies of the pubococcygeus muscle in the midline under laparoscopic surveillance. The blind end of the rectum is grasped with a blunt forceps through the transperineal opening and it is pulled down and exteriorized after sufficient dilatation of the anal orifice. The anastomosis between the rectum and the anus is completed with interrupted suture. At the end we perform a laparoscopic control that aims to verify the correct placement of the rectum (without rotations) with good vascularization and no bleeding.

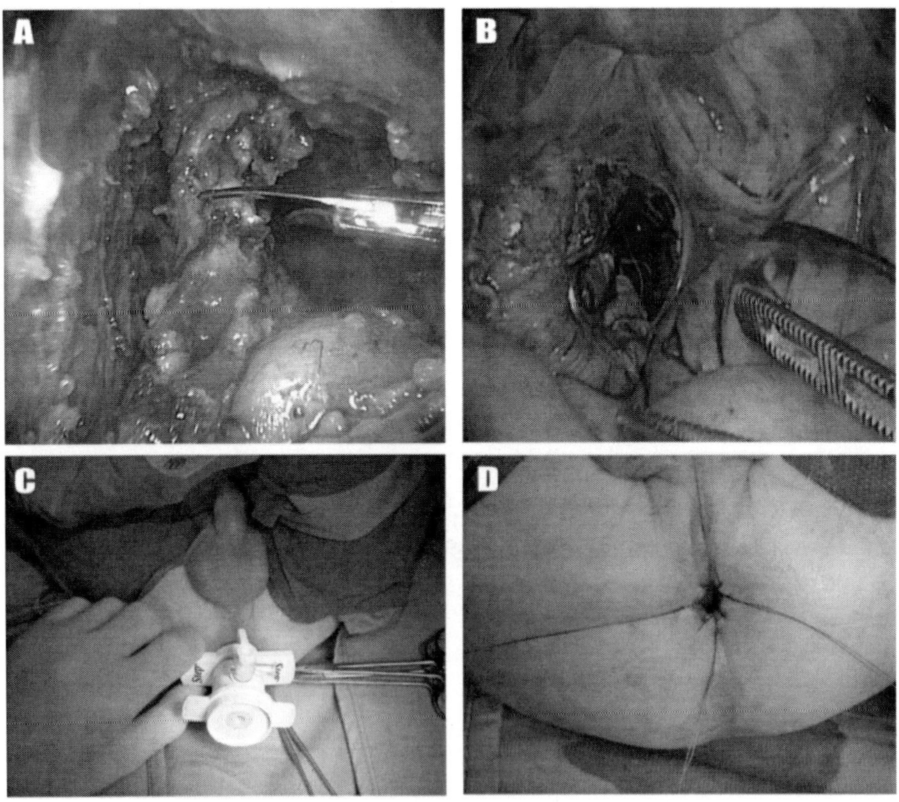

Figure 32. The fistula is isolated, ligated and sectioned (A). The intestine is pulled through (B) once the proper site has been identified with electrostimulators and the pathway has been created with a trocar inserted through the perineum (C). The anastomosis is completed during the perineal step (D).

Patients are fed on the first day after surgery and they are discharged on the 4th postoperative day. Anal dilatation is started after 15 days following a standard protocol and the colostomy is closed 2-3 months after the pull-through procedure is completed.

Complications

The most fearsome complication is the intra-operative hemorrhage that can require conversion to laparotomy. The technique allows for the centrality of the pull-through inside the muscle complex and it is associated with less scarring resulting in better rectal compliance but long-term follow-up for fecal continence should be better assessed.

References

Cho S, Moore SP, Fangman T. One hundred three consecutive patients with anorectal malformations and their associated anomalies. *Arch Pediatr Adolesc Med.* 2001 May;155(5):587-91.

Currarino G, Coln D, Votteler T. Triad of anorectal, sacral, and presacral anomalies. *AJR Am J Roentgenol.* 1981 Aug;137(2):395-8.

De Vries P, Peña A. Posterior sagittal anorectoplasty. *J Ped Surg*. 17:638-43,1982.

Georgeson KE, Inge TH, Albanese CT. Laparoscopically assisted anorectal pull-through for high imperforate anus--a new technique. *J Pediatr Surg.* 2000 Jun;35(6):927-30; discussion 930-1.

Lima M, Antonellini C, Ruggeri G, Libri M, Gargano T, Mondardini MC. Laparoscopic surgical treatment of anorectal malformations. *Pediatr Med Chir.* 2006;28(4-6):79-82.

Lima M, Tursini S. Pull through for high imperforate anus. In: Essential of Pediatric Endoscopic Surgery. A. K. Saxena, M. E. Hollwart (eds), 2009, *Springer*, Berlin.

Lima M, Tursini S, Ruggeri G, Aquino A, Gargano T, De Biagi L, Ahmed A, Gentili A. Laparoscopically assisted anorectal pull-through for high imperforate anus: three years' experience. *J Laparoendosc Adv Surg Tech A.* 2006 Feb;16(1):63-6.

Undescended Testes

Introduction

The term cryptorchidism is referred to the condition of abnormal testicular descent (TD). In this situation the testis is "hidden" and it cannot be identified in its normal position, which is inside the scrotum. Undescended testes carry the risk of malignant transformation and loss of fertility. It is thus mandatory to recognize this condition in order to plan the surgical correction. The lack of a unitary classification and the variability of nomenclature have always caused difficulties in comparing treatment results. A first distinction is between the non-palpable and the palpable testes that could be obtained after a physical examination. Palpable testis represents 92% of cases. The term refers to the testes that arrests along its normal descending path. It is further divided into palpable UDT, ectopic and retractile. Non-palpable testes represent 8% of cases: in 53% of cases the testes is absent (agenesy– blinding ending) or vanishing (atrophy), in 47% of cases although impalpable it is present (intra-abdominal or near the inguinal canal). Cryptorchidism is the most frequent abnormality of the uro-genital tract and it represents the most common congenital malformation. The testis originates early in foetal life. The testis formation is included in a process called sex determination during which the testis produces hormones that initiate and sustain normal male sexual differentiation with simultaneous regression of müllerian duct structures. The SRY gene on the Y chromosome seems to be responsible for male differentiation and it initiates testicular development. Testicular descent occurs in 10% at 24 weeks' gestation, in 50% at 27 weeks', in 75% at 28 weeks and in 80% at 34 weeks to birth. The descent can be illustrated in three different phases: transabdominal (that seems to be under AMH regulation); transinguinal (under androgen regulation) and extracanalicular (that include the descent from the external ring to the scrotum). The etiopathogenesis of undescended testis is still unknown and it involves many factors (endocrine, gubernalculum, epididymis, intra abdominal pressure, etc.).

Diagnosis

Cryptorchidism has specific features that make history and clinical examinations sufficient to diagnose the condition. Imaging and/or laboratory evaluation are rarely indicated and they are generally used for surgical planning. Parents should be questioned regarding previous history of normal descended testes during the first year of life or during different moments of the day (e.g. when the patient is relaxed in the bathtub, which may suggest excessive cremasteric reflex or retractile testes) and previous inguinal surgery (iatrogenic cryptorchidism). Cryptorchidism is usually an asymptomatic condition and only rarely does it give the feeling of mild pain or discomfort at the level of the inguinal region. The onset of symptoms may indicate the onset of complications. The aim of the clinical examination is the identification of a palpable gonad and of the lowest position that can be reached, and where the testicle can be placed without tension.

The follow laboratory tests should be performed in case of unilateral cryptorchidism associated with hypospadia and in case of bilateral cryptorchidism (suspected anorchia):

- LH
- FSH
- 17-OH progesterone
- Testosterone with or without hCG (human chorionic gonadotropin) stimulation
- Inhibin B
- Karyotype

Radiological evaluation is not superior to a physical examination in detecting the gonad and thus planning surgery. The rate of false negative and false positive of ultrasound, computed tomography and magnetic resonance is significant. Laparoscopy has now become the most common way to identify the position of an intra-abdominal testis and it permits a direct observation of the spermatic cord. Surgical exploration is mandatory and it is a key element in differentiating agenesy – atrophy and intra-abdominal testes.

Treatment

The goal of any intervention for cryptorchidism is to move the undescended testicle to a normal position in the scrotum, in the safest and least invasive way possible. Clinical decision-making about treatment is influenced by many factors such as the bilateralism, the palpability, the age at presentation and associated anomalies of medical conditions. If both testes are non-palpable the patient should be immediately referred to endocrinologic evaluation. In these cases laparoscopy is used to determine surgical therapy. Two or more stage procedures are performed in order to do one side at a time and to evaluate the results before proceeding to the other side. Testicular biopsy is usually not performed and it is reserved in case of ambiguous genitalia or chromosomal disorders. The optimal age for treatment should be established on the base of its influence on future spermatogenesis, hormonal production and risk for tumors. Actually there are no certain data but many studies report that early intervention is the most beneficial (< 1 years of age). Orchiopexy in patients born with UDT should not be performed before 6 months in order to allow the testes to descend.

Laparoscopy - Unilateral Non Palpable UDT

Laparoscopy is useful to determine which surgical approach should be taken.

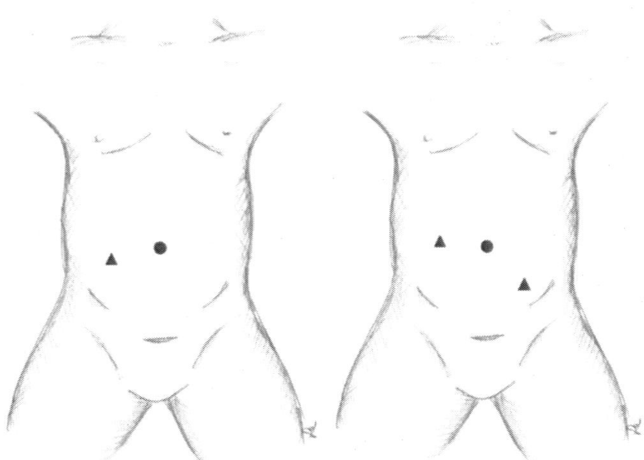

Figure 33. The lens in the umbilicus (circle) permits the abdominal exploration. The operative trocar (triangle) is inserted in the flank opposite to the pathological side (left). Three trocars (right) may be useful to exclude rare anatomical anomalies.

A 5 mm port is inserted through the umbilicus (subumbilical semicircular incision) for the 0° optic and the pneumoperitoneum is created with 0.5-1 L/min of flow and 8-10 mmHg of pressure. The abdominal cavity is explored starting from the internal inguinal ring. It is important to have the comparative image of the opposite side. The exploration proceeds to the pelvis and the iliac regions to the origin of the internal spermatic vessels. This is important especially in case of testicular agenesis where second or third trocars can be inserted to search for rare anatomical anomalies such as spleno-gonadic fusion.

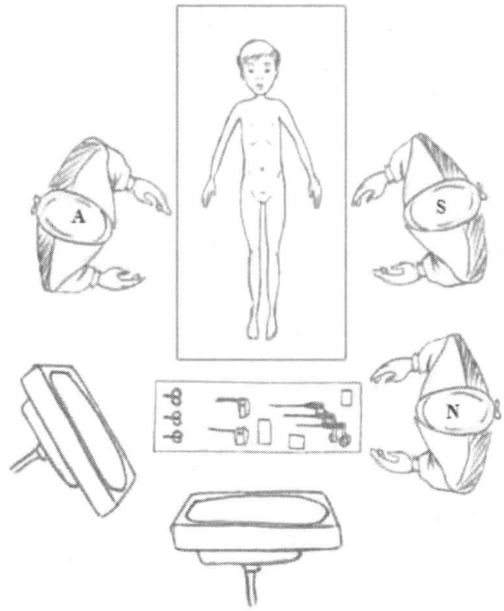

Figure 34. The patient lies supine with distended legs and arms. The trendelenburg position aids in better visualization of the lower abdomen and pelvis and a Foley catheter draining the bladder maximizes the operating space. S = surgeon (on the affected side); A = assistant; N = scrub nurse.

Laparoscopic findings can be different:

1) **Low abdominal testis** (< 2 cm from the inguinal ring) (Fig. 9 a-c): the testis is normal and it is near the internal inguinal ring (*iuxta-canalicular*); the ring is usually patent and the testis can intermittently enter the ring (*"peeping testis"*). In these cases the inguinal pressure pulls the testes in the abdomen while the scrotal traction takes it down the canal. Inguinal orchiopexy is performed at the same time.
2) **High abdominal testis** (> 2 cm from the internal inguinal ring) (Fig. 9 d-e): the testis usually lies on the posterior abdominal wall (retroperitoneal-iliac); rarely is it behind the bladder (pelvic). The internal inguinal ring is usually closed.
3) **Abdominal atrophy** of the testes (Fig. 10): hypoplastic vas and vessels are seen to end in a small-unformed testis (abdominal *"vanishing testis"*). If the testis is hypotrophic or atrophic an orchiectomy should be performed.
4) **Abdominal agenesis** of the testes (Fig. 11): the internal spermatic vessels are absent or hypotrophic and they end blindly in the abdomen (abdominal *"blind ending"*). The terminal part of the deferential artery is serpiginous and the vas is narrow. Pathological evaluation of the tip of the vessels may show remnants of testicular tissue or hemosiderin that are indicative of testicular resorption.
5) **Intracanalicular atrophy/agenesis** of the testes: there are hypoplastic vas and vessels going into the internal inguinal ring (intracanalicular "vanishing testis"). In these cases the need of an inguinal exploration may be useful to remove the atrophic testes and to reduce the risk of cancer even if the need of this operation is still debated. The complete absence of the vessels is typical of the intracanalicular testis

agenesis (intracanalicular "blind ending testis") that does not require an open inguinal exploration.

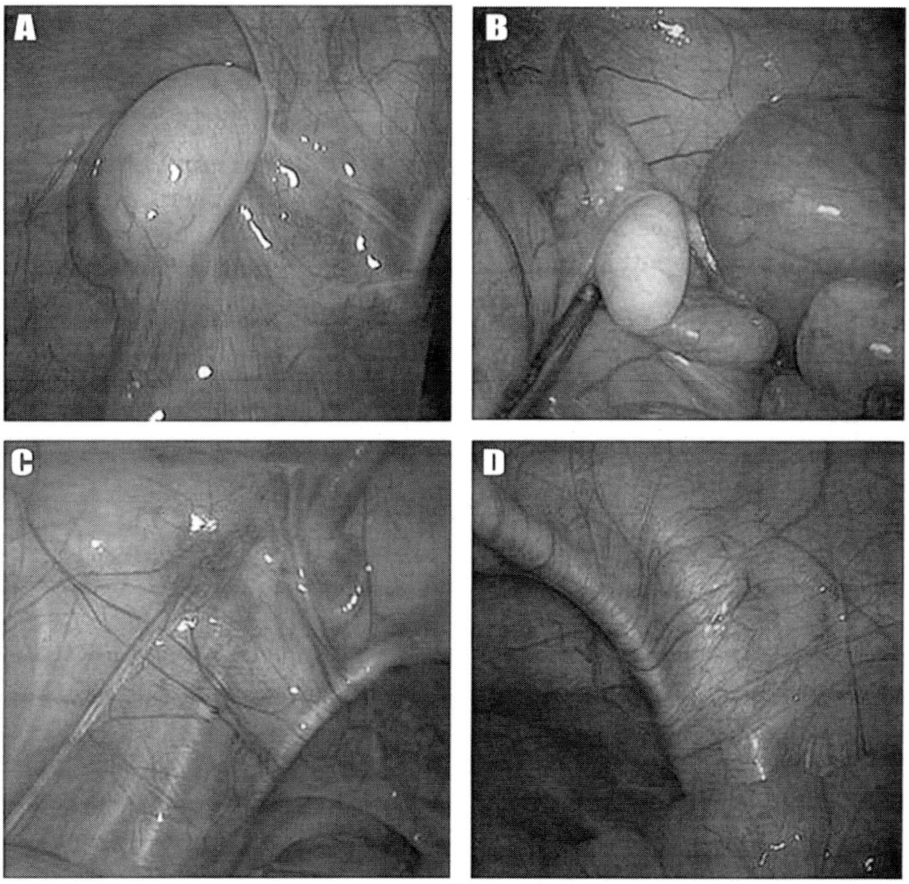

Figure 35. Intra-abdominal testes (A, B). Vanishing testes (C). Testicular agenesy (D).

The inguinal exploration after laparoscopy is recommended in case of obese children, opened internal inguinal ring (insufflations may have pushed the testis downward) and, as previously said, when the presence of an atrophic-hypotrophic testis is suspected.

The inguinal approach is unsuccessful in case of high abdominal testes. A two-stage orchiopexy is preferred when the vessels are too short. This procedure consists of mobilization and fixation of the testes as low as possible (e.g. at the pubic tubercle or inguinal ligament) followed by the second stage after 6-12 months. The advantage is that the testicular artery is preserved; the disadvantage is that some elements (the vas deferens, the epididymis and the testicular blood supply) may be injured during the second stage.

Fowler Stephens Orchiopexy – Unilateral Non Palpable UDT

The Fowler-Stephens orchiopexy is used in the case of high non-palpable testis (testes located more than 3 cm from the ipsilateral internal inguinal ring) and it consists of ligation of the spermatic vessels leaving the testicular vascularization to vassal, cremasteric and gubernacular arteries. The technique requires integrity of these collateral vessels and, for this reason it is not a good option after inguinal exploration, which may lead to vascular impairment. The technique is usually performed in two steps: vessels are first legated laparoscopically or by laparotomy. The second stage involves the section of the vessels and the completion of the orchiopexy. A waiting period of at least six months is required between the two steps in order to allow the collateral circulation to develop.

Koff Sethi - Unilateral Non Palpable UDT

The Koff and Sethi procedure is an alternative to the Fowler Stephens' (also called one-step Fowler-Stephens). The ligation of the spermatic vessels takes place in a lower position (at least 3-4 cm away from the testes) decreasing tension and enhancing viability. This maneuver is allowed thanks to the singular testicular vascular anatomy. Orchiopexy is thus performed in a single step procedure. Sometimes testes may be mobilized through a retroperitoneal dissection starting from a high suprainguinal incision. The main disadvantage is the risk of testicular atrophy due to possible vasospasm of small deferential vessels. The surgeon may also decide to leave the testes at the lower position reached and to conclude the procedure after a year, during a second operation.

Laparoscopic-Assisted Orchiopexy

This technique has been developed to preserve the spermatic vessels. The patient and trocar positions are the same as for a standard laparoscopy. The testicular vessels and the vas are mobilized from the posterior peritoneum in order to free the testes leaving the tissue between the spermatic vessels and vas intact. The testis is brought down to the scrotum through the internal inguinal ring or a neo-ring created between the umbilical artery and the inferior epigastric vessels. The creation of a neo-ring may also be useful in case of a short cord (Prentiss maneuver: a 12 mm expandable port or a blunt clamp is introduced through the base of the scrotum and it is used to create a neo ring medial to the epigastric vessels) because it shortens the path to the scrotum.

Microvascular Orchiopexy (Silber-Kelly) - Unilateral Non Palpable UDT

This technique was developed in order to preserve a better vascular testicular supply. It requires long operative times, special skills and dedicated instrumentation. This procedure should be performed around 3 years of age. Testicular vessels are divided and a microvascular asnastomosis between the testicular artery and vein and the inferior epigastric vessels is performed. It has a success rate of 80%.

An alternative procedure is the "ATTR" (literally "testicular wastewater autotransplantation") proposed by Lima and colleagues. It provides for the section of the vascular spermatic pedicle and the microsurgical venous anastomosis between the spermatic vein and the inferior epigastric vein. The gonad is then freed and brought down to the scrotum. The effectiveness of this technique is related to the fact that the deferential circle is able to offer a good supply of arterial blood but inadequate venous drainage when the spermatic circle is excluded. The venous anastomosis allows the surgeon to overcome this problem and it is safer than the Fowler-Stephens and simpler than the Silber-Kelly.

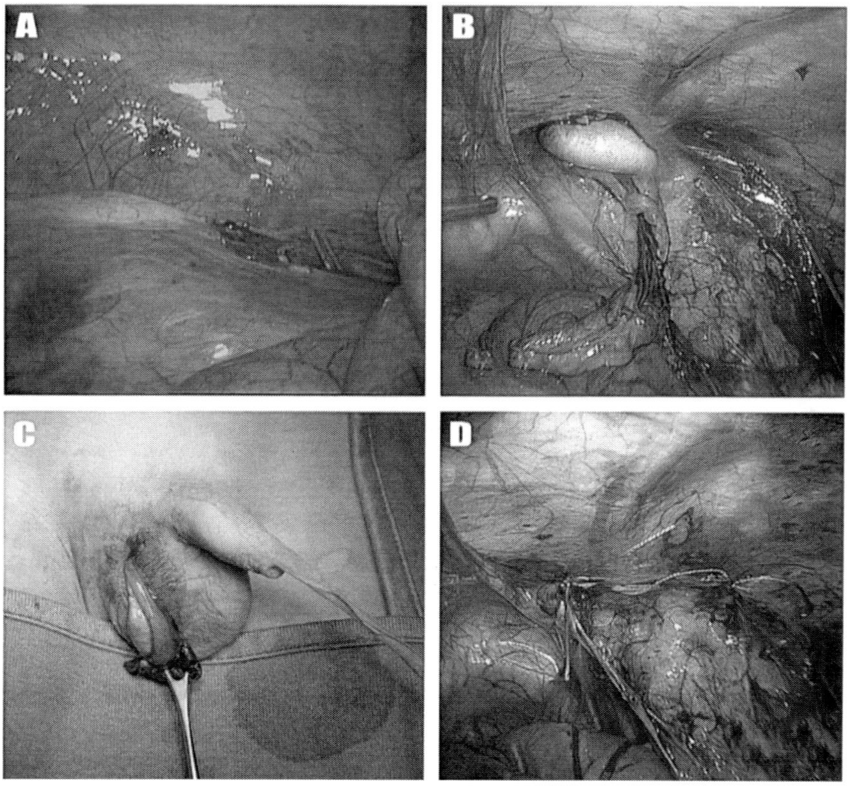

Figure 36. The undescended testes are identified during laparoscopy. The Fowler-Stephens orchiopexy is performed: vessels are clipped and the testis is brought down to the scrotum eight months after.

Complications

Wound infection and hemathoma are rare but described as immediate complications after orchiopexy. Recurrent cryptorchidism is possible and it is often related to inadequate inguinal hernia repair, to insufficient retroperitoneal dissection or patent processus vaginalis. Testicular atrophies or hypotrophies are the most important complications. They are related to ischemic injuries. Clinical follow-up should be done 12 months after surgery with ultrasound evaluation to define testicular volume. Re-evaluation at early puberty is necessary in bilateral cases. Patients with retractile testis require evaluation at 3, 5, 7 and 10 years old to detect later ascent. A close follow-up is also required in patients with spontaneous descent. Success of surgery is assessed by testicular position, presence of testicular atrophy and, later in life, by fertility and risk of cancer.

References

Esposito C. Laparoscopic Treatment of Non-Palpable Testis. In Endoscopic Surgery in Infants and Children. Bax K., Georgeson Ke, Rothemberg S, Valla JS., Yeung CK. 2008 *Sringer:* Cap101, 753-758.

Holcomb GW. Laparoscopy for the Non-Palpable Testis. In Pediatric Laparoscopy. Lobe TE. 2003. *Landes Bioscience:* Cap8, 83-89.

Ritzen EM. Undescended testes: a consensus on management. *Eur J Endocrinol.* 2008, (159): S87-S90.

Schleef J., Von Bismarck S. Groin exploration for non-palpable testes: laparoscopic approach. *J. Pediatr Surg.* 2002. 37: 1552-1555

Spinelli C, Lima M, Signoretti P, Bertelloni S, Franchi G. Il Criptorchidismo. Fisiopatologia, Clinica, *Terapia Medica e Chirurgica. Piccin,* 2001.

Inguinal Hernia

Introduction

Inguinal hernia is the protrusion of an abdominal organ into a patent processus vaginalis extending into the inguinal canal. It's a common condition of infancy and childhood. The processus vaginalis is an embryonic developmental outpouching of the peritoneum. In males, it precedes the testis in their descent. The processus vaginalis involutes by spontaneous obliteration, leaving a small remmant attached to the testis (the tunica vaginalis). Persistent patency of all or part of the processus vaginalis is the common element in the pathogenesis of both congenital inguinal hernia (if bowel or other organs enter the processus) and congenital hydrocele (peritoneal fluid passage only). In females the canal of Nuck corresponds to an open processus vaginalis; it's an out-pouching of peritoneum anterior to the round ligament.

Inguinal anomalies include:

- **Scrotal hernia**: processus vaginalis is completely opened and it permits the passage of abdominal content to the scrotum;
- **Inguinal hernia**: the distal part of the duct is obliterated but the proximal one remains patent;
- **Communicating hydrocele**: the duct has a narrow proximal opening at the internal ring with a distal sac;
- **Non communicating hydrocele**: complete obliteration of the proximal portion with distal patency of the processus vaginalis or isolated hydrocele of the tunica vaginalis;
- **Spermatic cord cyst**: hydrocele of the spermatic cord with small connection to the peritoneal cavity at the internal ring.

Congenital inguinal hernias are indirect hernias that result from the altered closure of the deep inguinal ring after testicle descent. The sac enters the inguinal canal through the internal ring (lateral to the epigastric vessels) and passes distally through the canal. Contrariwise in a direct hernia the defect is acquired and the sac enters the canal medial to the epigastric vessels through a weak point in the fascia of the abdominal wall.

Diagnosis

The most common presentation of inguinal hernias is a bulge in the groin or the scrotal sac that gets worse by activities that increase intra-abdominal pressure such as crying or straining. Palpation of the cord may elicit the "silk glove" sign (that is obtained by the rubbing of the opposing peritoneal membranes of the empty sac).

Infants should be examined both in supine and erect position. During clinical examination the mass usually reduces spontaneously.

In girls the most common structure to be palpated in the upper portion of the labia major is the ovary; in boys the examination should include an inspection of the testicles and scrotum to ascertain that the testis is within the scrotal sac (retractile testes may be diagnosed a hernias). The most common complication of inguinal hernia is bowel incarceration that causes pain, abdominal distension and emesis with the risk of vascular compromise to the incarcerated bowel within the sac. Once the diagnosis of inguinal hernia is made, elective treatment should be done as soon as possible because of the high risk of incarceration, especially in newborns.

Treatment

The treatment of inguinal hernia is surgery. The hernia sac is carefully separated from the vas deferens and the spermatic vessels. A high ligation is performed and after that the sac is opened and inspected. Recently laparoscopic inguinal hernia repair in children has become an alternative to the conventional open procedure with excellent results. Since the 1990s laparoscopy has been used for diagnosis and/or treatment of inguinal hernias in children. Advantages of laparoscopy are well known. In laparoscopic hernia repair, the structures of the spermatic cord are less manipulated and the risk of damage is reduced. The incarcerated organs are pulled with bowel forceps while performing external pressure on the inguinal region in order to put them back into the abdomen. It is possible to direct evaluate the effects on herniated organs. Laparoscopy also allows the identification of rare forms of hernias such as direct or femoral hernias and genital anomalies (Morris syndrome), which are easily identified.

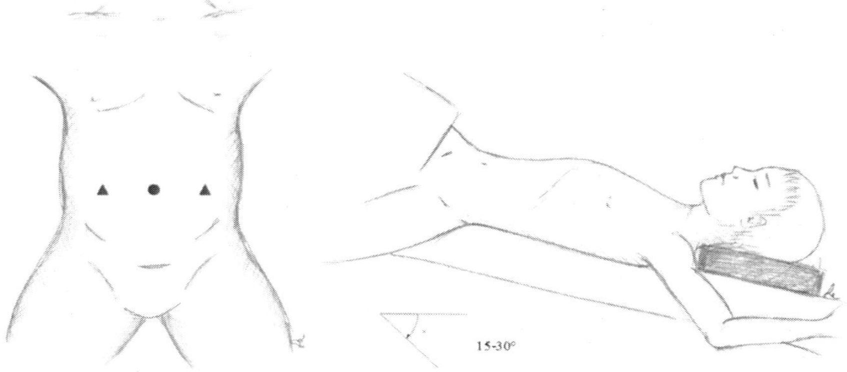

Figure 37. Trocars' position: lens (circle) and operative trocars (triangles). The patient is in the trendelenburg position.

A 5-mm trocar is placed through a sub-umbilical semi-circular incision and pneumoperitoneum is established with 0,5-1 L/min of flow and 8-10 mmHg of pressure. A laparoscopic inspection of the abdominal cavity is then performed. Two 2-3 mm operative trocars are inserted under direct vision in the right and left flank near the rectum muscle margin and on the transversal umbilical line. The distance between operative trocars is important to guarantee an adequate working chamber.

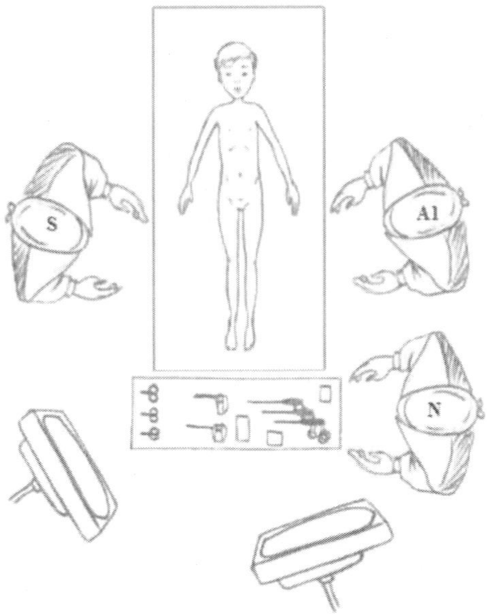

Figure 38. Operative set-up is the same as for cryptorchidism. S = surgeon (on the affected side); A = assistant; N = scrub nurse.

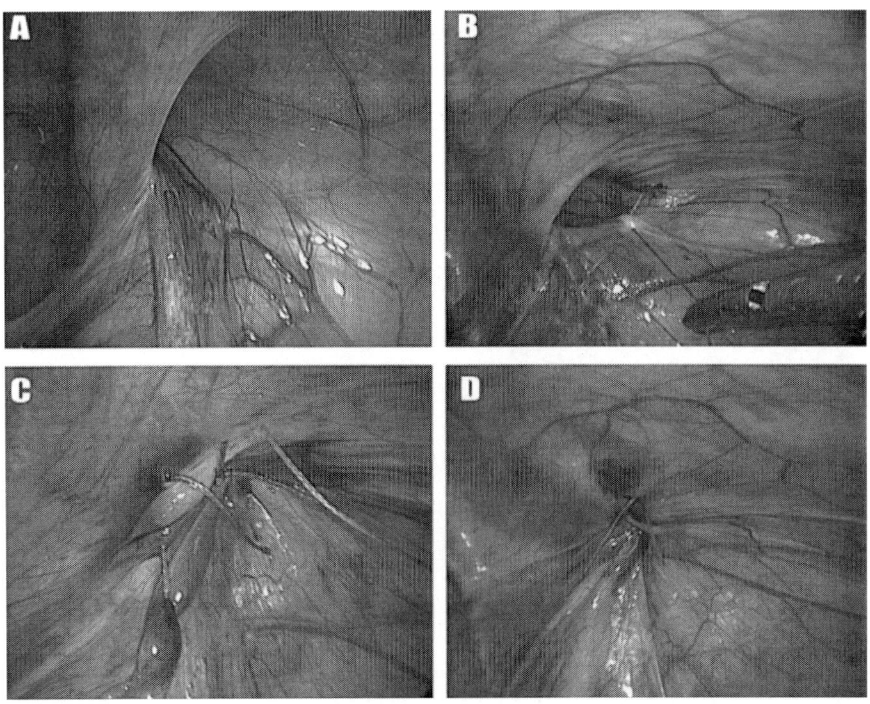

Figure 39. Patent peritoneal – vaginal duct (A). First passage of the "N" suture (B). Completed "N" suture (C). Closure of the duct (D).

If present, herniated organs should be reduced using the needle-holder. Laparoscopic reduction, supported by manual pressure from outside, is technically easier than pure manual reduction because the internal ring has been enlarged after insufflation. After reduction of herniated organs, the needle enters the abdominal cavity through the abdominal wall near the internal inguinal ring. The suture is performed with a continued "N-shaped" suture of the peritoneum starting laterally. Non-absorbable 4/0 or 3/0 braided sutures at least 12 cm long are employed.

Intracorporeal knotting is then performed. During the closure of the knot, external pressure on the inguinal region is created, especially in the case of high tension over the margins. The contralateral inguinal area is inspected and repaired during the same procedure. The needle is extracted through a port site after removing the instrument and the trocar.

The trocar wounds do not require suture closure but only SteriStrip™ and the umbilical port is closed with absorbable sutures.

In case of a spermatic cord cyst, it is possible to pull in the cyst through the internal ring and open it with scissors. The duct is then closed as described.

Laparoscopic inguinal hernia repair can be a routine procedure with results comparable to those of open procedures. It is gaining in popularity because of the potential advantages of faster recovery, attenuated pain and improved cosmesis. The most feared complication is recurrence, an incidence that should be better assessed with long-term studies. Other described complications are: spermatic vessels alterations with testicular atrophy or ipotrophy, ovaries injuries, vas cut.

References

Montupet P, Esposito C. Laparoscopic treatment of congenital inguinal hernia in children. *J Pediatr Surg.* 1999 Mar;34(3):420-3.

Schier F, Montupet P, Esposito C. Laparoscopic inguinal herniorrhaphy in children: a three-center experience with 933 repairs. *J Pediatr Surg.* 2002 Mar;37(3):395-7.

Treef W, Schier F. Characteristics of laparoscopic inguinal hernia recurrences. *Pediatr Surg Int.* 2009 Feb;25(2):149-52.

Yang C, Zhang H, Pu J, Mei H, Zheng L, Tong Q. Laparoscopic vs open herniorrhaphy in the management of pediatric inguinal hernia: a systemic review and meta-analysis. *J Pediatr Surg.* 2011 Sep;46(9):1824-34.

Zani A, Eaton S, Hoellwarth M et al. Management of pediatric inguinal hernias in the era of laparoscopy: results of an international survey. *Eur J Pediatr Surg.* 2014 Feb;24(1):9-13.

Varicocele

Introduction

The term varicocele refers to the dilatation of testicular veins in the pampiniform venous plexus. The venous reflux causes sperm modifications, hormonal changes and testicular cell alterations. All these elements lead to male infertility ("seminal stress syndrome"). The varicocele can be primitive or secondary. Primitive varicocele seems to be related to the specific anatomical pathway of the left spermatic internal vein, which explains the higher frequency on the left side, lack of venous valves, disruption of the venous pump, compression of the left renal vein between the superior mesenteric artery and the aorta, and vascular spasm due to adrenalin release. Secondary varicocele is due to an extrinsic obstruction of the internal spermatic vein. In 1980 Coolsaet proposed an etiopathogenetic classification system for primitive varicocele.

Table 7. Coolsaet classification

VARICOCELE – COOLSAET ETIOPATHOGENETIC CLASSIFICATION	
Type I	Reno-spermatic reflux (the left renal vein is squeezed between the aorta and the superior mesenteric artery). Anterior varicocele
Type II	Iliaco-testicular reflux (the left iliac vein is squeezed by the right common iliac artery). Posterior varicocele
Type III	Association of type I and II varicocele

Diagnosis

Varicocele presents as a soft, distensible mass in the scrotum. Physical examination should be performed in the supine position (redundant hemiscrotum) and on stand ("bag of worms" appearance). The condition is usually asymptomatic. Sometimes the boy feels discomfort and a dragging sensation. Clinical classifications are the Dubin-Amelar, Steeno and Horner (see Table 8).

Table 8. Clinical classification of varicocele

VARICOCELE – CLINICAL CLASSIFICATION
DUBIN-AMELAR • Grade I = palpable varicocele after Valsalva maneuver • Grade II = palpable varicocele • Grade III = visible varicocele
HORNER • Grade I = palpable and invisible varicosities • Grade II = palpable and visible varicosities • Grade III = palpable varicosities that alter scrotal symmetry
STEENO • Grade I = small, difficult to palpate • Grade II = moderate, easy to palpate • Grade III = severe, palpable and visible

Ultrasound evaluation with Doppler allows evaluation of both the testes and the spermatic cord veins. A reflux longer than 2 seconds under the Valsalva maneuver is considered pathological. On the base of radiological findings, the varicocele is classified as follows.

Abdominal US is required in case of uncommon ages of presentation or when a secondary varicocele is suspected.

Table 9. Radiological classification of varicocele

VARICOCELE – RADIOLOGICAL CLASSIFICATION
SARTESCHI • Grade I = prolonged reflux only during Valsalva; scrotal varicosity is not evident in the standard US study • Grade II = posterior varicosities that extend to the superior pole of the testis. Their diameters increase and venous reflux is seen in the supratesticular region only during the Valsalva maneuver. • Grade III = Vessels appear enlarged at the inferior pole of the testis when the patient is evaluated in a standing position; no enlargement is detected if the patient is examined in a supine position. Reflux observed only under during the Valsalva maneuver. • Grade IV = Vessels appear enlarged even when the patient is studied in a supine position; the dilatation is more marked in the upright position and during the Valsalva maneuver. Testicular hypotrophy is common at this stage. • Grade V = Venous ectasia is evident even in the prone decubitus and supine positions. Reflux is observed at rest and does not increase during the Valsalva maneuver.

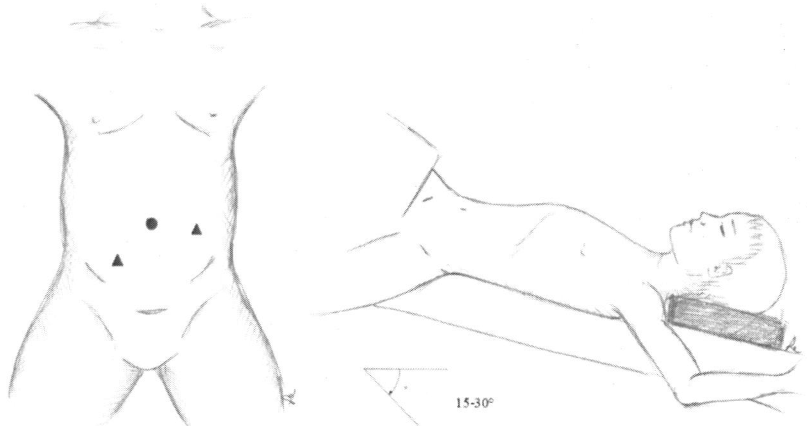

Figure 40. Lens (5mm, 0 degree) is inserted in the umbilicus (subumbilical semicircular incision; circle in the figure). Trocars (5 mm; triangles in the figure) are placed in the right iliac fossa and in the left flank under direct vision. The patient is in the trendelenburg position.

Treatment

Surgery is required in case of symptomatic varicocele, testicular hypotrophy or high grade (II-III clinical grade). Abdominal US is required in case of uncommon ages of presentation or when it is secondary. Many techniques have been proposed to correct the varicocele. The most common are the Ivanissevich (internal spermatic vessels isolation and ligation with artery sparing) and the Palomo (venous ligation without artery sparing) that are also performed by laparoscopy or retroperitoneoscopy. We perform the "en bloc" laparoscopic internal spermatic vessels ligation that has a low recurrence rate because it includes small spermatic veins that run near the artery, often left during the artery sparing. Compared to retroperitoneoscopy, the laparoscopic approach has a wider operative chamber.

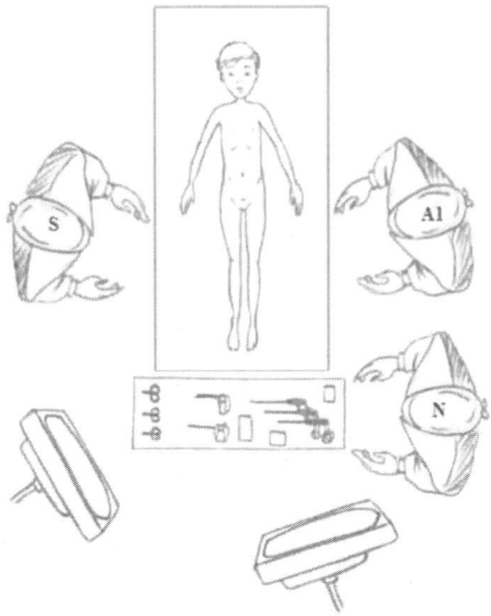

Figure 41. Operative set-up is the same as for cryptorchidism and hernia. S = surgeon; A = assistant; N = scrub nurse. The surgeon is on the affected side.

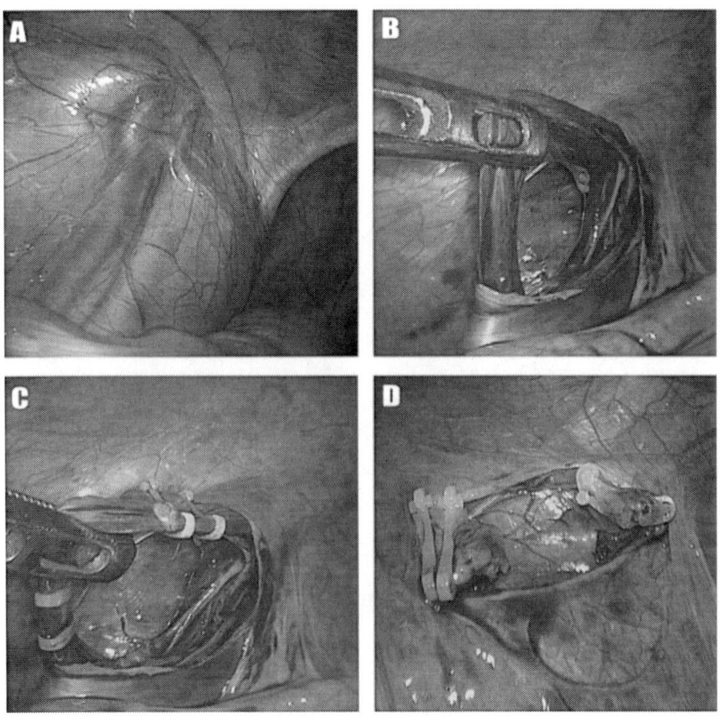

Figure 42. Laparoscopic view of dilated spermatic vessels (A). Spermatic vessels isolation after the creation of a window in parietal peritoneum (B). Clips placement (C). Vessel section between the clips (D).

Once trocars have been placed, the abdominal cavity is inspected and the parietal peritoneum above the spermatic vessels is carved at a few centimetres far from the inguinal ring. Vessels that are beneath the peritoneum are isolated from the retroperitoneal fat with scissors and “L-shaped” dissecting forceps. The aim is to avoid lymphatic vessels that run in the fat and to create a window for clips placement. A total of four clips are applied (2 proximally and 2 distally) after the vessels are grasped in the central part. At this time vessels are sectioned between the clips. Small collateral vessels can be closed by cauterization. At the end of the procedure the tip of the sectioned vessels is placed under the peritoneum. Laparoscopy also allows the treatment of deferential varicoceles (isolation and ligation of the deferential vein after vas isolation). The urinary catheter is removed at the end of the procedure. Liquid intake is allowed after 2 hours and feeding after 3 hours. Limitation of physical activities is suggested for 2-3 weeks after surgery.

Complications

There are early and late complications:

- Early = scrotal edema and temporary hydrocele due to lymphatic stasis, inguinal hematoma and paresthesias of the internal tight and scrotum
- Late = recurrence, persistent hydrocele and testicular atrophy. Recurrences may be related to internal spermatic vein duplicity or the presence of Coolsaet grade II-III. Hydrocele is often seen after Palomo technique.

References

Diamond DA, Gargollo PC, Caldamone AA. Current management principles for adolescent varicocele. *Fertil Steril.* 2011 Dec;96(6):1294-8.

Dòmini R., Belbusti R., Lima M., Signoretti P., Jasonni V., Argomenti di Andrologia Chirurgica Pediatrica, Piccin Editore, *Padova* 1998; cap 2; 75-115.

Esposito C, Monguzzi GL, Gonzalez-Sabin MA, Rubino R, Montinaro L, Papparella A, Amici G. Laparoscopic treatment of pediatric varicocele: a multicenter study of the Italian society of video surgery in infancy. *J Urol.* 2000 Jun;163(6):1944-6.

Varlet F, Becmeur F; Groupe d'Etudes en Coeliochirurgie Infantile. Laparoscopic treatment of varicoceles in children. Multicentric prospective study of 90 cases. *Eur J Pediatr Surg.* 2001 Dec;11(6):399-403.

Choledochal Cyst

Introduction

A choledochal cyst is a rare congenital malformation characterized by dilatation of the common bile duct with a potential risk of malignant transformation. The incidence is about 1 in 10,000 live births in America and Europe, the rate is remarkably higher in Asian populations compared with their western counterparts, particularly in Japan.

The classification of the choledochal cyst was introduced for the first time in 1959 by Alonso-Lej et al. who described three types of bile duct dilatation. Later, this system was modified and extended to 5 types by Todini et al. in 1977.

Table 10. Classification

Choledochal cyst classification	
Type I	cyst of the common bile duct
Type II	cystic diverticulum coming off of the common bile duct
Type III	cyst in the intraduodenal portion of the common bile duct
Type IV	multiple cysts in the intra- and extrahepatic biliary tract
Type V	single or multiple cysts in the intrahepatic ducts alone

The etiology of this malformation is still not clear, several theories over the years have been proposed. The most popular theory is the one postulated by Babbitt in 1969. According to the author at the bottom of this malformation there is an abnormal junction between the pancreatic duct and the common bile duct. These two anatomical structures meet outside of the papilla of Vater and form a long common channel. The formation of a long common biliary pancreatic channel makes the sphincter of Oddi ineffective, causing pancreatic reflux into the biliary tract. The mixing of pancreatic juice and bile results in the activation of pancreatic enzymes. These active enzymes cause inflammation and deterioration of the bile duct wall, determining dilation, inflammation and the risk of malignant transformation.

The V-type, or Caroli disease, is considered a separate entity. This is a multiple saccular or cystic dilatation of the intrahepatic bile ducts. Simple Caroli disease is isolated biliary dilation, whereas Caroli syndrome is cystic disease associated with congenital hepatic fibrosis.

Diagnosis

The clinical picture of a choledochal cyst depends primarily on the age at onset. Symptoms occur in 85% of cases in childhood, the remaining in adulthood. In the case of prenatal diagnosis, the patient may be asymptomatic and it is necessary to intervene before the onset of complications. The classic triad of symptoms includes palpable abdominal mass, abdominal pain and intermittent cholestatic jaundice with hypo-acolia fecal and dark urine. Only less than 20% of children present all three symptoms. The disease has a chronic course, but an acute onset with cholangitis, pancreatitis or peritonitis. In some cases the diagnosis may be prenatal or resulting from an abdominal ultrasound performed for other reasons.

All patients with clinical suspicion of choledochal cysts should undergo blood tests and abdominal ultrasound. Blood tests will highlight a typical picture of cholestasis with elevated levels of total and conjugated bilirubin, increased gamma-glutamyl transpeptidase and moderately elevated transaminases. The first step is to confirm the diagnosis with an abdominal ultrasound. After US evaluation MRCP is considered the gold standard for the diagnosis of coledochal cysts, with a high sensitivity (90-100%). Endoscopic retrograde cholangiopancreatography (ERCP) is a sensitive diagnostic modality for coledochal cysts, but it is an invasive procedure that may cause cholangitis and pancreatitis. In addition it exposes the patients to the risks of radiation.

Treatment

Since its first report by Farello et al. in 1995, the laparoscopic choledochal cyst excision with Roux-en-Y hepaticojejunostomy (LCE) in children has gained worldwide attention.

A 10 mm umbilical trocar for 5-10 mm and 0° optic is inserted with open technique. The carbon dioxide pneumoperitoneum is created at the pressure of 8 to 10 mm Hg and 0.5-1L/min of flow depending on the patient's age. Three additional 3-5 mm trocars are then placed under direct vision at the right hypochondrium, epigastrium, and left hypochonduim.

The gallbladder is raised and the liver retractor is placed in order to expose the choledochal cyst. Under laparoscopic guidance, the gallbladder is punctured for performance of intraoperative cholangiography.

Then the dissection of the dilated common bile duct (choledochal cyst) is started at its lower anterior part with the use of monopolar electrocautery and continued distally to the posterior wall of the cyst toward the hepatic hilum. The choledochal duct is legated distally and sectioned, as well as the cystic duct.

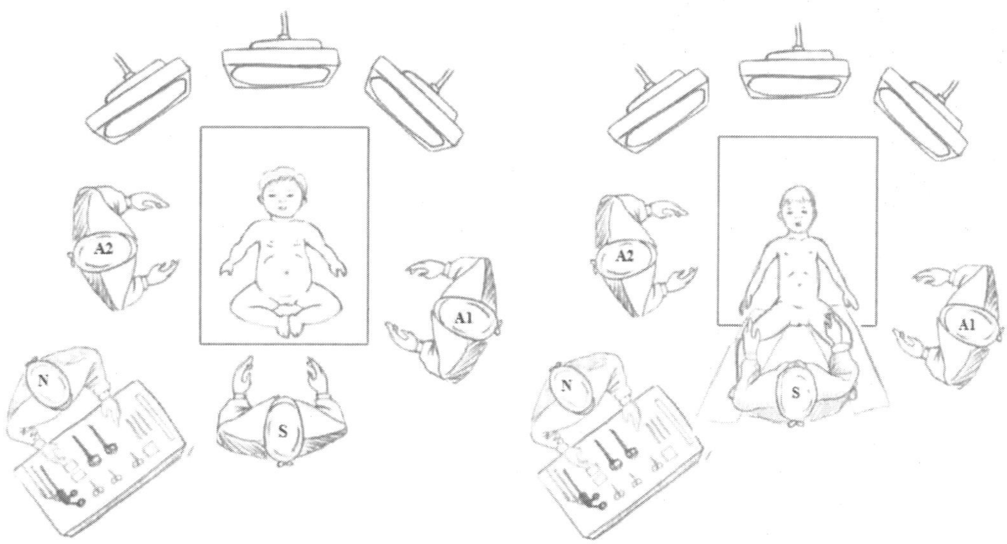

Figure 43. The patient is supine at the end of the operating table (left = infants; right = children). S = surgeon; A1 = assistant 1; A2 = assistant 2; N = scrub nurse.

Subsequently the cholecystectomy is performed. The cyst can be exteriorized with the gallbladder in an endo-bag. The ligament of Treitz was identified under laparoscopy and the proximal jejunum 15 cm distal to the ligament was captured and exteriorized through umbilical trocar site. Previously, the loop can be marked so as to distinguish the proximal from the distal margin.

Outside the abdomen the Roux loop is created. The jejuna loop is brought to the porta hepatis via the retrocolic route. The hepatic duct is sectioned and anastomosed laterally to the jejunal loop intracorporeally using interrupted suture (5.0 monofilament) starting from the posterior wall. The mesenteric defects were closed with interrupted sutures. Through access trocar you place two drains, one under the liver and the other near the anastomosis.

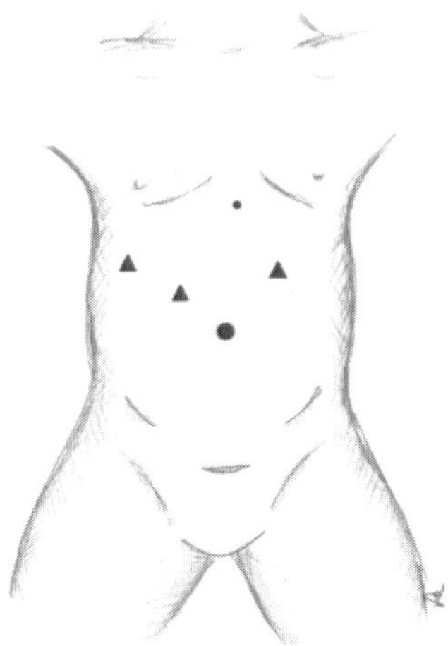

Figure 44. The lens is inserted by open technique at the umbilicus (circle). 3-5 mm operating trocars (triangles) are placed under direct vision in the right and left hypocondrium and on the right anterior axillary line (hypocondrium). The hepatic retractor is inserted in the epigastrium (small circle).

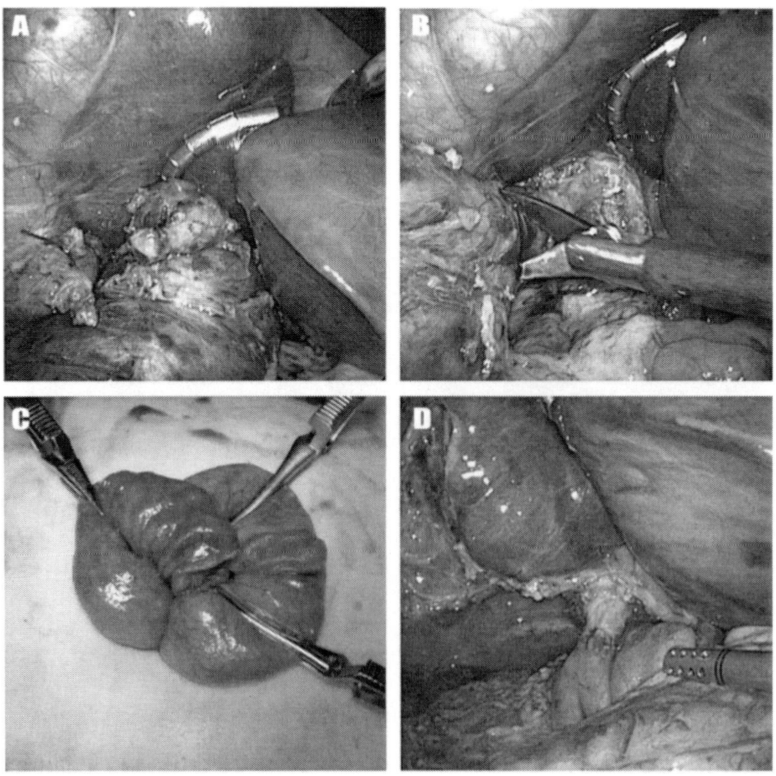

Figure 45. Section of the cystic duct (A). Section of the common hepatic duct (B). Completed extracorporeal Roux (C). Completed hepatico-entero-anastomosis (D).

Complications

The complications of surgery for CC consist of bile leakage, anastomotic failure, cholangitis, pancreatitis, adhesive bowel obstruction and wound infection. In the literature, there are no significant differences in terms of postoperative complications between the laparoscopic and open surgery. The minimally invasive surgery is important. The laparoscopic approach can relieve and even eliminate tissue adhesion, early postoperative pain, and can promote resumption of peristalsis, excellent esthetics, and resumption of activities.

References

Babbitt DP. Congenital choledochal cyst: new etiological conceptbased on anomalous relationships of the common bile duct and pancreatic bulb. *Ann Radiol* (Paris) 1969;12:231-40.

Farello GA, Cerofolini A, Rebonato M, Bergamaschi G, Ferrari C, Chiappetta A. Congenital choledochal cyst: video-guided laparoscopic treatment. *Surg Laparosc Endosc.* 1995;5:354–358.

Keane F, Hadzic N, Wilkinson ML, et al. Neonatal presentation of Caroli's disease. *Arch Dis Child Fetal Neonatal Ed* 1996;77:F145-6.

Lipsett PA, Pitt HA. Surgical treatment of choledochal cysts. *J Hepatobil Panc Surg.* 2003;10:352–359.

O'Neill JA Jr. Choledochal cyst. *Curr Probl Surg* 1992;29:361-410.

Park DH, Kim MH, Lee SK, Lee SS, Choi JS,Lee YS, et al. Can MRCP replace the diagnostic role of ERCP for patients with choledochal cysts? *Gastrointest Endosc* 2005;62:360-6.

Todani T, Watanabe Y, Narusue M, et al. Congenital bile duct cysts: classification, operative procedures, and review of thirty-seven cases including cancer arising from choledochal cyst. *Am J Surg* 1977;134: 263-9.

Wang DC, Liu ZP, Li ZH, Li DJ, Chen J, Zheng SG, He Y, Bie P, Wang SG. Surgical treatment of congenital biliary duct cyst. *BMC Gastroenterol.* 2012 Mar 30;12:29.

Gallbladder Disease

Introduction

Laparoscopic cholecystectomy has become a viable, safe and effective alternative to open surgery in adult patients. Its benefits are now well known in the pediatric age.

The main indications for cholecystectomy are: symptomatic cholelithiasis, complicated obstructive disease and biliary dyskinesia. Other indications include: cholecystitis without calculi, gallbladder polyps and persistent right upper quadrant abdominal pain of unknown etiology.

Cholelithiasis is considered an uncommon disease in childhood, but recently several studies have documented an increase in the incidence rate of this disorder. The proportion of cholecystectomies performed for gallstones in hematologic disorders remain stable but there has been an increase in cases of biliary dyskinesia and non-hemolytic (cholesterol) cholelithiasis.

Treatment

A nasogastric tube and Foley urinary catheter were used to decompress the stomach and bladder, respectively. A 10 mm umbilical trocar for 5-10 mm and 0° optic is inserted with open technique. The carbon dioxide pneumoperitoneum is created at the pressure of 8 to 10 mm Hg and 0.5-1L/min of flow depending on patient's age. 3-5 mm trocars are then placed under direct vision at the left hypochondrium, right flank and epigastrium. (Figure 3)

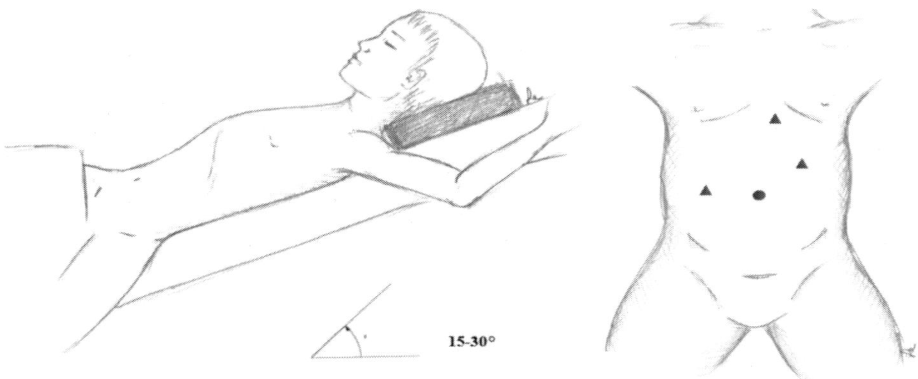

Figure 46. The patient is in the anti-trendelenburg position. The optic (circle) is inserted by open technique at the umbilical level. 3-5 mm operating trocars (triangles) are placed under direct vision in the right flank, left hypocondrium and epigastrium.

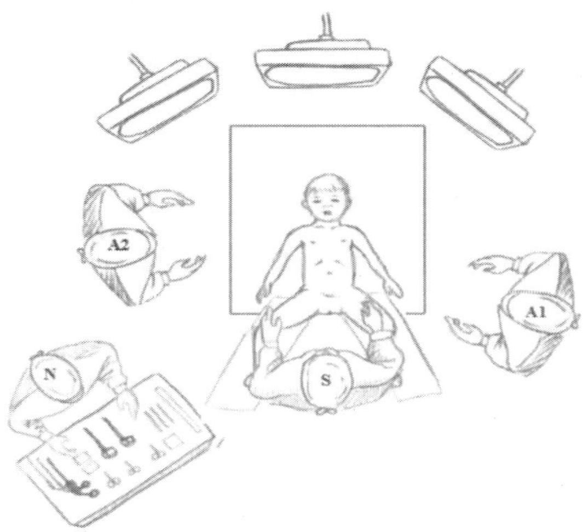

Figure 47. The patient is placed on the operating table in the supine position with the legs spread apart. S = surgeon; A1 = assistant 1; A2 = assistant 2; N = scrub nurse.

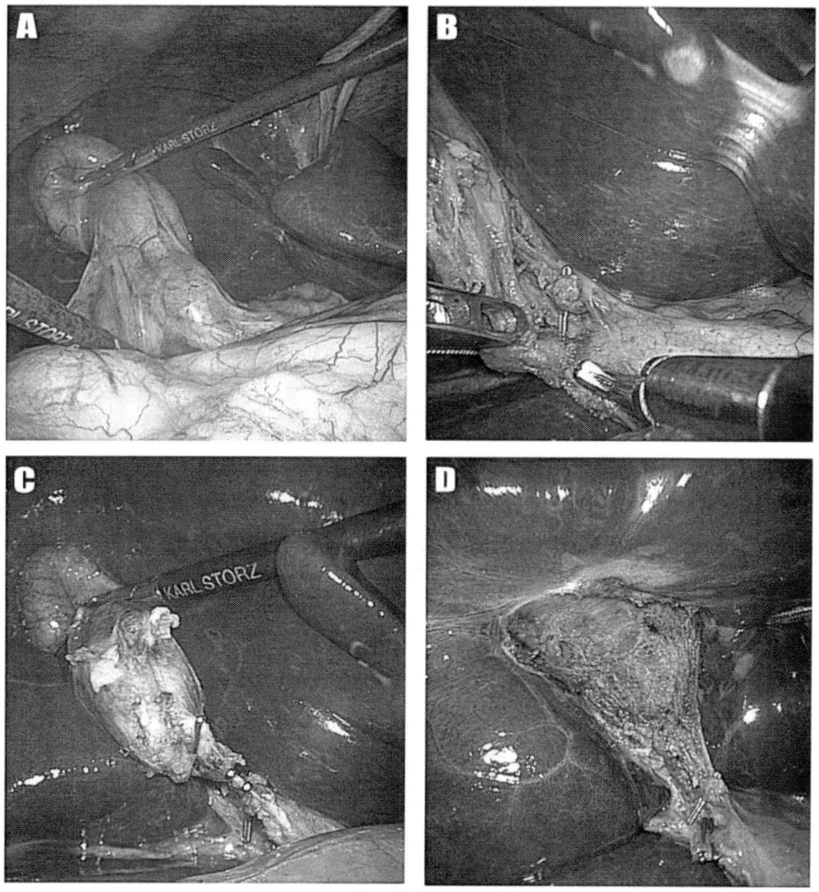

Figure 48. Gallbladder exposition (A); isolation of vessels and cystic duct and clip placement (B, C); appearance at the end of the procedure (D).

Through the trocar in the epigastrium the liver is retracted to expose the infundibulum of the gallbladder. The gallbladder must be grasped lower, toward Calot's triangle, and retracted in caudal direction.

We proceed to the dissection starting from the head of the gallbladder to the cystic duct opening the triangle of Calot. Hedging against all structures especially the cystic artery and the cystic duct is important. Placing three clips two proximal and one distal to the cystic duct, it is then dissected. The same procedure is performed to load the cystic artery. It isolates the gallbladder infundibulum starting towards the bottom using a monopolar hook. Clearing the gallbladder, it is removed through the umbilical port. At the end of the procedure the nasogastric tube and urinary catheter are removed. Two hours after surgery, the patient begins to take clear liquids and resumes after five hours to feed. The abdominal drain is usually removed in 1-2 days post-surgery and antibiotic therapy is practiced for five days after surgery.

Complications

The complication rate of the approach is similar to that of open laparoscopy. The conversion rate is uncommon, determined by the need to control the bleeding. Laparoscopic cholecystectomy is a safe technique that also allows us to reduce the need for post-operative analgesia, and at the same time to reduce the length of hospital stay.

References

Bailey PV, Connors RH, Tracy TF, Jr, Sotelo-Avila C, Lewis JE, Weber TR. Changing spectrum of cholelithiasis and cholecystitis in infants and children. *Am J surg.* 1989;158:585–8.

Miltenburg DM, Schaffer R, 3rd, Breslin T, Brandt ML. Changing indications of Pediatric cholecystectomy. *Pediatrics.* 2000;105:1250–3

Peter C.W Kim, David Wesson, Riccardo Superina, Robert Filler Laparoscopic cholecystectomy versus open cholecystectomy in children: Which is better*? Journal of Pediatric Surgery,* Volume 30, Issue 7, July 1995, 971-973.

Wesdrop I, Bosman D, de Graaff A, Aronson D, vander Blif FM, Taminiau J. Clinical presentations and predisposing factors of cholelithiasis and sludge in children. *J Pediatr Gastroenterol Nutr.* 2000;31:411–7.

Biliary Atresia

Introduction

Biliary atresia (BA) is the most common cause of neonatal cholestasis. It is characterized by progressive fibro-obliterative cholangiopathy affecting varying degrees of both the extra- and intra-hepatic biliary tree resulting in obstructive bile flow, cholestasis and icterus in neonates.

The incidence of biliary atresia ranges from 1 in 10,000, to 1 in 16,700 live births, with a stable incidence over the past several decades. (95, 126) The incidence of BA is higher in Japan, China and probably south Asia (~1 in 8-9 000) than in Europe and in the USA (~ 1 in 12 - 15 000 live births).

About 10-20% of cases have other congenital abnormalities, specifically, an association that we have called the Biliary Atresia Splenic Malformation (BASM) syndrome. These patients are more often female and they have variable combinations of associated malformations including asplenia/polysplenia, situs inversus, preduodenal portal vein, absent inferior vena cava, intestinal malrotation, cardiac malformations and pancreatic malformations. However, genetic etiology has not been proven in these patients. The remaining 80% of cases of BA are isolated. The pathogenesis of BA is unknown. It is likely to be multifactorial, related to the interaction of genetic and environmental factors. Hypotheses have included viral, autoimmune and immune-mediated pathogeneses as well as damage to the biliary tract by toxic monohydroxy bile acids. BA is classified on anatomical bases, referring to the level and severity of the obstruction. The more commonly used is the Japanese and Anglo-Saxon classification that describes the 3 main types.

Table 11. Classification

Biliary atresia classification	
Type I	Atresia is limited to the common bile duct, and the gallbladder and hepatic ducts are patent;
Type II	Atresia affects the hepatic duct, but the proximal intrahepatic ducts are patent. • Type IIa = patent gallbladder and patent common bile duct are present • Type IIb = the gallbladder as well as the cystic duct and common bile duct are also obliterated.
Type III	There is discontinuity of not only the right and left intrahepatic hepatic ducts, but also of the entire extrahepatic biliary tree.

The most common form is the complete AB (type III) with a percentage of 73%, followed by subcomplete form (IIb) that is found in 18% of cases, while the III and IIa forms are very rare.

Diagnosis

The infant with biliary atresia is born at term, weight is appropriate for gestational age and the infant is in good general health. The classic clinical presentation of BA is constituted of jaundice (conjugated, and persisting beyond two weeks of life), acholic (white) stools, dark urine, and hepatomegaly. Only in the most advanced stage of the disease, clinical signs related to portal hypertension such as ascites and splenomegaly, or the lack of absorption of vitamin K, appear.

Physiologic jaundice (unconjugated hyperbilirubinemia) occurs in up to 90% of healthy neonates and it is defined as a temporary inefficient hepatic excretion of bilirubin. Given the need of an urgent surgical repair in patients with BA, it is advised that all infants who remain jaundiced after 14 days of age should have urinalysis for bilirubin and measurement of total and direct bilirubin in serum. Physiologic jaundice usually disappears by this time except in a small number of breasts fed infants. If conjugated bilirubin is present and the stools are non-pigmented, investigations for biliary atresia should proceed immediately.

The diagnosis of biliary atresia involves the exclusion of other known causes of neonatal cholestasis. There is not a blood test pathognomonic for biliary atresia but discrimination between parenchymal and extrahepatic ductal disease is usually possible. In cases of BA, biochemical liver function tests are typically those of cholestasis, with elevated levels of total and conjugated bilirubin (>20 umol/L total bilirubin, of which >20% is conjugated), increased gamma-glutamyl transpeptidase and alkaline phosphatase, and sometimes slightly higher than normal transaminases. In case of clinical suspicion and laboratory BA, to reach the diagnosis, the patient may be subjected to: abdominal ultrasound, radioisotope excretion scan, liver histology, and intraoperative cholangiography.

Typical BA findings in the ultrasound include: absent, hypoplastic or contracted gallbladder; hyperechogenic liver hilum, known as the triangular cord sign, anatomically corresponding to the extrahepatic ducts replaced by fibrous mass; liver with increased volume and echogenic; polysplenia and other signs of Biliary Atresia Splenic Malformation Syndrome (BASM).

Hepatobiliary scintigraphy using technetium-labeled iminodiacetic acid derivatives aims at offering a dynamic, objective assessment of both parenchymal liver function and biliary excretion. In BA this exam will reveal a lack of excretion of the radioisotope into the intestine; however, this can also be observed in any severe neonatal non-obstructive cholestasis.

Liver histology is obtained by percutaneous ultrasound guided biopsy. Typical histological findings in BA include varying degrees of portal fibrosis, bile duct proliferation, cholestasis and inflammation. The degree of liver fibrosis varies from mild portal tract fibrosis to bridging fibrosis and cirrhosis. Occasionally, giant cell transformation is observed, impeding the differential diagnosis between BA and neonatal hepatitis, which can be especially difficult early in the course of the disease due to the dynamic nature of liver histology in BA. Intraoperative cholangiography is performed before portoenterostomy if there is any doubt of the diagnosis at the time of operation.

Treatment

The surgical treatment of biliary atresia (BA) is still a great challenge for pediatric surgeons. Conventional surgery for extrahepatic bile duct atresia (EHBDA), introduced by Kasai in 1957 usually requires a large, painful, muscle-cutting laparotomy, dislodgment of the liver, and wide manipulations, followed by adhesions and possible complications that may disturb the postoperative course and hamper liver transplantation (LT). The incidence of all these complications could be minimized by minimally invasive access via laparoscopy.

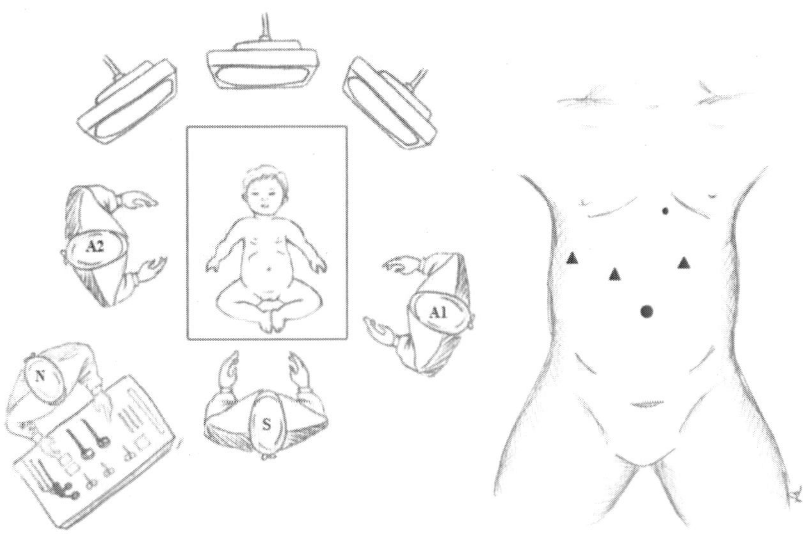

Figure 49. The patient is in the supine position at the end of the operating table. S = surgeon; A1 = assistant 1; A2 = assistant 2; N = scrub nurse. The lens is inserted in the umbilicus (circle); 3 mm trocars (triangles) are placed under direct vision in the right and left hypocondrium and on the right anterior axillary line (hypocondrium). The hepatic retractor is inserted in the epigastrium (small circle).

An incision is made in the internal umbilical ring and the peritoneum is opened under direct vision. A 10 mm trocar is introduced by an open technique into the abdomen and you create the pneumoperitoneum 8-10 mmHg with insufflation speed to 0.5-1 L / min. This port is used to introduce the 30° optic. Three additional operative trocars to 3 mm are placed under direct laparoscopic vision in the right hypochondrium, left hypochondrium and epigastrium. This port is used to introduce liver retractor in order to allow an adequate exposure of the porta hepatis. After the exploration of the abdominal cavity and adequate exposure of the hepatic hilum, in doubtful cases, the surgeon may perform an intraoperative cholangiography. Once confirmation of the presence of biliary atresia is initiated dissection of the gallbladder begins using monopolar unicino 3 mm. The atresic gallbladder and cystic duct are dissected from the liver and dissection is extended until the portal vein and the left and right hepatic arteries to reach the plate portal. In the next step we proceed to the removal of the plate portal in order to prepare the porta hepatis.

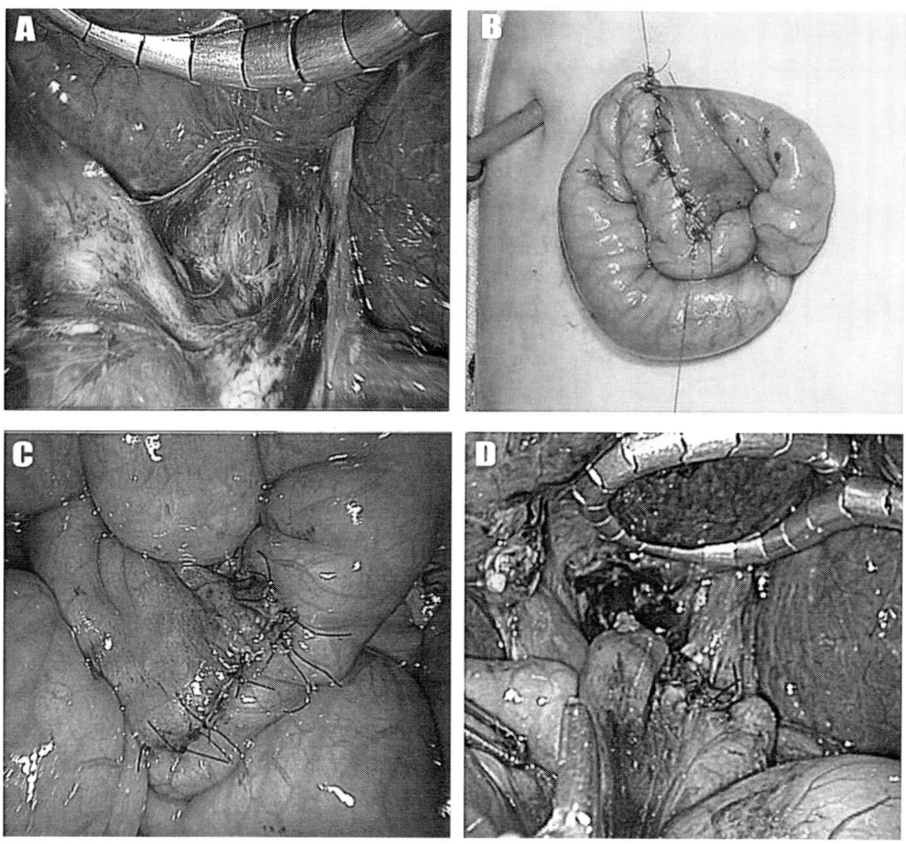

Figure 50. Exposed porta hepatis (A). Completed extracorporeal Roux loop (B). Laparoscopic control of the anastomosis (C). Hepatico-entero-anastomosis (D).

Laparoscopically easily identifies the ligament of Treitz. The proximal jejunum is gripped 20-40 cm distal to the ligament and exteriorized through the umbilical port. The Roux loop is created; the jejunal loop is inserted through the mesocolon to reach the hepatic hilum, passing in front of or behind the colon.

It then proceeds to execute the porto entero anastomosis. It is a termino-lateral intracorporeal anastomosis packed with sutures in PDS 5/0, starting from the posterior wall. The mesenteric defects were closed with 5-0 PDS. Finally you place the abdominal drain below the liver and near the anastomosis. The patient postoperatively keeps the nasogastric tube until recovery of intestinal peristalsis and subsequently feeding is gradually introduced, usually in the 3rd – 4th post-operative day. Antibiotic therapy and steroids are administered for two weeks.

Complications

Surgical complications related to an intervention of porto entero anastomosis are rare and are the standard complications of abdominal surgery. These include the formation of adhesions, intestinal anastomotic dehiscence, or intussusception in the foot point of the limb Roux-en-Y, as well as internal hernia.

The minimal invasive approach, compared to traditional open surgery, reduces the incidence of incisional hernias and in particular the formation of postoperative intestinal adhesions that can hinder the subsequent liver transplant.

References

Basset MD, Murray KF: Biliary atresia. Recent progress. *J Clin Gastroenterol* 2008;42:720–729

Davenport M, Savage M, Mowat AP, Howard ER. The Biliary Atresia Splenic Malformation syndrome. *Surgery* 1993; 113: 662 – 668.

Dutta S, Woo R, Albanese CT. Minimal access portoenterostomy: Advantages and disadvantages of standard laparoscopic and robotic techniques. *J Laparoendosc Adv Surg Tech A* 2007;17:258–264

Hartley JL, Davenport M, Kelly DA: Biliary atresia. *Lancet* 2009;374:1704–1713

Hussein, M.,Howard, E. R.,Mieli-Vergani, G. et al. Jaundice at 14 days of age: exclude biliary atresia. *Arch. Dis. Child.* 1991; 66:1177–1179.

Jenner, R. E. & Howard, E. R. Unsaturated monohydroxy bileacids as a cause of idiopathic obstructive cholangiopathy. *Lancet* 1975; 2:1073–1074.

Karrer FM, Lilly JR, Stewart BA, Hall RJ. Biliary atresia registry, 1976 to 1989. *J Pediatr Surg*. 1990;25:1076-80.

Martinez-Ferro M, Esteves E, Laje P. Laparoscopic treatment of biliary atresia and choledochal cyst. *Semin Pediatr Surg* 2005;14:206–215

Muraji T, Suskind DL, Irie N: Biliary atresia: A new immunological insight into etiopathogenesis. *Expert Rev Gastroenterol Hepatol* 2009;3:599–606

Nio M, Ohi R, Miyano T et al. Five and 10-year survival rates after surgery for biliary atresia: a report from the Japanese Biliary Atresia Registry. *J Pediatr Surg* 2003; 38: 997-1000.

Takaya J, Nakano S, Imai Y, Fujii Y, Kaneko K. Usefulness of magnetic resonance cholangiopancreatography in biliary structures in infants: a four-case report. *European Journal of Pediatrics.* 2007;166(3):211–214.

Laparoscopic Splenectomy

Introduction

The first laparoscopic splenectomy was performed in an adult in 1991, and then in 1993, the first childhood case in was reported

Since then, advances in minimally invasive laparoscopic surgery have made this approach safe and effective in children. Now laparoscopic splenectomy is preferred compared to open surgery in many cases.

The advantages of the laparoscopic approach include less postoperative pain, reduced need for anesthesia after surgery, rapid recovery and supply activities, and better cosmetic results. The conversion rate reported is less than 10 %, due to bleeding and parenchymal injury.

Currently the limitations to laparoscopic splenectomy are a massive splenomegaly and severe comorbidities. "Massive" splenomegaly is defined as a spleen larger than four times normal for age.

The most frequent indications for splenectomy in children are many malignant and benign hematologic disorders, hereditary spherocysosis and idiopathic thrombocytopenic purpura for the majority of cases. Other indications are: thalassemia, hemolytic disorders, leukemia, and lymphoproliferative disorders.

Pre-operative diagnostic imaging, especially ultrasound, it is important to define the size and volume of the spleen and the possible presence of an accessory spleen.

The splenectomized patient is at high risk of infectious diseases, especially lung, and reach out to sepsis. The rate of sepsis in children is between 0.13% and 8.91% compared with 0.28% to 1.9% in the adult. The rate of infection appears to be related to the age that the splenectomy is performed; it is in fact equal to 13.8% before the age of 5, decreasing 0.5% if the surgery is performed after 5 years. Since many studies indicate sepsis as the risk after splenectomy, adequate immunization is recommended both before and after surgery to reduce this risk. Therefore it is important that the patient receive vaccinations against pneumococcus, meningococcus and H. influenzae B two weeks before surgery.

Treatment

The approach to splenectomy may be anterior or lateral. The anterior or "supine" approach allows good access to the omental pouch and splenic hilum. It is valid especially in case you need to perform concomitant procedures such as cholecystectomy. The patient can then be placed in a semi-lateral position to facilitate access to the spleen. The lateral approach involves placing the patient at a 90° angle to the operating table. The spleen and viscera fall medially due to gravity, facilitating the dissection of the ligaments and hilar structures. Thereby allowing a safe vascular control and optimal visualization of the pancreatic tail, reducing the risk of pancreatic insult.

A 10 mm umbilical trocar for 5-10 mm and 0° optic is inserted with the open technique. The carbon dioxide pneumoperitoneum is created at the pressure of 8 to 10 mm Hg and 0.5-1L/min of flow depending on the patient's age. Three additional 5-mm trocars are then placed under direct vision at the right hypochondrium, left flank and epigastrium. The latter is used to introduce the liver retractor. (Fig. 2)

To access the epiploon cavity in order to see the ileum liver, we proceed to the section of colonosplenic ligament, gastro-splenic ligament, phrenoslenic ligament and short gastric vessels.

The dissection is performed through Ultracision or LigaSure. View of the splenic hilum, carefully isolating the artery and vein spleen, which are then cut with clips, staplers or energy devices (Ligasure^{TM}, Ultracision^{TM}). The spleen thus mobilized can be extracted through the umbilical port using an endobag that contains the spleen during the splitting. During this process it is important to ensure that there is diffusion of splenic tissue within the abdominal cavity.

In case of splenomegaly extraction can take place alternately through the Pfannenstiel incision. After splenectomy controlling hemostasis, abdominal drainage is placed in the splenic lodge.

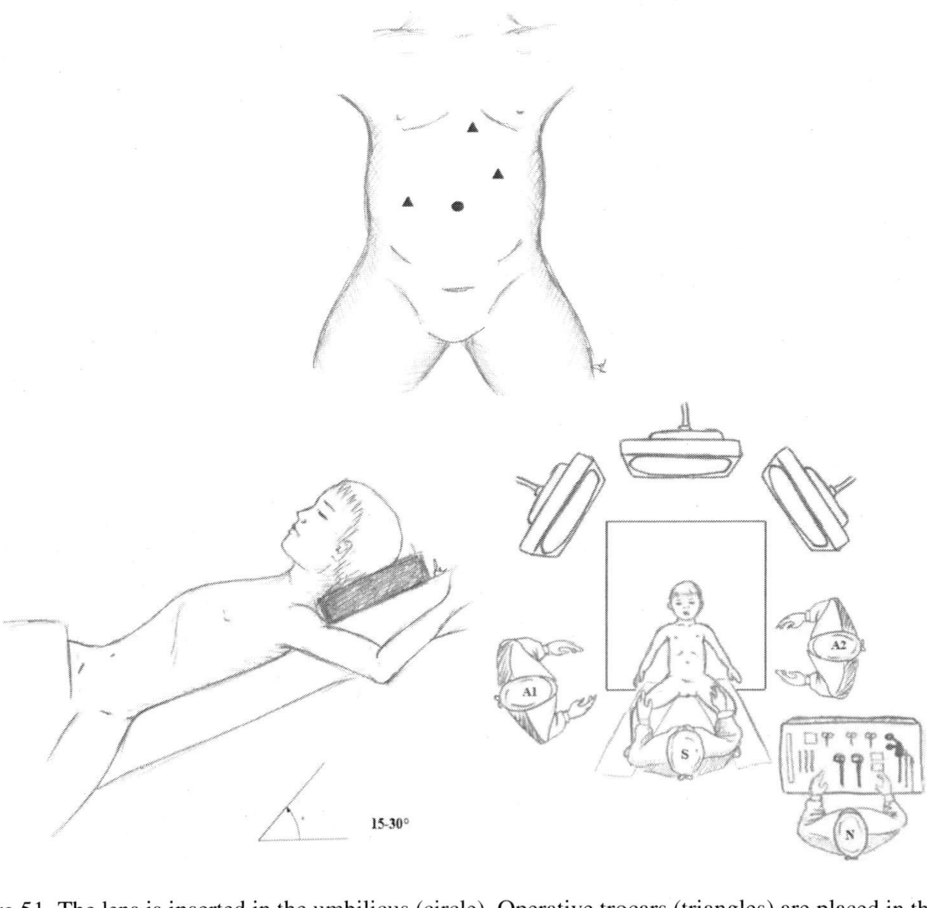

Figure 51. The lens is inserted in the umbilicus (circle). Operative trocars (triangles) are placed in the right hypocondrium, left flank and epigastrium. The patient is in the anti-trendelenburg position. Operative set-up (S = surgeon; A1 = assistant 1; A2 = assistant 2; N = scrub nurse).

Laparoscopic Partial Splenectomy

The partial splenectomy aims to remove about 80-90% of the splenic parenchyma. This is an advantage especially in children where the residual normal spleen can continue to play its immunological function.

It was initially applied for hemolytic anemia, and can now be applied in the case of Gaucher's disease, Hodgkin's disease staging, splenic cyst (congenital or post traumatic), hamartomas and hemangiomas.

The procedure is performed with an anterior approach. After an adequate statement of the splenic hilum the splenic artery is identified. Depending on the location of the lesion, branches of the splenic artery of the upper or lower pole are preserved. The remaining branches are dissected through clips, staplers or energy devices. The same procedure is carried out to the splenic vein.

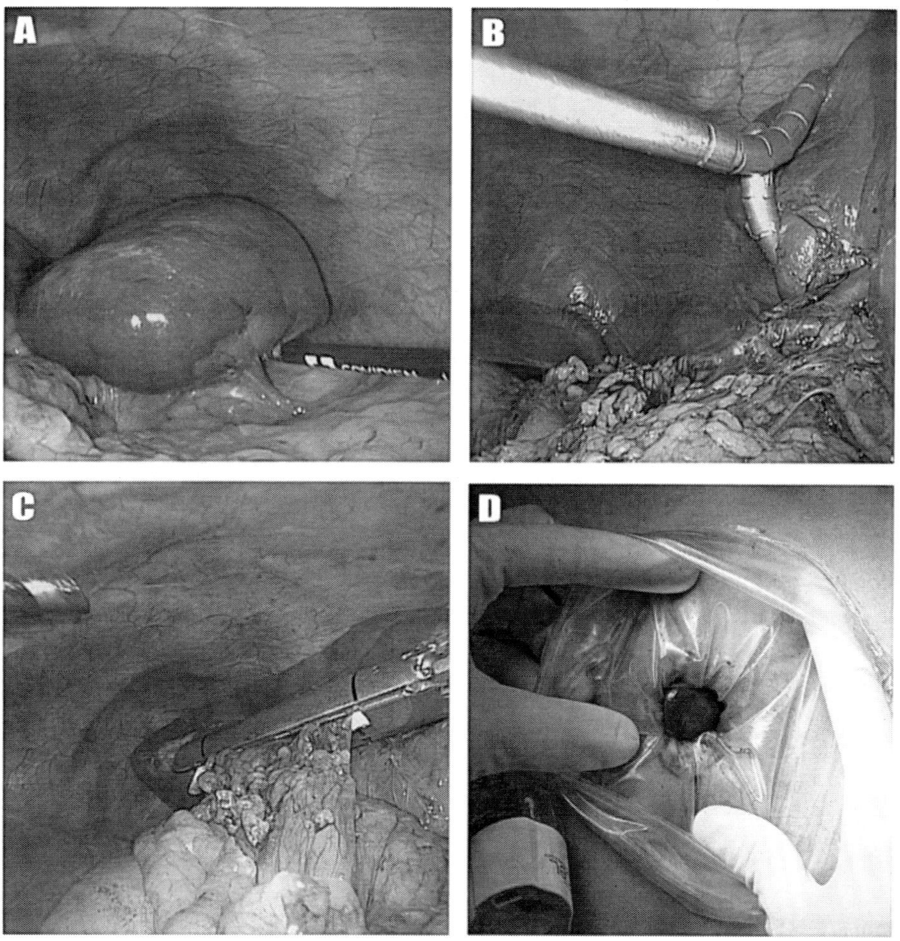

Figure 52. Splenectomy. Identification of the spleen (A); vessels isolation (B) and legation (C); exteriorization of the removed spleen through the Endobag.

The ischemic tissue is demarcated and separated from the healthy parenchyma through harmonic scalpel or stapling device. In cases of excessive mobilization, the residual parenchyma is fixed to the retroperitoneum to prevent torsion. The removal of the spleen is performed through an endobag or through Pfannenstiel incision after carefully controlled hemostasis with ultracision, ligasure or aragon. An abdominal drain is placed in the splenic lodge near the residual parenchyma.

Complications

The rate of complication of laparoscopic splenectomy is approximately 15%, compared with 26% in open approach. Laparoscopic splenectomy results in a significant reduction in pulmonary, wound, and infectious complications.

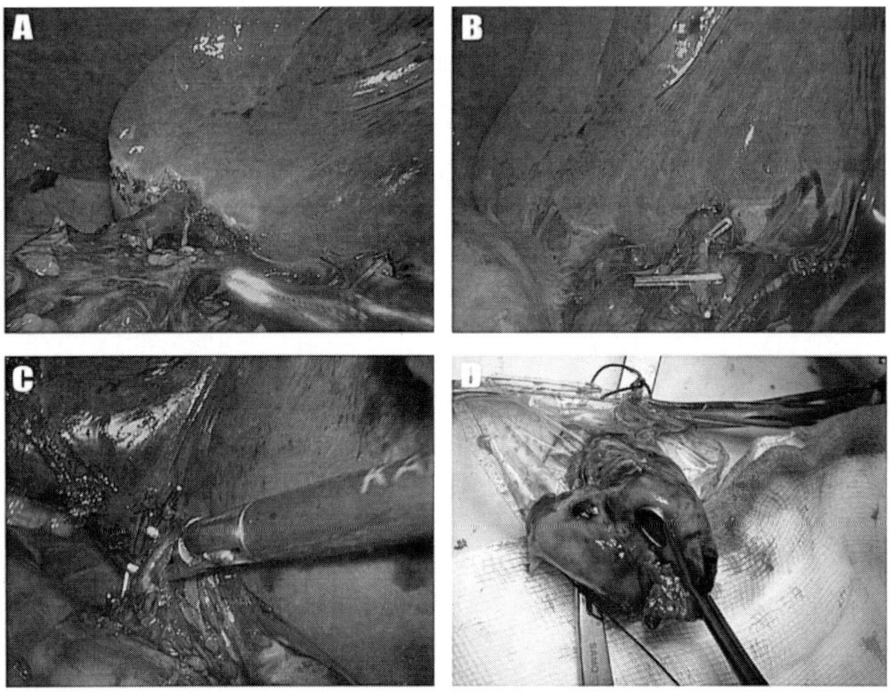

Figure 53. Partial splemectomy. Identification and isolation of splenic hilum (A). Clips placement (B). Section of the splenic vessels (C) and exteriorization through an endobag (D).

References

Basset MD, Murray KF: Biliary atresia. Recent progress. *J Clin Gastroenterol* 2008;42:720–729.

Davenport M, Savage M, Mowat AP, Howard ER. The Biliary Atresia Splenic Malformation syndrome. *Surgery* 1993; 113: 662 – 668.

Dutta S, Woo R, Albanese CT. Minimal access portoenterostomy: Advantages and disadvantages of standard laparoscopic and robotic techniques. *J Laparoendosc Adv Surg Tech A* 2007;17:258–264.

Hartley JL, Davenport M, Kelly DA: Biliary atresia. *Lancet* 2009;374:1704–1713.

Hussein, M.,Howard, E. R.,Mieli-Vergani, G. et al. Jaundice at 14 days of age: exclude biliary atresia. *Arch. Dis. Child.* 1991; 66:1177–1179.

Jenner, R. E. & Howard, E. R. Unsaturated monohydroxy bileacids as a cause of idiopathic obstructive cholangiopathy. *Lancet* 1975; 2:1073–1074.

Karrer FM, Lilly JR, Stewart BA, Hall RJ. Biliary atresia registry, 1976 to 1989. *J Pediatr Surg*. 1990;25:1076-80.

Martinez-Ferro M, Esteves E, Laje P. Laparoscopic treatment of biliary atresia and choledochal cyst. Semin Pediatr Surg 2005;14:206–215.

Muraji T, Suskind DL, Irie N: Biliary atresia: A new immunological insight into etiopathogenesis. *Expert Rev Gastroenterol Hepatol* 2009;3:599–606.

Nio M, Ohi R, Miyano T et al. Five and 10-year survival rates after surgery for biliary atresia: a report from the Japanese Biliary Atresia Registry. *J Pediatr Surg* 2003; 38: 997-1000.

Takaya J, Nakano S, Imai Y, Fujii Y, Kaneko K. Usefulness of magnetic resonance cholangiopancreatography in biliary structures in infants: a four-case report. *European Journal of Pediatrics*. 2007;166(3):211–214.

Acute Abdomen: Acute Appendicitis and its Complications, Meckel's Diverticulum, Intussusception

Acute Appendicitis

Introduction

Acute appendicitis is the most common emergency in children and should always be considered among the differential diagnosis in cases of abdominal pain. The first laparoscopic appendectomy in children was carried out in 1988 and since then has spread among pediatric surgeons who are more interested in minimally invasive approaches.

Diagnosis

Clinical presentation includes pain in the right iliac fossa preceded by pain in the periumbilical region, mild fever, and nausea or vomiting. Children do not have the same compliance of adults, so it is necessary to consider all the factors that may affect the clinical evaluation such as crying and fear. If the baby cries it's important to wait for the inspiratory phase to execute palpation. In older children, it is appropriate to distract the patient from pain to obtain a more accurate evaluation. To date there are no specific investigations and the diagnosis is based on history, physical findings, laboratory results (neutrophilic leukocytosis and increased inflammatory markers) and diagnostic imaging techniques available in emergency such as ultrasonography or sometimes CT scan.

Treatment

Minimally invasive appendectomy can be performed with two main techniques: laparo-assisted and laparoscopic. Both techniques will be described.

Laparo-assisted appendectomy is a single incision technique. A subumbilical or transumbilical incision is performed and a 12 mm Hasson's trocar is inserted. CO2 pneumoperitoneum is established at pressure and flow is adjusted according to the weight of the patient (traditionally includes between 0,8-12mmHg of pressure and 0,5-1,5L/min of flow). A 10mm, 0° telescope with 5mm operative channel is used to explore the abdominal cavity. If abdominal effusion is found, a vacuum cleaner is used before starting the appendectomy. Anti-trendelenburg position can be useful in this phase to avoid bacterial spread in the abdominal cavity. After this maneuver the patient is placed in trendelenburg position and the operating room table is rotated towards the surgeon. Instruments can be inserted through the operative channel and used to find and mobilize the appendix. We usually use graspers, swabs and hooks in case of adhesions. The appendix is taken with a grasper and exteriorized through the umbilical wound. The skeletonization and removal are carried out as in the open technique. At the end of the procedure we always check the presence of a Meckel's diverticulum exteriorizing the terminal ileum.

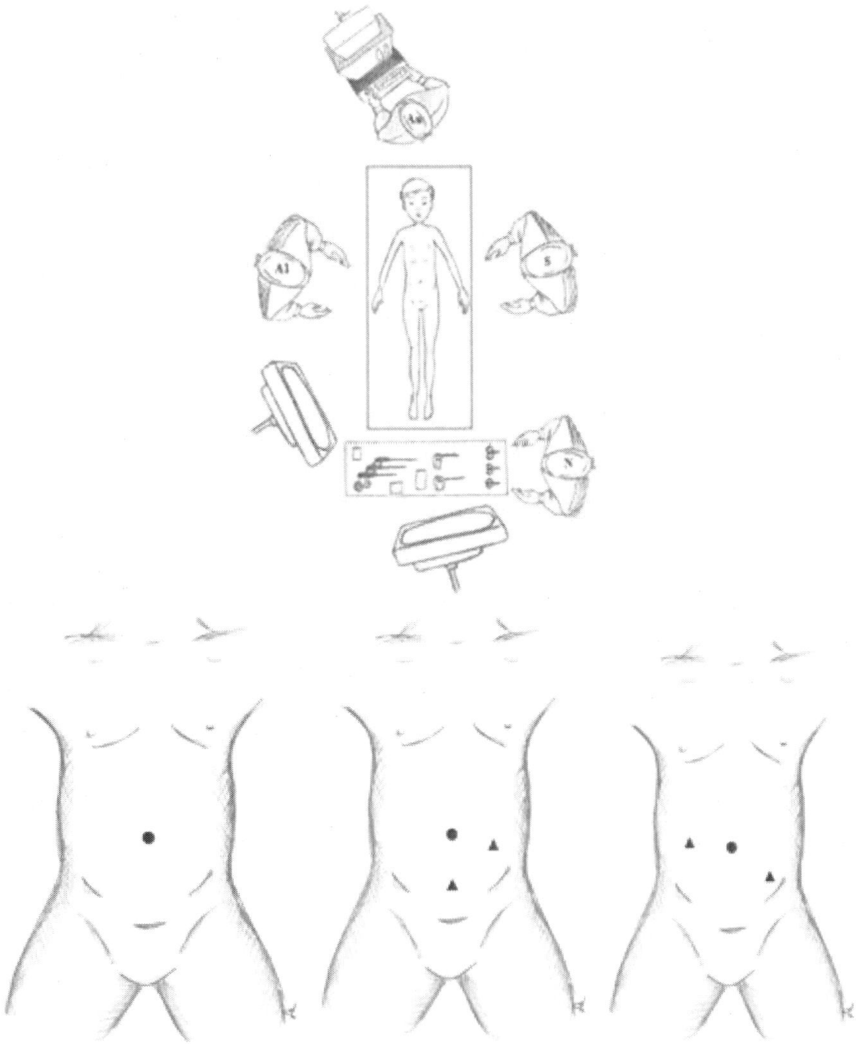

Figure 54. Operative room set-up for appendectomy (S = surgeon; A1 = assistant 1; An = anesthesiologist; N = scrub nurse); trocars position for laparo-assisted appendectomy (operative trocar in the umbilicus: circle in left figure) or laparoscopic appendectomy (additional trocars are inserted: triangles in central and right figures).

The laparoscopic appendectomy requires the use of a 5mm telescope and two 5mm operating trocars in addition to the umbilical one (12mm Hasson trocar). The positions of the trocars can be different. The most used are: in the left iliac fossa and in the right flank or in the left iliac fossa and suprapubic. Skeletonizing of the appendix is performed retrogradely using hook, bipolar instrument or harmonic scalpel and the appendix is ligated with two preformed loops. Alternatively, the appendix can be closed using a stapler. Once cut, the appendix is removed through the umbilical wound. Drainage is carried out in case of appendicular abscess or peritonitis. Usually we resort to the laparoscopic approach only if technical difficulties have prevented the laparo-assisted one. In both cases, before concluding the procedure, a last check is mandatory to make sure that hemostasis is good and that there is no residual purulent effusion. After removing the trocar under vision, wounds can be closed with absorbable sutures.

The nasogastric tube and urinary catheter are left only in case of gross peritonitis or in patients younger than five years. Intravenous broad-spectrum antibiotics are used in case of appendicular abscess or peritonitis and must be continued orally after discharge for 4-6 days. Feeding is started after resumption of intestinal transit.

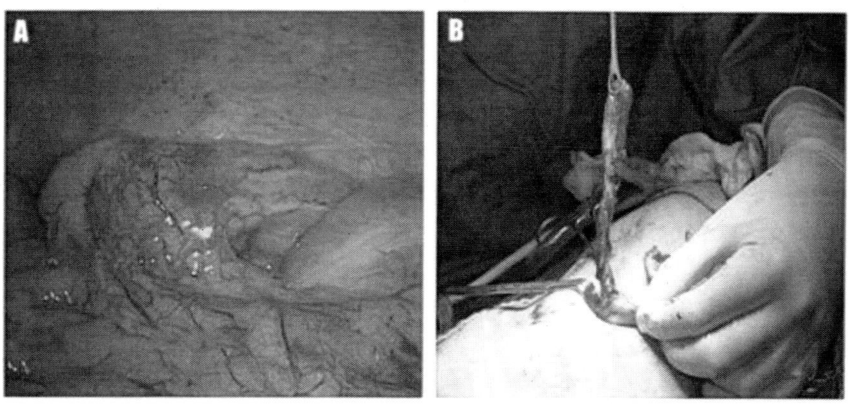

Figure 55. Laparoscopic view of acute appendicitis (A). Appendix skeletonization after exteriorization (B).

Complications

Complications may be different and range from benign conditions to conditions than can influence the long-term quality of life. Umbilical port site infection is frequent especially in peritonitis. Its incidence can be reduced by a good disinfection before suturing or protecting the wound. For example, the appendix can be inserted into a specimen retrieval bag or into the umbilical trocar and extracted with it. If a too thin suture is used, herniation may occur in the post-operative. This is more frequent in the umbilical port site because of its greater caliber. In any case, the patient is advised against excessive physical exertion for 3 weeks/a month after surgery.

In the case of an appendicular abscess or peritonitis is important to irrigate the abdominal cavity with saline and remove it to minimize the bacterial load. Abscesses may form from residues of purulent effusion and are usually located in the right iliac fossa or in the recto-vesical or recto-uterine pouch. Clinical manifestation is characterized by pain and mild fever in the 5-6th post-operative day. Diarrhea and dysuria may also be present. Abscesses are generally treated conservatively, with intravenous antibiotic therapy (based on antibiogram, if possible) and only rarely require surgical treatment.

Appendicitis of the stump is a rare entity, but its diagnosis is very difficult because of the history of an appendectomy in the patient's history. To avoid this risk it is necessary for the residual stump to be as small as possible. In the case of gross peritonitis, the patient may develop adhesions that lead to subocclusive/occlusive episodes or, in the female, to Fallopian tube dysfunction and sterility.

Meckel's Diverticulum

Introduction

Meckel's diverticulum is an embrionic remnant of the omphalomesenteric duct, which normally regresses after the sixth week of gestation. Its presence is estimated in 2% of the population and the symptomatic cases range from 4% to 35%. It is located in the antimesenteric side of the ileum, between 30 and 100 cm from the ileocecal valve. Its length ranges from 1 to 10 cm and may have a broad or a narrow base. Areas of ectopic gastric or pancreatic epithelium may be present inside the diverticulum.

Diagnosis

The most common presentation is painless rectal bleeding due to ulceration of intestinal mucosa adjacent to the ectopic one. The bleeding can be consistent and may require transfusions. Another clinical presentation is diverticulitis. In this case the symptoms are the same as acute appendicitis, which often represents the preoperative diagnosis.

Meckel's diverticulum can also be inverted like a glove finger into the lumen and act as a lead-point for intussusception. If the distal end of the diverticulum is connected to the umbilical scar by a fibrous cord, a volvulus may occur.

In asymptomatic patients, Meckel's diverticulum can be founded during a laparoscopy performed for other reasons. Its removal is controversial but in literature, degeneration in adult life is reported. Scintigraphy with technetium pertechnetate can highlight the ectopic gastric mucosa confirming a suspected diagnosis. It should be noted that this study has a false-negative rate of 5-10%. However, some authors argue that laparoscopy, with its potential diagnostic and therapeutic, exceeded scintigraphy.

Treatment

If there is a diagnostic suspicion of Meckel's diverticulum, we use an umbilical 12mm Hasson trocar for a 10mm or 5 mm, 0° telescope and two 3mm or 5mm operative trocars according to the patient's weight. Those that can be used are graspers, hook, bipolar instrument, harmonic scalpel etc. The goal is resection of the diverticulum but the procedure varies according to the clinical picture. We always prefer to exteriorize the diverticulum through the umbilical wound using the instrument to free it. It may be necessary to lyse inflammatory adhesions with graspers or with a buffer, or to reduce an intussusception or to cut a fibrous band to solve a volvolus.

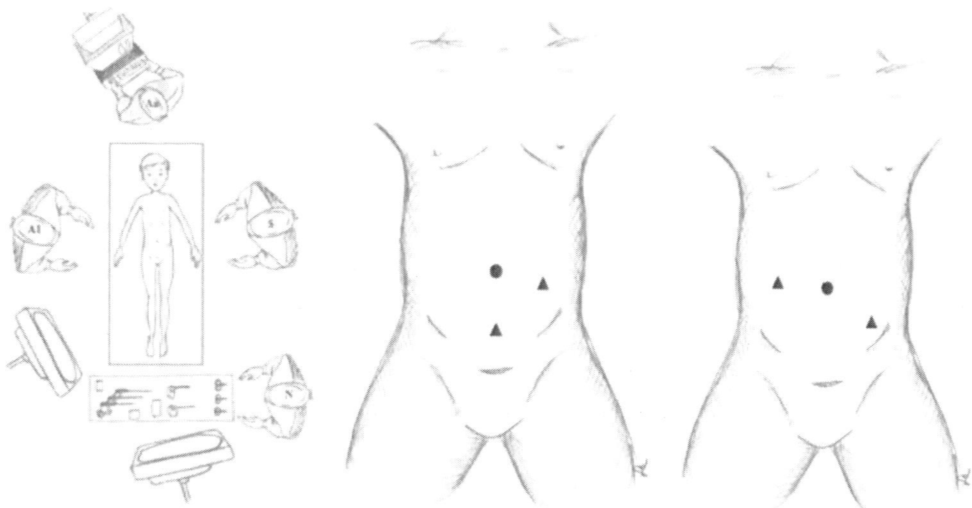

Figure 56. Operative room set up (S = surgeon; A1 = assistant 1; An = anesthesiologist; N = scrub nurse) and possible trocars position.

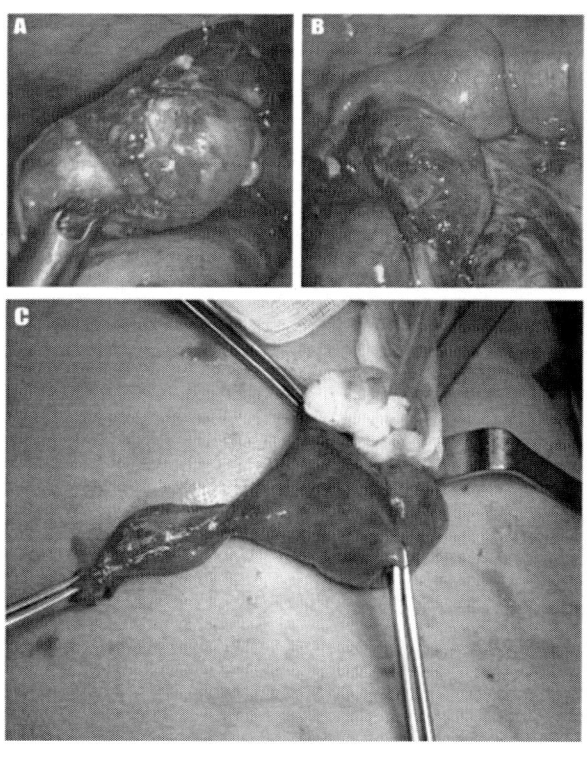

Figure 57. Laparoscopic view of Meckel's diverticulitis (A). Meckel's diverticulum is freed and grasped (B). Exteriorization through the umbilical wound allows removal as in open technique (C).

Once exteriorized, the diverticulum can be removed. Many authors argue that in case of narrow based diverticulum, a stapler can be used for a complete removal with a very low risk of leaving ectopic mucosa. Alternatively, you can perform a wedge resection followed by transversal suturing.

In the case of broad-based diverticulum, it is always necessary to perform resection of the adjacent bowel (about 5 cm). After the suture it is mandatory to check that no stenosis has been created. The umbilical wound is closed with an absorbable suture and the lateral ones with cutaneous strips. Antibiotic administrations depend on intraoperative findings. A nasogastric tube is required in case of bowel resection. Parenteral feeding is necessary until intestinal transit can be resumed.

Complications

Complications consist of the theoretic possibility of stenosis or recurrent bleeding for the persistence of ectopic mucosa but to our knowledge no post-operative complications are reported in literature.

Intussusception

Introduction

Intussusception occurs when a segment of intestine (intussusceptum) enters an adjacent distal segment (intussuscipiens). Transitory intussusception is physiological especially in small bowel but becomes pathological when it persists. The incidence is 1-4% and the main age ranges between 3 and 12 months. This is probably due to hypertrophic Peyer's plaques (frequently found in infants especially during upper airways phlogosis or enteritis) that act as a leading point.

A pathological lesion such as Meckel's diverticulum, polyps, duplications or neoplastic lesions must be checked in older patients. Intussusception is ileo-colic in 80-90% of cases and ileo-ileal in 15% of cases. Typically, the terminal ileum enters the cecum and goes on thanks to the peristalsis. In this way the mesentery is stretched within the lumen causing venous congestion at first and than ischemia.

Diagnosis

The patient is usually a well-nourished infant who complains of cramps typically at the rate of regular peristalsis (about 20 min). As time passes, the patient may become lethargic and evacuate currant jelly-like stools. On palpation, a sausage-shaped mass can be found in the right abdominal quadrants.

In advanced stages, signs of occlusion appear, such as bilious vomiting, abdominal distention, and dehydration. Laboratory data reveal electrolytic anomalies and increase in inflammatory parameters.

Diagnosis is based on ultrasounds that reveal a target sign (if seen transversally), or doughnut or pseudo-kidney sign (if seen longitudinally). A contrast enema is undertaken to confirm the diagnosis and to try to reduce the intussusception. A Foley catheter is inserted into the rectum and the contrast is injected holding the buttocks tight to prevent leakage. With the fluoroscope it is possible to follow the path of the retrograde contrast and evaluate the resolution of intussusception.

The attempts of reduction are currently performed with saline or air under ultrasound control. The reduction rate of non-surgical treatment ranges between 75% and 90%. In the other case surgical approach is necessary.

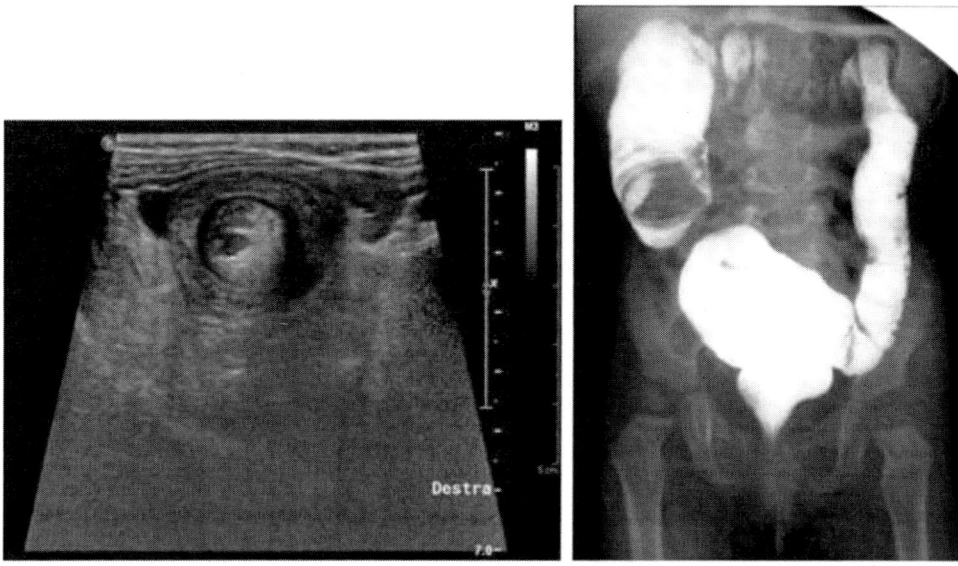

Figure 58. Diagnostic imaging. Ultrasounds reveal a target sign, while in a contrast enema the medium doesn't reach the cecum and the terminal ileum.

Treatment

A subumbilical incision is made and a 12mm Hasson trocar is inserted. CO2 pneumoperitoneum is established at pressure and flow is adjusted according to the weight of the patient. We use a 10 or 5 mm 0° telescope to explore the abdominal cavity.

The reduction is performed by an intracorporeal gentle traction of the proximal segment combined with the squeezing of the distal one with the aid of atraumatic graspers. After resolution of the intussusception, the involved segment is exteriorized through the umbilical wound and explored manually to exclude pathological leading points.

If pathological lesions are present, the involved segment can be resected as in an open technique. If the laparoscopic approach is unsuccessful, conversion is required. In severe cases, manual reduction is impossible and it is necessary to perform a bowel resection followed by end-to-end anastomosis.

Antibiotics are administered according to the intraoperative findings. A nasogastric tube is recommended in case of bowel resection.

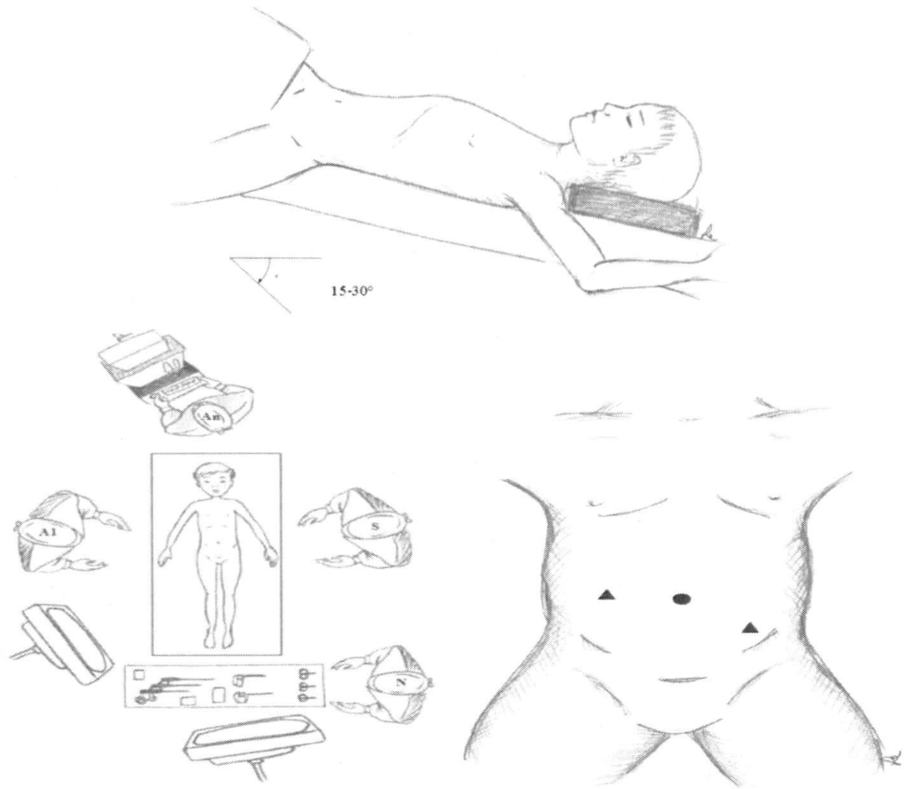

Figure 59. Operative room set up (S = surgeon; A1 = assistant 1; An = anesthesiologist; N = scrub nurse) and trocar position (The lens in inserted in the umbilicus. Two other 3-5mm trocars are positioned under vision on the right and left flank).

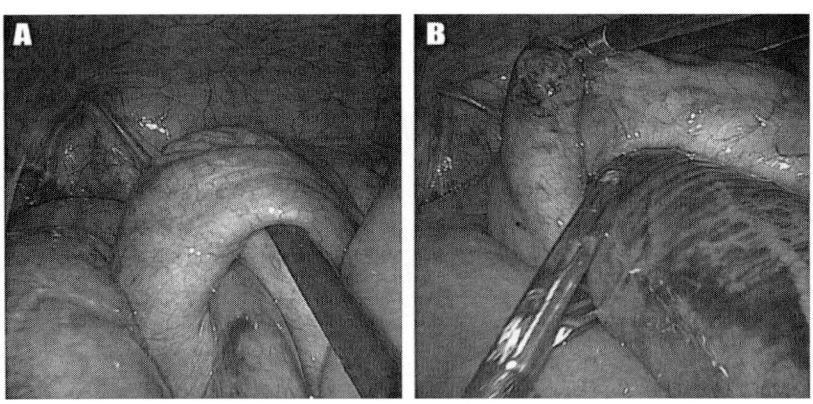

Figure 60. Laparoscopic view of intussusception (A). Laparoscopic reduction of the intussusception (B).

References

Guys JM, Hery G, Haddad M, Intestinal disease. In Zachariou Z (ed) Pediatric Surgery Digest 2009 *Springer* Ch 23 pp 439-450

Jasonni V, Appendectomy. In Puri P, Hollwarth ME (eds) Pediatric Surgery. *Springer* Ch 29 pp321-326

Lesquereux-Martínez L, Macías-García F, Beiras-Sarasquete C et al. Adenocarcinoma arising in Meckel's diverticulum: a case report and literature review. *Gastroenterol Hepatol.* 2011 Mar;34(3):137-40.

Lloyd D Omphalomesenteric Duct Remnant. In Puri P, Hollwarth ME (eds) Pediatric Surgery. *Springer* Ch 30 pp327-332

M. Lima, T. Gargano M. Maffi. An unusual case of intramural Meckel's diverticulum as a lead point for ileoileal intussusception – Laparoscopically assisted management *J of Pediatr Surg Case Reports* Volume 1, Issue 5, May 2013, Pages 111–113

Mazziotti MV, Langer JC, Meckel Diverticulum, Duplications, Small Bowel Obstruction and Intussusception. In Langer JC, Albanese CT (eds) Pediatric Minimal Access Surgery (2005) *Taylor and francis group* Ch 17 pp 217-223

Naffis D, Laparoscopic appendectomy in children. Semin Pediatr Surg 1993; 2(3):174-177

Rothemberg SS, Laparoscopic Treatment of Ileocolic Intussusception. In: Lobe TE (ed) Pediatric Laparoscopy (2003) *Landes Bioscience Georgetown*, Texas USA Ch 17 pp 148-150

Schier F, Laparoscopic Treatment of Meckel's Diverticulum. In: Bax KMA, Geogeson KE, Rothemberg SS, Valla J-S, Yeung CK (eds) Endoscopic Surgery in Infants and Children (2008) *Springer* Ch 42 pp 309-313

St-Vil D, Brandt ML, Panic S et al. Meckel's diverticulum in children: a 20 year review. *J Pediatr Surg* 1991; 26:1289

Waag KL, Intussusception. In: Puri P, Hollwarth ME (eds) Pediatric Surgery. *Springer* Ch 28 pp 313-320

Walton JM, Fitzgerald P, Laparoscopic appendectomy. In Langer JC, Albanese CT (eds) Pediatric Minimal Access Surgery (2005) *Taylor and francis group,* Ch 16 pp 209-216

Nephrectomy

Introduction

The first laparoscopic nephrectomy was performed by Clayman et al. in an adult in 1991, through a transperitoneal approach. One year later Erlich et al. reported the first series of pediatric cases. The laparoscopic nephrectomy can be performed either transperitoneal or retroperitoneal. Which of the two approaches is the more beneficial is still a topic of discussion. The retroperitoneal approach is advantageous in that: it is a short distance from the kidney, it reduces the risk of contamination of the peritoneum from kidney disease and it does not have the problem that organs, such as liver, spleen and bowels do to obstruct the surgical field. The retroperitoneum is a virtual space, and for many surgeons in laparoscopy it is difficult to work in a space so small. To overcome this drawback One Trocar Assisted Nefrectomy (OTAN) was introduced. The procedure provides a single access to an operative optic through which the kidney is exteriorized.

The indications for nephrectomy are:

- Congenital renal dysplasia
- Multicystic renal dysplasia associated with systemic hypertension or who in the follow up had no involution
- Reflux-associated nephropathy
- Intractable protein loss associated with nephrotic syndrome

Treatment

The patient is placed in a lateral decubitus position. A roll is placed between the costal arch and the iliac crest in order to exhibit the affected side.

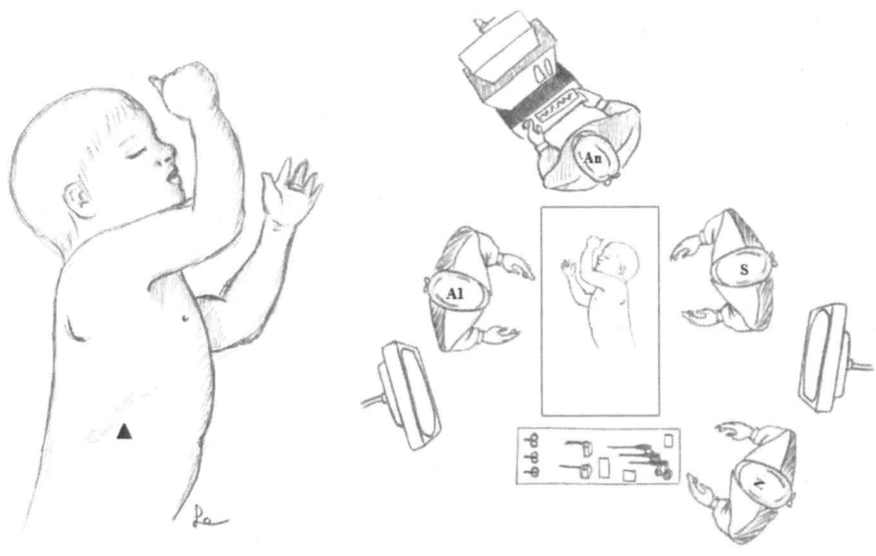

Figure 61. The lens (triangle) is inserted along a line drawn from the apex of the XII rib. Operative set-up. S = surgeon; A1 = assistant 1; An = anesthesiologist; N = scrub nurse.

A single skin incision is performed to a trocar 10 mm below the XII rib at the point where the axillary line intersects a horizontal imaginary line passing through the umbilicus.

The fascia was opened longitudinally. The dissection was carried out through the muscle to Gerota's fascia, which was then opened to the peri-renal space. A 10 mm trocar with pneumatic anchorage is inserted. The trocar was connected with CO_2 and the retroperitoneal space was developed with a pressure of 8-10 mm Hg at a speed of insufflation of 0.5-1 L / min.

The lower pole renal appears gliding along the anterior margin of the psoas muscle ileum and the rear part of the kidney is freed. Subsequently, the kidney is completely separated from the retroperitoneal fat and the parenchyma is isolated. It is important at this stage to accurately identify the renal hilum and the ureter.

The trocar was removed and then the kidney was retrieved through the trocar's incision. The renal vessels may be cauterized if hypoplastic in retroperitoneoscopic, while the vessels of normal caliber can be externalized and tied to the outside of the body. The ligation of the ureter is carried proximally so as to avoid the onset of vesico ureteral reflux. The section of the ureter may occur inside or outside the body. It then performs a check retroperitoneoscopic and finally a lodge is positioned in the penrose type renal drainage.

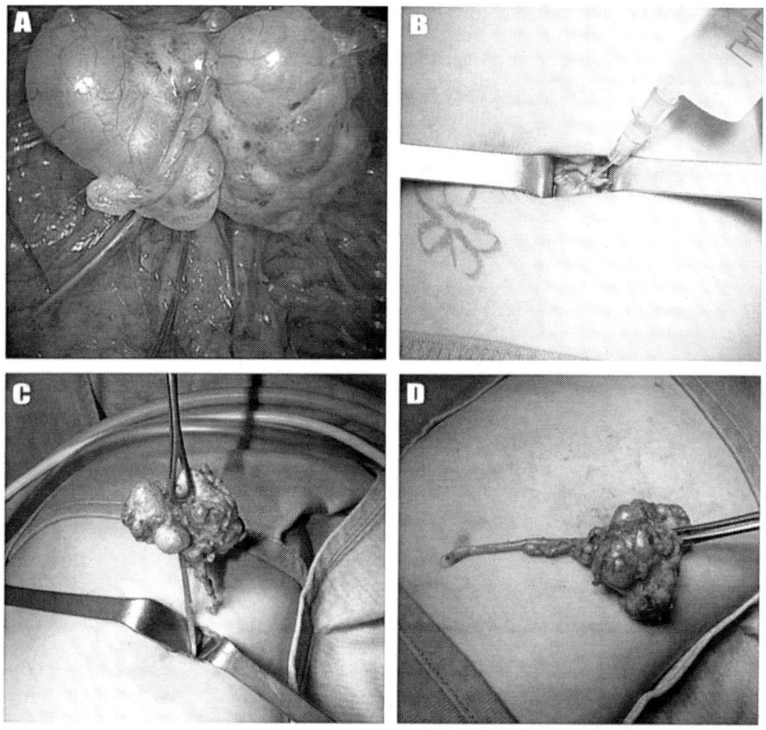

Figure 62. Nephrectomy for multicystic kidney. The cysts are emptied in order to extract the kidney through the skin incision.

Heminefrectomy

Introduction

Partial nephrectomy is usually done in children to remove a non-functioning upper or lower pole secondary to complicated duplex anomalies of the kidney. The usual pathology of the upper pole is obstruction associated with a ureterocele or incontinence secondary to an ectopic ureter. The lower pole is dysplastic due to reflux nephropathy. Laparoscopic partial nephrectomy can be performed using a retroperitoneal or transperitoneal approach.

Treatment

The patient was placed in a lateral decubitus position. In order to sufficiently exhibit the side, a roll is positioned between the costal arch and the iliac crest. The operating area extends laterally from the spinal cord to the mid-line; longitudinally extending the internal mammary line that goes from the iliac crest. A skin incision is performed with a trocar 5 mm below the twelfth coast at the point where the axillary line intersects a horizontal imaginary line passing through the umbilicus. The fascia was opened longitudinally. The dissection was carried out through the muscle to Gerota's fascia, which was then opened to the peri-renal space. The lens is inserted by open technique and connected with CO2 and the retroperitoneal space was developed with a pressure of 8-10 mm Hg at a speed of insufflation of 0.5-1 L / min. Two operating trocars were inserted under direct vision, one at the level of the cost vertebral angle and the other 2 cm from the iliac crest.

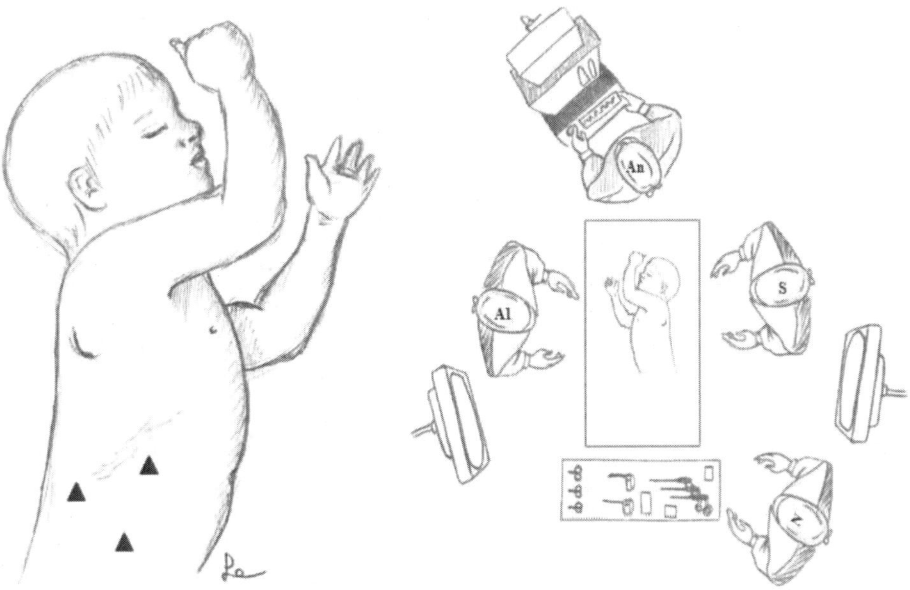

Figure 63. Operative trocars (triangles) are placed 2 cm over the iliac crest (over the middle axillary line) and at the costo-vertebral angle (just over the paravertebral muscle margin). Operative set-up: S = surgeon; A1 = assistant 1; An = anesthesiologist; N = scrub nurse. The lens (circle) is inserted on the prolongations of the XII rib.

Polar vessels to the dysplastic are identified and sectioned with Ligature or Ultracision or they can be closed with clips and then dissected. The upper pole ureter is identified at the lower pole of the kidney and dissected very close to its wall to avoid injury to the vascular supply of the lower pole ureter. The lower pole ureter should be ligated close to the bladder to avoid postoperative reflux into a long ureteral stump.

The parenchyma that is to be removed is ischemic after the section of the vessel and therefore well-marked from the healthy one. It proceeds to its section along the line of demarcation with ischemic Ligature or Ultracision. The hemi kidney is exteriorized through the optic access. It then performs a check retroperitoneoscopic and is finally lodged in positioned in the penrose type renal drainage.

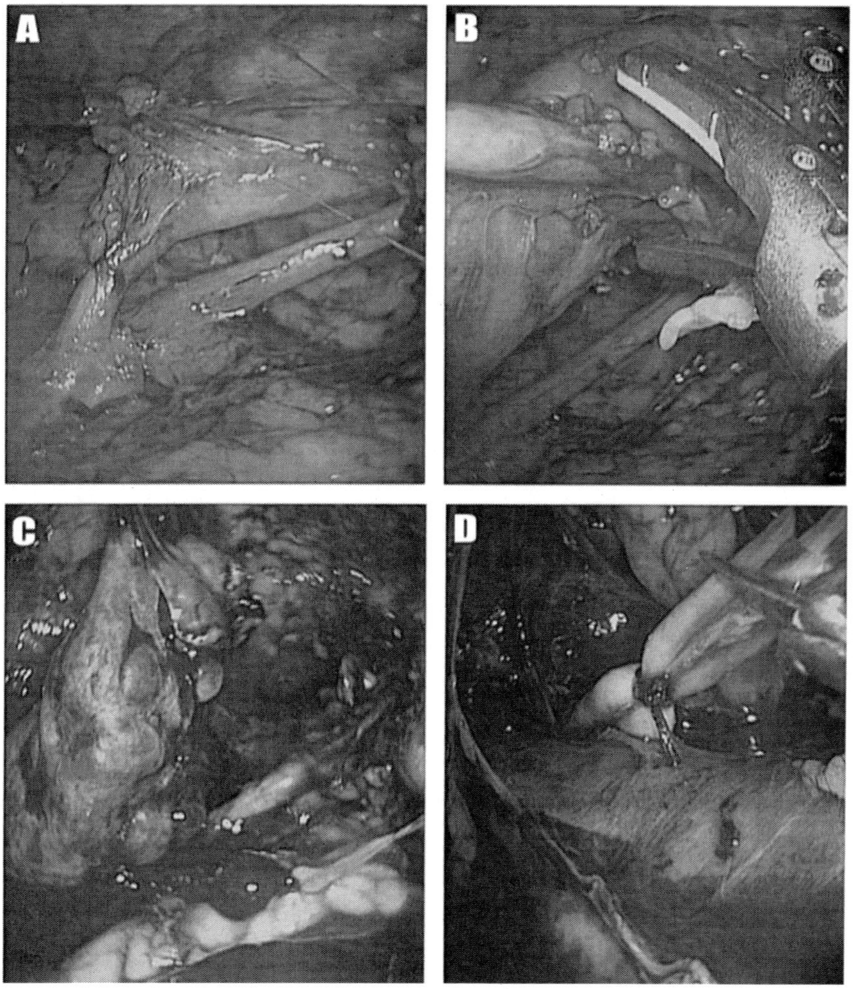

Figure 64. Heminephrectomy. The non-functioning hemi kidney is removed after the identification of its vessels and ureter.

Pelvi-Ureteric Junction Obstruction

Introduction

Pelvi-ureteric junction (PUJ) obstruction is characterized by a functionally significant impairment of urinary transport caused by intrinsic or extrinsic obstruction in the area where the ureter joins the renal pelvis. The symptoms differ by age group. The newborn or infant may present with symptoms related to a urinary tract infection, and an abdominal mass may be palpated. Children, more than one year of age, may present gastro intestinal symptoms (nausea, vomiting, growth retardation) associated with flank pain. In older age, the clinical picture is typical of renal colic with or without hematuria. The first diagnostic approach is renal ultrasound, which showed a pielica ectasia, with glasses more or less dilated, while the ureter appears normal. The patient must then be placed in cystography to exclude abnormalities in the urethra and bladder, and in particular to exclude that pyelectasis is secondary to a vesico ureteral reflux. Finally, with diuretic renal dynamic scintigraphy (Tc-99m-MAG 3) it is able to confirm the diagnosis by evaluating whether the pelvic extension is actually due to an obstructive barrier. The Anderson – Hynes pyeloplasty is still the gold standard for surgical treatment of the ureteropelvic junction obstruction (UPJO). The first laparoscopic pyeloplasty in children was reported in 1995 by Peters et al. (37). Transperitoneal pyeloplasty and retroperitoneal approaches not have been used to perform laparoscopic pyeloplasties in children. The retroperitoneal approach is advantageous in that: it is a short distance from the kidney, it reduces the risk of contamination of the peritoneum from kidney disease and does not have the problem that organs, such as liver, spleen and bowels do to obstruct the surgical field.

Treatment

We currently place the patient in a lateral position on the healthy flank.

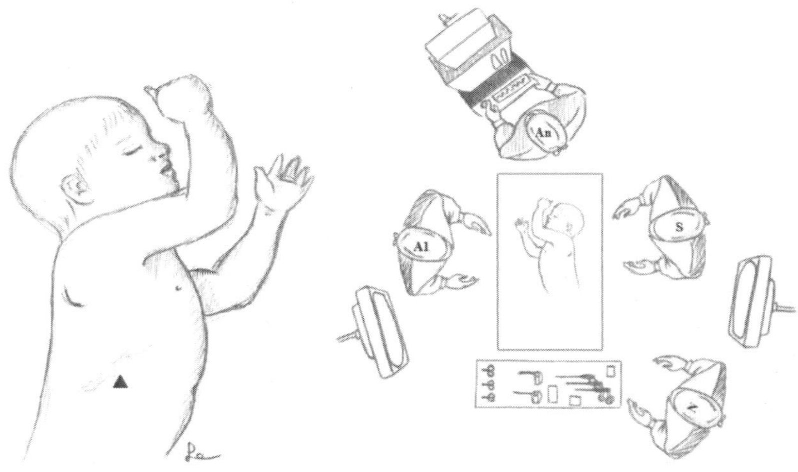

Figure 65. The operative trocar is placed on the apex of the XII rib (triangle). Operative set-up (left): S = surgeon; A1 = assistant 1; An = anesthesiologist; N = scrub nurse.

A 12 mm long incision is made on the 11th – 12th rib and a 10 mm balloon anchorage trocar is inserted after the opening of the Gerota's fascia (blunt dissection). The retroperitoneal working space is created by moving the telescope or with an endo peanut. Once the lower renal pole is identified the pelvis and the proximal ureter are isolated and exteriorized. The pelvis can be emptied with a needle if required. Once a traditional dismembered pyeloplasty is performed and a double-J® stent is inserted through the anastomosis, the pelvis is put back in the retroperitoneal space and the anastomosis is checked (Fig. 3). In case of extrinsic obstruction (crossing vessels – Fig.4) vessels are de-crossed before completing the anastomosis. At the end of the procedure a prefascial penrose drain is left.

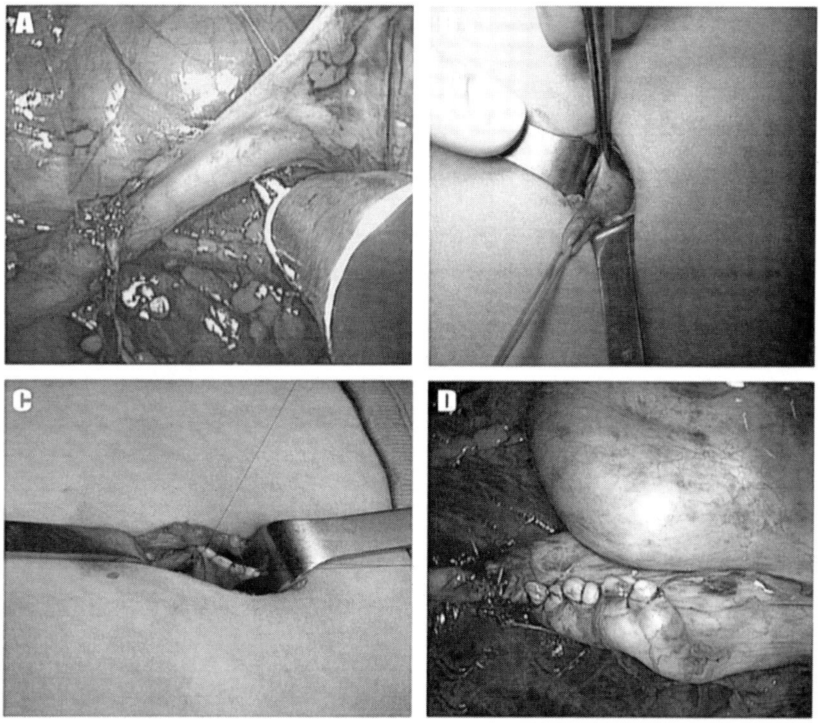

Figure 66. Identification and isolation of the stenosic pyelo ureteral junction (A). Exteriorization of the stenotic tract, dilated pelvis and ureter (B). Completed pyeloplasty (C). Final laparoscopic control (D).

Complications (Retroperitoneal Approach)

The complications associated with these mini-invasive retroperitoneal approaches are mostly due to the risk of peritoneal perforation, which is the first cause of conversion. In the literature the risk of iatrogenic urinoma is also reported. In hemi nephrectomy there is an additional risk of ischemia parenchyma residue linked to the section of the vessels.

References

Clayman RV, Kavoussi LR, Soper NJ, Diekers SM, Meretyk S, Roemer FD, Pingleton ED, Thomson PG, Long SR. Laparoscopic nephrectomy: initial case report. *J Urol* 1991; 146:278–282.

Ehrlich RM, Gershman A, Mee S, Fuchs G. Laparoscopic nephrectomy in a child: expanding horizons for laparoscopy in pediatric urology. *J Endourol* 1992; 6:463.

El-Ghoneimi A, Valla JS, Steyaert H, Aigrain Y. Laparoscopic renal surgery via a retroperitoneal approach in children. *J Urol* 1998;

Hamilton BD, Gatti JM, Cartwright PC, et al. Comparison of laparoscopic versus open nephrectomy in the pediatric population. *J Urol.* 2000;163:937–939.

Johnston JH, Evans JP, Glassberg KI, Shapiro SR. Pelvic hydronephrosis in children: a review of 219 personal cases. *J Urol.* 1977 Jan;117(1):97-101.

Kumar M, Kumar R, Hemal AK, Gupta NP. Complications of retroperitoneoscopic surgery at one centre. *Brit J Urol Int* 2001; 87:607–612.60:1138–1141.

O'Reilly PH, Brooman PJ, Mak S, et al.: The long-term results of Anderson-Hynes pyeloplasty. *BJU Int*. 87:287-289 2001

Peters CA, Schlussel RN and Retik AB: Pediatric laparoscopic dismembered pyeloplasty. *J Urol*. 1995 Jun;153(6):1962-5.

Snyder HM 3rd, Lebowitz RL, Colodny AH, Bauer SB, Retik AB. Ureteropelvic junction obstruction in children. *Urol Clin North Am*. 1980 Jun;7(2):273-90.

Zhang X, Li HZ, Ma X, et al.: Retrospective comparison of retroperitoneal laparoscopic versus open dismembered pyeloplasty for ureteropelvic junction obstruction. *J Urol*. 176:1077-1080 2006

Uterovaginal Anomalies

Introduction

Uterovaginal anomalies are relatively common congenital malformations derived from the altered development of the genital tract. They are often associated with urinary anomalies (eg: Wunderlich-Heryn-Werner syndrome: double uterus with an obstructed hemi vagina and ipsilateral renal agenesis) and sometimes with anorectal malformations. The overall incidence of these defects is approximately 0.001 – 10% of women in the general population and 8-10% in women with a history of adverse pregnancy outcomes. These abnormalities comprise a wide spectrum of genital tract defects that are classified in the American Society for Reproductive Medicine (formerly Fertility Society – AFS 1988, Fig 51) classification, modified by John Rock's according to embryologic considerations (Tjaden and Rock 1992). The anatomical and clinical characteristics are resumed in Table 11.

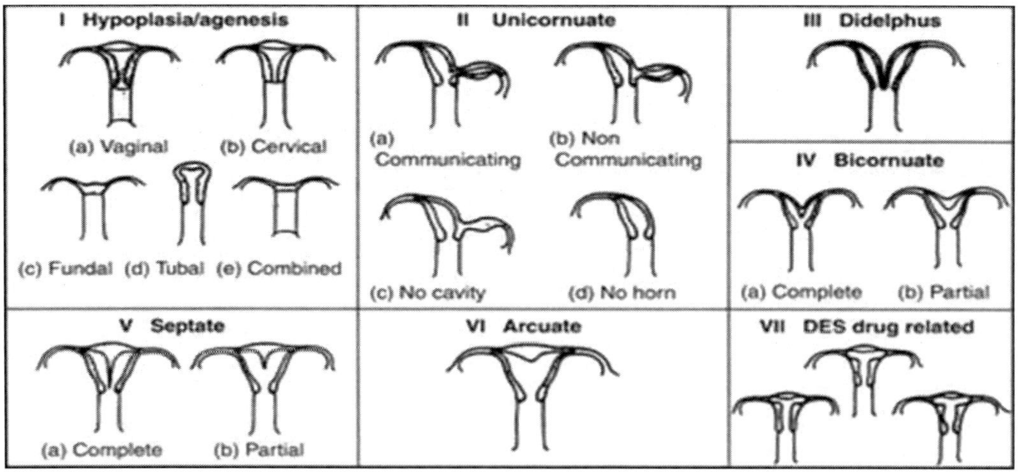

Figure 67. AFS Classification.

Table 12. Embryological, anatomical and clinical aspects of the four Classes of the Uterovaginals anomalies classification modified by John Rock's

Class	Embryologic origin	Anomalies defect	Clinical presentation	Use of laparoscopy
I	Dysgenesis of the müllerian ducts	*Mayer-Rokitansky-Küster-Hauser syndrome:* Absence of vagina with/without uterine remnants	Primary amenorrhea; Cyclic abdominal pain for detection of blood in the rudimentary uterine	*Laparoscopic sigmoid vaginal replacement*
II	Disorders of vertical fusion of the müllerian ducts	Atresia of a portion of the vagina: *Transverse vaginal septum (obstructed / unobstructed)* *Cervical agenesis or dysgenesis*	Acute or subacute abdominal pain; Abdominal tumor; Hydromucocolpos; Hematocolpos in peripuberal period; Endometriosis;	*Define the anatomy;* *Detect and tract secondary endometriosis;* *Perform complete hysterectomy in patient with cervical agenesis*
III	Disorders of lateral fusion of the müllerian ducts	<u>Asymmetric-obstructed disorder of uterus or vagina usually associated with ipsilateral renal agenesis:</u> - *Unicornuate uterus* with a non communicating rudimentary anlagen or horn - Unilateral obstruction of a cavity of a *double uterus* - *Unilateral vaginal obstruction* with double uterus <u>Symmetric-nonobstructed:</u> - *Didelphic uterus* (with/without vaginal complete or partial vaginal septum) - *Septate uterus* (complete or partial; with or without complete or partial vaginal septum) - *Bicornuate uterus* (complete or partial; with or without complete or partial vaginal septum) - *Unicornuate uterus* - *T-shaped uterine cavity* (DES drug-related)	Severe dysmenorrhea; Hematosalpinx; Hematometra; Hematocolpos: Lower abdominal pain; Intermenstrual bleeding; Regular menses (sometimes); Perivaginal mass; Endometriosis	*Define the anatomy;* *Detect and tract secondary endometriosis;* *Combined hysteroscopic and laparoscopic treatment*
IV	Unusual configurations of vertical and lateral fusion defects	Combined lateral and vertical fusion defects together cloacal as well as urogenital sinus anomalies.	Variable	*Complex treatment*

Diagnosis

These abnormalities are often recognized after the onset of puberty. Clinical examination is often unremarkable (external genitalia are normal and there is a patent vagina). Ultrasounds are more manageable and they find their role in the initial evaluation and in future follow-up; this exam is useful to detect associated renal defects. Pelvic magnetic resonance imaging is the technique of choice for evaluation of these females. It provides important details regarding not only the uterus but also other pelvic structures (fallopian tubes and ovaries) and it helps to differentiate various uterine malformations. It is also harmless for the patient. Hysterosalpingography can be useful to evaluate the cervical canal, uterine cavity and Fallopian tubes but does not allow the visualization of the external uterine anatomy.

Laparoscopic is indicated in case of:

- **Vaginal agenesis (Mayer-Rokitansky-Kuster-Hauser syndrome**) *diagnostic purposes:* explorative laparoscopy to understand the internal genital anatomy in patients with primary amenorrhea; *therapeutic purpose:* laparoscopic vaginal reconstruction with the intestine (sigmoid neovagina) has been described;
- **Disorders of vertical fusion of the müllerian ducts:** *diagnostic purposes*: explorative laparoscopy to understand the internal genital anatomy, detect secondary endometriosis; *therapeutic purpose:* perform complete hysterectomy in patient with cervical agenesis and treat secondary endometriosis;
- **Lateral fusion Mullerian duct defects**: *diagnostic purposes*: laparoscopy allows the diagnosis confirmation and permits to exclude endometriotic foci; *therapeutic purposes*: laparoscopy aims at reducing the risk of uterine perforation during operative hysteroscopy. Inveterate obstruction leads to Fallopian tube damage that requires salpingectomy.

Treatment

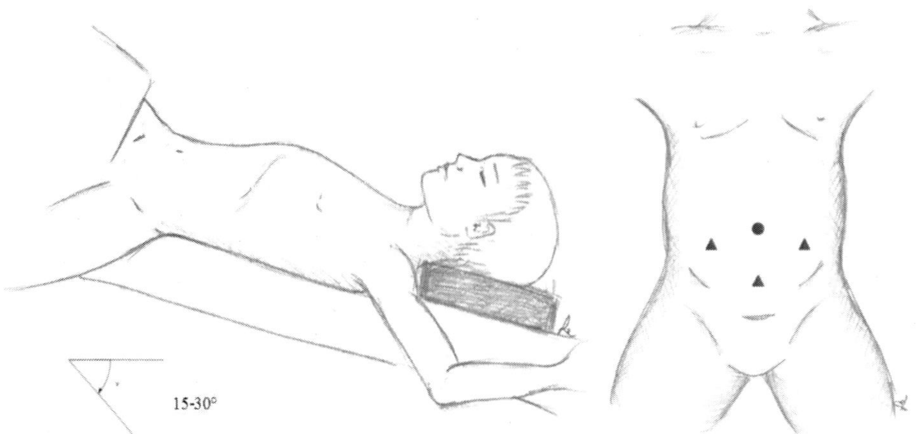

Figure 68. The patient lies in the supine trendelenburg position. Operative trocars (triangles) are in the right and left iliac fossa and in the hypogastrium. Lens is in the umbilicus (circle).

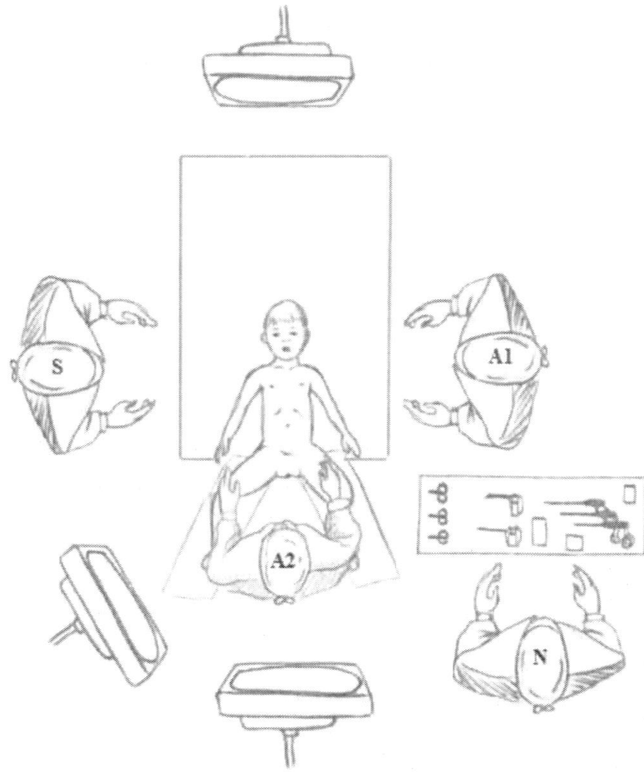

Figure 69. Operative set-up. S = surgeon; A1 = assistant 1; A2 = assistant 2; N = scrub nurse.

Combined Hysteroscopic and Laparoscopic treatment of Obstructed Uterine Duplication

At first hysteroscopy examination is performed to confirm the diagnosis. There are various endoscopic elements to evaluate: the vaginal canal (normal or abnormal), the uterine cervix (single or double), the presence of a protruding uterine canal wall that corresponds to obstructing uterine septum and tubaric ostium (unique or double). The endoscopic evaluation is followed by laparoscopy. A 5 mm port for the 0° optic is inserted through the umbilicus with open technique (sub-umbilical semi-circular "smile" incision). Pneumoperitoneum is created with 10 mmHg of pressure and 0.5-1 L/min of flow (depending on patient's size). Operative trocars are inserted under direct vision. Laparoscopic exploration allows the diagnosis confirmation (hematometra and/or hematosalpinx). Moreover it is useful to search for endometriotic foci. When operative endoscopy is required, the laparoscope is left in place to monitor the hysteroscopic operation. This way the risk of perforation is reduced. The operative hysteroscopy is performed in order to resect the septum cranially, thus creating one single uterine cavity.

After obtaining cervical dilatation with Hegar, to allow the insertion of the hysteroscope, the septum is incised and resected through scissor and wire loop cautery. The septum is very thick and it may difficult to reach the obstructed cavity. When the hysteroscopic light is uniformly distributed on the uterine surface (laparoscopic view) the resection is completed.

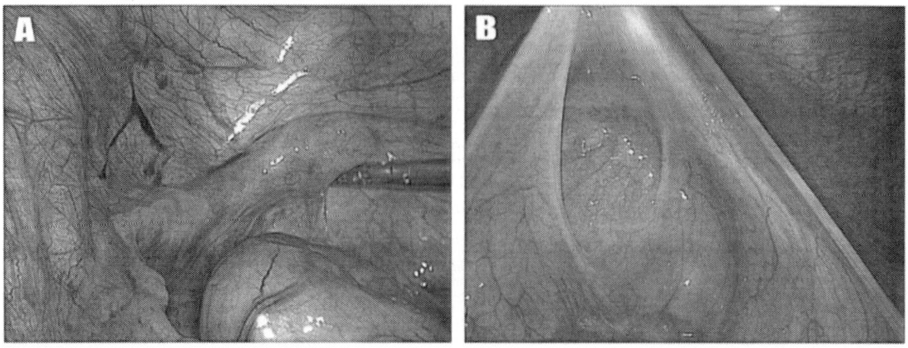

Figure 70. Vaginal agenesy with rudimentary uterus (A) and utero-vaginal agenesy (B).

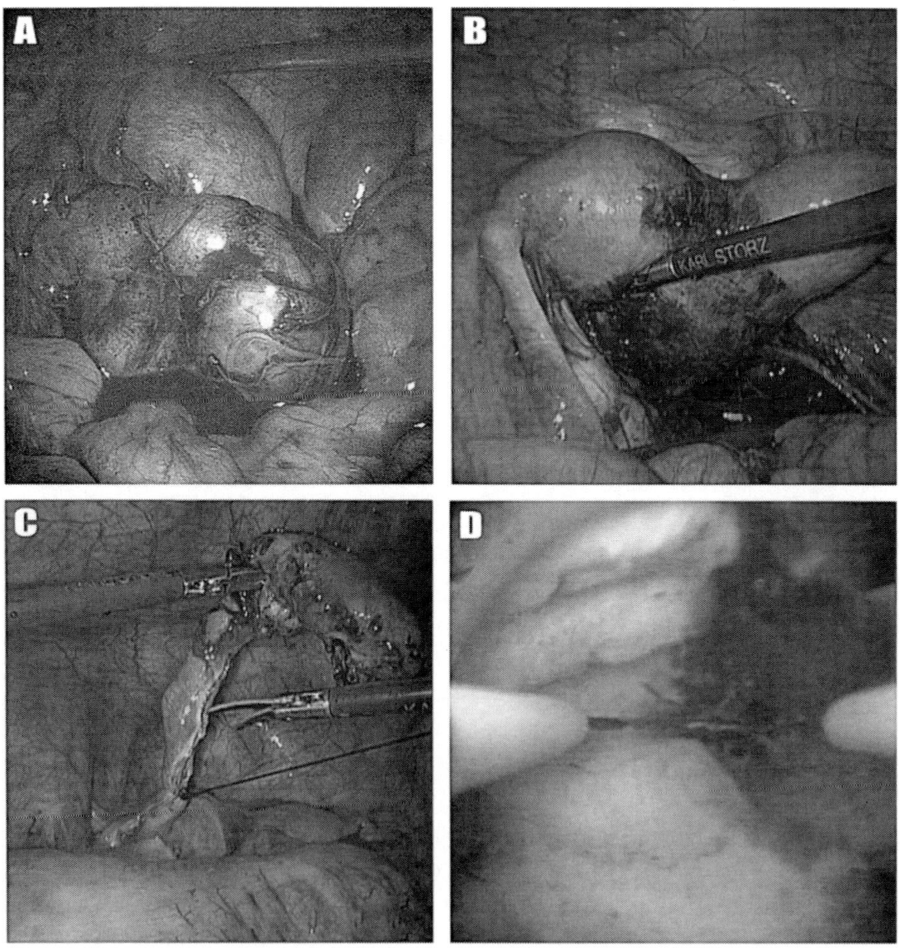

Figure 71. Examples of uterovaginal anomalies: didelphic uterus with dilated tuba (A); bicornuate uterus with distended left hemi-uterus and left tube due to obstructing cervical septum (B). The damaged tuba is removed (C) and the septum is resected endoscopically under laparoscopic surveillance (D).

Complications

The experience is limited due to the rarity of the pathology. Even if hysteroscopy is classically described as a safe procedure it is not completely free from the risk of uterine perforation (the wall of the non-obstructed uterus is very thin). The main cause of conversion is the lack of dilatation of the uterine cervix, which does not make the hysteroscopic procedure possible.

References

Alborzi S, Asadi N, Zolghadri J, Alborzi S, Alborzi M. Laparoscopic metroplasty in bicornuate and didelphic uteri. *Fertil Steril.* 2009 Jul;92(1):352-5.

Bailez MM. Laparoscopy in uterovaginal anomalies. *Seminars in Pediatric Surgery* (2007) 16, 278-287.

Ribeiro SC, Tormena RA, Peterson TV, Gonzáles Mde O, Serrano PG, Almeida JA, Baracat EC. Müllerian duct anomalies: review of current management. *Sao Paulo Med J.* 2009 May;127(2):92-6. Review.

Rock JA, Baramki TA, Parmley TH, et al: A unilateral functioning uterine anlage with müllerian duct agenesis. *Int J Gynaecol Obstet* 18:99, 1980

Ruggeri G, Gargano T, Antonellini C, Carlini V, Randi B, Destro F, Lima M. Vaginal malformations: a proposed classification based on embryological, anatomical and clinical criteria and their surgical management (an analysis of 167 cases). *Pediatr Surg Int.* 2012 Aug;28(8):797-803.

Spitzer RF, Caccia N, Kives S, Allen LM. Hysteroscopic unification of a complete obstructing uterine septum: case report and review of the literature. *Fertil Steril.* 2008 Nov;90(5):2016.e17-20. Epub 2008 Mar 6. Review.

The American Fertility Society classifications of adnexal adhesions, distal tubal occlusion, tubal occlusion secondary to tubal ligation, tubal pregnancies, müllerian anomalies and intrauterine adhesions. *Fertil Steril.* 1988 Jun;49(6):944-55.

Ovarian Lesions

Functional Ovarian Cysts

Introduction

Functional lesion cysts are usually benign and self-limiting. They occur mostly in neonatal and pubertal age.

They represent the most common abdominal tumors detected in female fetuses and newborns. Their origin is related to maternal and placental follicular stimulation, with spontaneous resolution in 90% of cases by three months of age. An ovarian cyst is present in 80% of pre-pubertal girls and it is frequent in adolescents. The lesions appear as small cystic lesions (90% of cases), follicular and corpus luteal cysts. Luteal cysts are typical of adolescents with ovulatory cycles. They are frequently bilateral lesions that can reach considerable size and regress with the decline in the level of serum progesterone.

Paraovarian cysts are more rare and they have a mesothelial, paramesonephric or mesonephric origin.

Diagnosis

The prenatal US diagnosis is possible after the 30 weeks of gestation. The suspicion arises when a female fetus has a cystic mass in the abdomen that does not derive either from the gastrointestinal nor the urogenital tract (differential diagnosis includes mesenteric cyst, duplication, hematometra, urachal cyst, etc.). At birth the diagnosis is confirmed by postnatal-US. We can identify “simple” cysts (completely anechogenic, unilocular, with thin walls) and “complex” cyst (with septa, fluid/debris, calcification) on the base of US appearance. In later ages diagnosis is often made occasionally by US evaluation performed for other causes. When present, symptoms are related to the onset of complications (torsion, rupture, hemorrhage, necrosis) or the presence of a large cyst (intestinal obstruction, respiratory distress, dysmenorrhea in peripuberal children).

It is important to rule out a neoplasm cyst, which is rare in neonatal age and more frequent in the peri-puberal period. Tumor markers (alfafetoproteina, betaHCG, CA 125) and pelvic MRI are useful in doubtful cases (e.g. complex cyst).

Treatment (See Neoplastic Ovarian Lesions for Surgical Technique)

The treatment depends on dimensions, clinical presentation and ultrasound pattern. Simple cysts up to 40-45 mm of diameter are managed conservatively. Surgery is indicated in case of:

- Large simple cyst: > 40-45 mm in neonatal age, > 5cm in older patients if it persists for more than 4-8 weeks (the hormonal stimulation isn’t useful). In this case US guided needle aspiration can be a first therapeutic option but surgery is necessary in case of recurrence. The aspiration of the ovarian cyst during fetal life is controversial due to the high associated risks (preterm delivery, infection, unclear diagnosis).
- Complex cyst: 50% of them are neoplastic, benign in most cases (dermoide cyst or mature teratoma) and rarely malignant (malignant teratoma, gonadoblastomas).
- Symptomatic and complicated cysts.

Neoplastic Ovarian Lesions

Introduction

Ovarian neoplasms are very rare in the pediatric age, especially in the neonatal age. Malignant tumors represent 10-25% of all ovarian tumors and 1% of all malignant lesions in this age range. Moreover, ovarian cancers have a good prognosis in children. There is a precise correlation between age and histological types of ovarian tumors. Although germ cell tumors may develop in all ages, the sex cord and stromal tumors prevail in patients less than 4 years old, while epithelial tumors are more common in adolescents.

The most common ovarian neoplasm is the benign cystic teratoma, with a prevalence of 50% of all ovarian neoplasms in childhood. The other forms are summarized in Table 12.

Table 13. Ovarian neoplasms

Embryological origin	Denomination	Natural history	Hormonal activity	Comments
Epithelial tumors	*Cystoadenoma* (serous/mucinous) *Cystoadenocarcinoma*	Benign Malignant	None None/CA 125	Frequent Rare
Germ cell tumors (GCT)	*Yolk sac tumors*	Malignant	α-fetoprotein	Rare
	Choriocarcinoma	Malignant	β-hCG	Isosexual precocious pseudopuberty
	Immature Teratoma *Mature Teratoma*	Malignant Benign	Normally none	Teratoblastoma, Teratocarcinoma, Rarely feminizing
	Dysgerminoma	Malignant	Normally none	5-10% bilateral, Dysgenetic (ovotestis)
	Gonadoblastoma	Potentially Malignant	Androgenic	Chromosomal abnormalities, Virilizing
Sex cord stromal tumors	*Juvenile granulose cell tumors*	Rarely malignant	Estrogenic, Inhibin, anti- Müllerian (AMH) hormone	Isosexual precocious puberty
	Sertoli/Leydig cell tumors	Potentially Malignant	Androgenic/CA125, α-fetoprotein	Virilizing
	Theca cell tumors	Rarely malignant	Estrogenic	Isosexual precocious puberty
Secondary neoplasms	Hodgkin's disease Neuroblastoma Rhabdomyosarcoma Nephroblastoma Etc.			

Diagnosis

Diagnosis is based on age and hormonal status, imaging features and biological markers. The malignant nature of the tumor is rarely obvious. Ovarian lesions are frequently asymptomatic; symptoms are nonspecific: abdominal pain (50-70%), palpable abdominal mass (2-35%), irregular menstrual bleeding (8-18%). Solid ovarian masses on US are more likely to be malignant (30-40%) than complex (10%) or pure cystic (3%) lesions. Laboratory studies and tumor markers are very specific when positive, but they are frequently negative. The absence of metastasis on CT or MRI scans does not exclude a malignant origin. An ovarian lesion found in a prepubertal or teenage girl should be considered malignant until proven otherwise. Laparoscopy is a very useful diagnostic and staging tool. Contrarily, its therapeutic role remains a matter of debate for the risk of chemical peritonitis, adhesions and peritoneal granulomas in case of rupture. These complications were reduced after the introduction of laparoscopic Endobags. The aim of surgery should be the preservation of ovarian function and of future fertility. Small (< 5cm), cystic and well-marked lesions can be enucleated with gonadic real sparing. Complete resection is mandatory in case of malignancies: open surgery is often necessary (salpingo-oophorectomy). Laparoscopic biopsy is performed when the tumor can't be resected.

Treatment

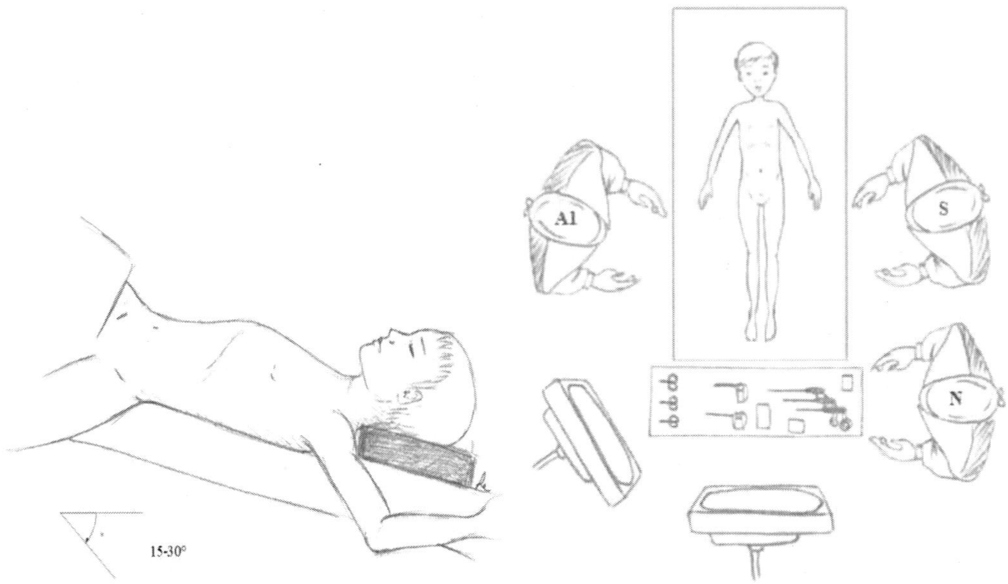

Figure 72. Trendelenburg is used for older patients but not in neonates. Operative set-up for right ovarian lesion. The surgeon is opposite of the affected side (S = surgeon; N = scrub nurse; A1 = assistant 1).

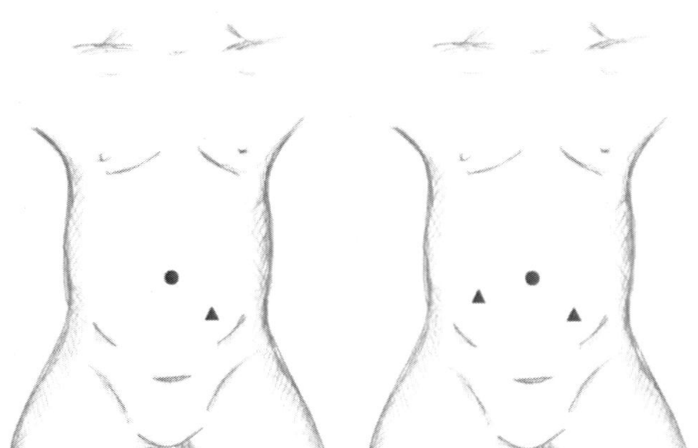

Figure 73. In the neonate we perform a video assisted procedure using only a 3mm trocar placed in the flank opposite to the ovarian lesion. After emptying the cyst, the ovary is easily pushed through the umbilical wound thanks to umbilical elasticity. In older children we perform a laparoscopic procedure using two additional trocars that are placed in the right and left iliac fossa – flank in case of right lesions (triangles).

A sub-umbilical semi-circular "smile" incision is made with open technique. We use a 5 – 10 mm trocar/optic 0°, depending on the aim of laparoscopy (diagnostic or therapeutic). The optic may be replaced during the procedure. Pneumoperitoneum is created with 1 L/min of flow and 10-12 mmHg of pressure for adolescent patients and 0.5 L/min of flow and 6-8 mmHg of pressure for neonates and infants. Operative trocars are placed under direct vision. A laparoscopic careful exploration is performed (ovaries, peritoneum and omentum should be inspected):

- In case of *functional cystic lesion*, an incision is made in the thinnest part of the cyst wall along the ovarian longitudinal axis after its careful isolation with blunt dissection. It may be useful to pull up the cyst wall and the ovary in opposite directions to expose the cleavage plane: a grasper is used to gently hold the gonad whereas instruments must only push tubes. When the cleavage plane between the cyst wall and the ovary is created, the cyst can be punctured and emptied under laparoscopic surveillance, avoiding the spillage. After blunt isolation of the cyst, it is extracted through the umbilicus and any residual cyst walls or redundant ovarian cortex are removed. The excised cyst and collected fluids are sent for examination. The procedure is the same in cases of meso-sapingeal cysts: the cyst is incised parallel to the longitudinal tubaric axis. A cleavage plane is created between the peritoneum and the cyst. The cyst is then emptied and extracted by stripping. In the neonate the video-assisted procedure is the treatment of choice when surgery is required.
- In case of *benign ovarian lesion* (homogeneous surface, no adhesions), a laparoscopic ovarian-sparing surgery is accepted. The technique has been mentioned above. The extraction is performed placing the piece into an endobag that avoids the spillage; the mass can be extracted through the umbilical wound with minimal widening. In case of a mass larger than 3 cm or a solid tumor, we prefer to extract the tumor through a Pfannenstiel incision.
- In case of *malignant lesion*, a careful exploration of the abdominal cavity is performed. The pathological and the contralateral ovary surface are inspected as the peritoneal surface and the omentum to exclude suspicious granulations and lymphadenopathies. Laparoscopy allows the collection of samples for staging. Laparoscopic or video-assisted enucleation, ovariectomy or salpingo-ovariectomy is performed when it is possible. Laparoscopic ovariectomy or salpingo-ovariectomy requires the ovarian suspensor ligament (containing ovarian vessels) to be sectioned with Ligasure or Ultracision; during the ovariectomy the ovarian ligament (containing the ovarian branch of uterine arteries) is also sectioned; during salpingo-ovariectomy the ovarian ligament and the tuba are both legated with an endoloop, placed at the tubaric isthmus. Attention should be paid to avoid mass rupture. The extraction is performed into an endobag through the umbilical wound or through a Pfannestiel incision.
- In case of *torsion*, the treatment changes with the degree of ovarian vascular compromise: the mass can be emptied by transparietal puncture under laparoscopic surveillance to facilitate the ovary and the vascular pedicle to be extracted through the umbilical wound. In case of necrosis it is necessary to perform a radical surgery

(ovariectomy with or without the salpingectomy). Conservative treatment (cystectomy or tumor excision) may be performed when there is no necrosis.

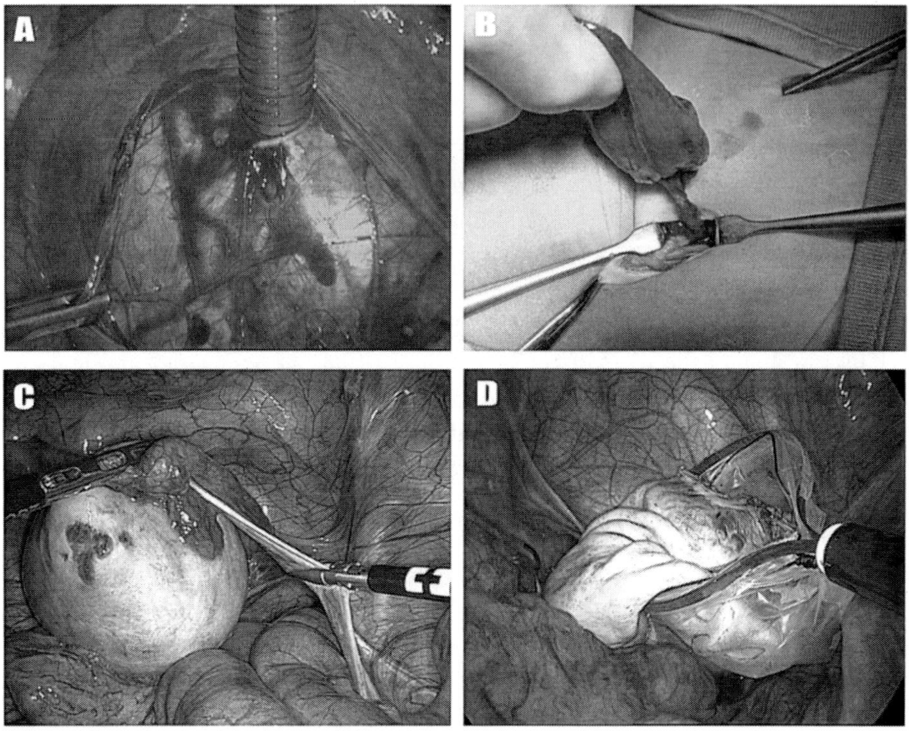

Figure 74. Example of mass emptied during laparoscopy (A). The torted ovary is extracted after emptying the associated cyst (B). In older patients the mass is resected laparoscopically (C) and removed in an endobag (D).

Complications

Intraoperative rupture, failure to complete resection, inadequate surgery for a malignant condition or failure to recognize such a condition must be considered major complications. The risk of intra-peritoneal spillage is greater compared to that of the classical laparotomy.

Laparoscopy does not worsen the prognosis, even with unexpected malignancies.

References

Amies Oelschlager AM, Sawin R. Teratomas and ovarian lesions in children. *Surg Clin North Am.* 2012 Jun;92(3):599-613. Review.

Billmire DF. Malignant germ cell tumors in childhood. *Semin Pediatr Surg.* 2006. Feb;15(1):30-6. Review.

Le´curu F, Desfeux P, Camatte S, et al. Stage I ovarian cancer: comparison of laparoscopy and laparotomy on staging and survival. *Eur J Gynaecol Oncol* 2004;25(5):571–6.

Luzzatto C, Midrio P, Toffolutti T, Suma V. Neonatal ovarian cysts: management and follow-up. *Pediatr Surg Int.* 2000;16(1-2):56-9

Medeiros LR, Fachel JM, Garry R, et al. Laparoscopy versus laparotomy for benign ovarian tumours. *Cochrane Database Syst Rev* 2005;3:CD004751.
Yuen PM, Yu KM, Yip SK, et al. A randomized prospective study of laparoscopy and laparotomy in the management of benign ovarian masses. *Am J Obstet Gynecol* 1997;177(1):109–14.
Sarnacki S, Brisse H. Surgery of ovarian tumors in children. *Horm Res Paediatr.* 2011;75(3):220-4. Review.

Disorders of Sex Differentiation

Introduction

The sex of an individual is the result of a differentiating process that includes chromosome complement, gonads, external and internal genitalia. The embryo development into a male or female individual depends on the differentiation of the bipotential embryonic gonads into either the testes or ovaries. In a XY embryo the Y-linked *SRY* (sex determining region in Y) gene starts a process resulting in a functional testis and ultimately a male phenotype. In an embryo with 2 X chromosomes the undifferentiated gonad develops as an ovary resulting in a female phenotype. Chromosomal defects, abnormalities of gonadal development or defects in the synthesis of sex hormones or relevant receptor, result in congenital *disorders of sex differentiation* (DSDs): chromosomal DSD, gonadal DSD or phenotypic/anatomical DSD.

The word *intersex* has conventionally been used to refer to the appearance of the external genitalia being at variance with normal development for either sex. In 2005, in Chicago, a multidisciplinary meeting of medical and nonmedical experts (the Consensus Statement on management of intersex disorders) revised the classification of these pathologies, replacing terms such as of *intersex*, *hermaphroditism*, and *pseudohermaphroditism*, with the newly term *disorders of sex differentiation* (DSDs). The new classification separates DSDs with sex chromosome abnormalities (sex chromosome DSD: 53.0%) from DSDs with a normal chromosome complement (46,XX DSD: 29.9% and 46,XY DSD: 17.1%).

- **46, XY DSD (previous male pseudohermaphrotism):** the presence of normal testicular tissue histology and total or partial defect of masculinization of the external genital and secondary sexual features. In this case laparoscopy has a diagnostic and therapeutic role: the detection of undescended testes and the execution of orchidopexy; the resection of müllerian residual in deficiency of müllerian inhibiting substance (MIS); gonadectomy in presence of high risk of malignancies.
- **46 XX (previous female pseudohermaphrotism):** the presence of normal ovarian tissue histology and external genitals with different degrees of virilization and masculine development of the urogenital sinus. Laparoscopy is an uncommon surgical approach. The majority of these patients have congenital adrenal hyperplasia.
- **45 X0/46 XX – 46 XX/46 XY – Gonadal dysgenesis:** the presence of variable karyotype and external genitals, of both gonads (one undescended testes on one side

and one gonadal stria on the other side). The frequency of the sexual ambiguity and the high risk of malignancies (gonadoblastoma), justify the laparoscopic removal of müllerian residual and gonad.

- **Ovotesticular DSD (previous true hermaphroditism):** the presence of altered karyotype and external genitalia with both ovarian and testicular tissues. These may be present separately or in the same gonad (ovotestis). Laparoscopy is the gold standard surgical technique for gonadectomy or the selective resection of the testicular tissue present in the ovotestis, for the risk of degeneration.

The overall incidence of DSDs is one in 5,500. Congenital adrenal hyperplasia (CAH: 29.9%) and mixed gonadal dysgenesis are the most common causes of ambiguous genitalia, constituting approximately over 50% of all cases of genital ambiguity in the newborn period.

Table 14. DSD classification

Sex chromosome DSD	46, XY DSD	46, XX DSD

• 45, X Turner syndrome and variants
• 47, XXY Klinefelter syndrome and variants
• 45, X / 46 XY (mixed gonadal dysgenesis, ovotesticular DSD)
• 46 XX / 46 XY (chimeric, ovotesticular DSD)
	• Disorders of gonadal (testicular) development
	  ◦ Complete gonadal dysgenesis (Swyer syndrome)
	  ◦ Partial gonadal dysgenesis
	  ◦ Gonadal regression
	  ◦ Ovotesticular DSD
	• Disorders in androgen synthesis or action
	  ◦ Androgen biosynthesis defect (17-OH dehydrogenase deficiency, 5α-reductase deficiency)
	  ◦ Defect in androgen action (complete or partial androgen insensitivity – e.g. Morris syndrome)
	  ◦ LH receptor defects (Leydeg cell hypoplasia)
	  ◦ Disorders of AMH (anti müllerian hormone) and AMH receptor (persistent müllerian duct syndrome)
	• Other (severe hypospadias, cloacal extrophy)
		• Disorder of gonadal (ovarian) development
		  ◦ Ovotesticular DSD
		  ◦ Testicular DSD (XRY+, dup SOX9)
		  ◦ Gonadal dysgenesis
		• Androgen excess
		  ◦ Fetal (21 or 11 hydroxylase deficiency)
		  ◦ Fetoplacental (aromatase deficiency)
		  ◦ Maternal (luteoma)
		• Other (cloacal extrophy)

Diagnosis

Most DSDs are diagnosed in the neonatal period. Presentations in older children include: previously unrecognized genital ambiguity, inguinal hernia in a girl (e.g., complete androgen insensitivity), delayed or incomplete puberty, primary amenorrhea or virilization in a girl, breast development in a boy and gross or cyclic hematuria in a boy. The evaluation and management of DSDs is complex and requires a multidisciplinary team (geneticist, neonatologist, endocrinologist, gynecologist, psychiatrist, pediatric urologist and a social worker). There are not only medical issues but also psychological, social, and ethical aspects.

Gender identity is a multifactorial process involving both prenatal and postnatal variables. Pre- and postnatal hormonal conditions, sex rearing, timing of sex reassignment and corrective surgery appear to be important components for the development of gender-role behavior and gender identity in DSD patients.

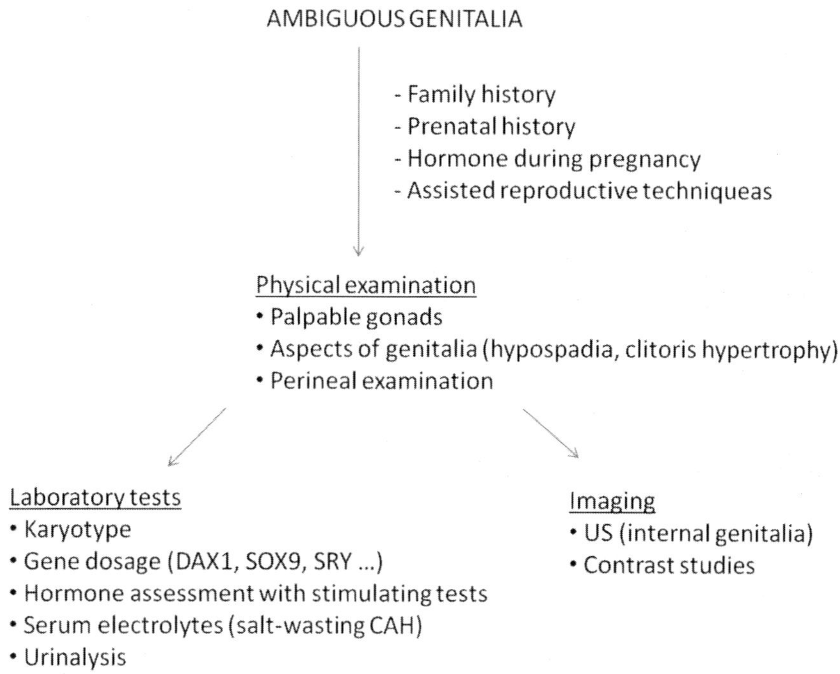

Figure 75. Patients' management.

Treatment

Laparoscopic exploration is necessary when a definite diagnosis cannot be determined and in cases of intra-abdominal or non-palpable testes in suspected DSDs. A few years ago, surgical correction was aimed at making ambiguous genitalia compatible with the assigned gender. The gender was not necessary genetically determined but determined in the way that parents reared their babies. Nowadays surgery is planned when sexual identity has developed.

The laparoscopic technique has a diagnostic and therapeutic role allowing the overview of the abdominal cavity and the identification of internal genitalia. The indications for laparoscopy are: the removal of non-functional dysgenetic gonads or contrary to the assigned gender (older patients), the removal of müllerian remnants and gonadal biopsy.

Gonadectomy and Gonadal Biopsy

Gonadectomy is indicated to prevent testicular malignancy.

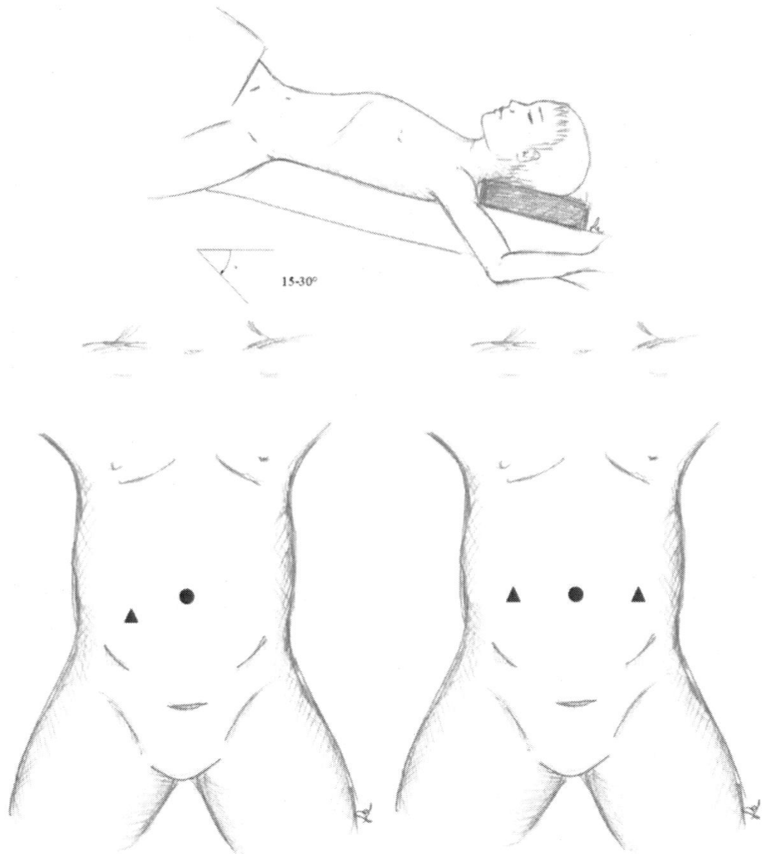

Figure 76. The patient lies in the supine trendelenburg position (left figure). Video-assisted procedures are performed with a single 3-5 mm additional trocar in the flank opposite to the affected side (triangle in central figure). Two 3-5 mm operative trocars in the right and left flank are used during laparoscopy (right figure). Lens is inserted in both cases through the umbilical wound (circle).

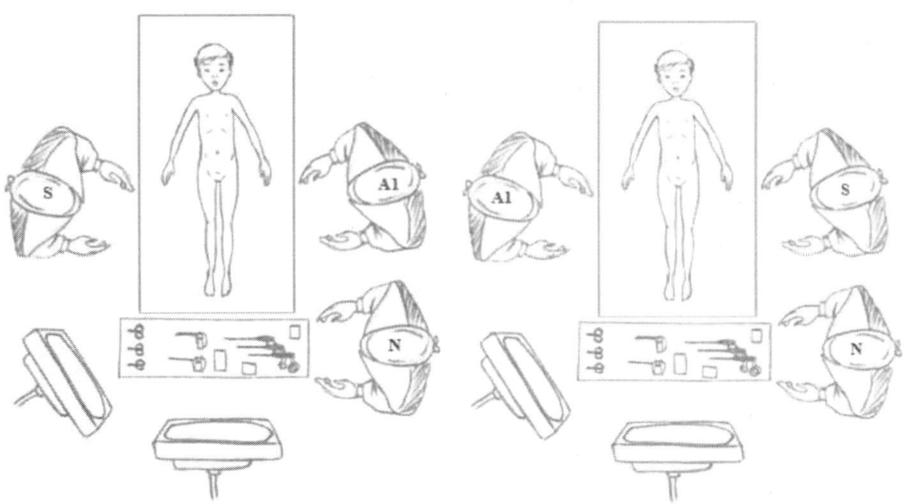

Figure 77. Operative set-up. The surgeon changes his position on the base of the laterality. S = surgeon, A1 = assistant 1; N = scrub nurse.

The trocar for the 0° optic of 5-10 mm is inserted into the abdomen with open procedure through a sub-umbilical semi-circular incision. The pneumoperitoneum is created with 0.5-1 L/min of flow and 8-10 mmHg of pressure. After the exploration of the abdomen, two operative trocars (3-5 mm) are inserted under direct vision.

The first step is the identification of the gonad or the gonadal streak. The tubo-ovarian ligament is then sectioned with Ligasure or Ultracision and the utero-ovarian ligament is closed with an endoloop. A fallopian tube can be legated with the same endoloop prior to resection. The vas is cut in case of peripheral androgen insensitivity if the gonad is in the abdomen. Whereas it is pulled into the abdomen through the inguinal ring and it is removed if the gonad is in the inguinal canal. The gonad is held and the vascular peduncle is cauterized or tied with the endoloop and then dissected. The sample is removed in a finger glove (5 mm trocar) or in an endobag (10 mm trocar). The video-assisted technique is preferred in babies < 10 Kg. Gonads are exteriorized through the umbilicus and biopsy or gonadectomy is performed outside the abdomen. It requires the insertion of a single operative trocar (5 mm) in the right iliac fossa through a semi-circular incision. This trocar is used to identify and exteriorize the gonad. Testicular biopsies are indicated in case of suspected carcinoma or undifferentiated intratubular germ cell neoplasia (premalignant lesion).

Laparoscopic **biopsies** are performed in the same abovementioned way. The biopsy is performed sectioning the gonad with curve scissors over the longitudinal axis on the avascular side. Ligasure or Ultracision may cause tissue alteration. Bleedings are controlled with bipolar cauterization, Argon gas or interrupted suture. The sample is then exteriorized in a finger glove (5 mm trocar) or in an endobag (10 mm trocar).

The video-assisted procedure consists of gonadal exteriorization through the umbilical port. The residual gonad is sutured (interrupted, non-absorbable suture) and replaced into the abdomen.

Müllerian Remnant

Laparoscopy permits the visualisation of the müllerian remnant with a low risk of iatrogenic damage. A cystoscopy can be performed during the procedure to facilitate the identification and the isolation of the remnant.

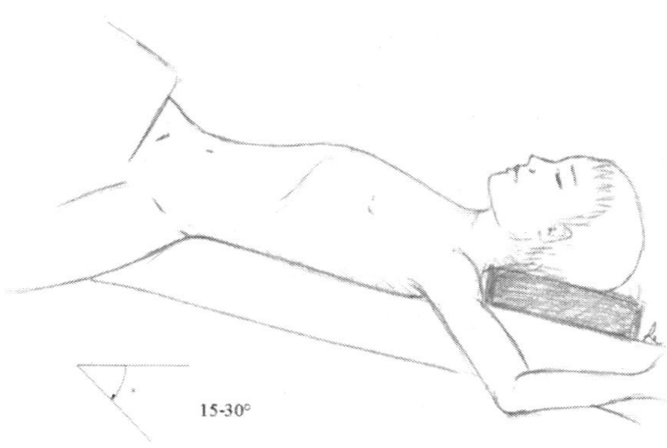

Figure 78. (Continued).

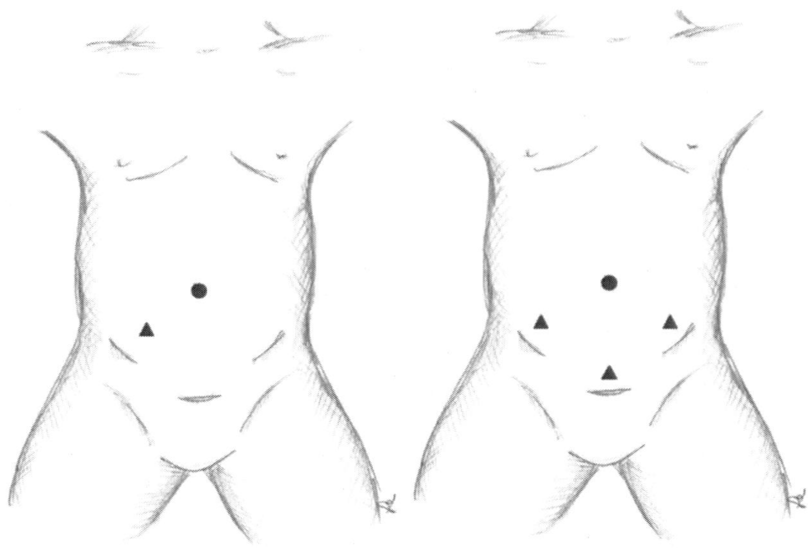

Figure 78. The trendelenburg position is also used in this case (left). The 3 mm operative trocar is inserted in the flank opposite to the affected side in case of video-assisted procedures (triangle on the central figure). The lens is inserted in the umbilicus (circle on the right figure) and 3-5 mm operative trocars in the right and left fossa and in the sovrapubic region (triangles) in case of laparoscopy.

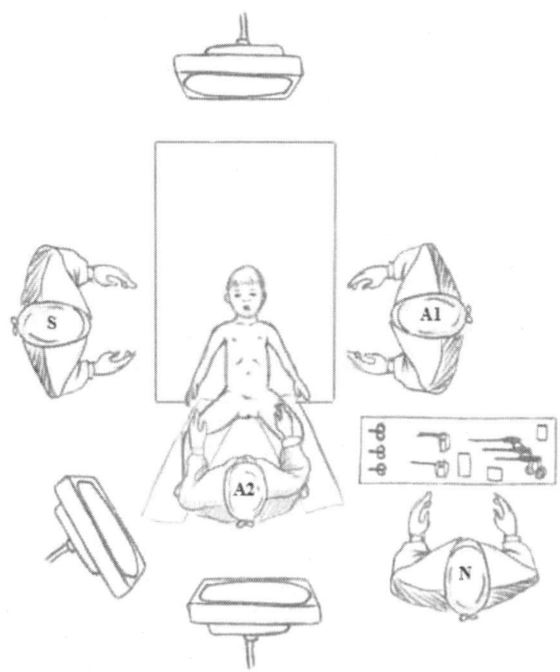

Figure 79. Operative set-up. S = surgeon, A1 = assistant 1; N = scrub nurse.

Instruments' insertion has been previously described (see gonadectomy and biopsy). The first step is the identification of the müllerian remnant under cystoscopic guidance. The peritoneum over the remnant roof is opened. The remnant is isolated with a hook coagulator, Ligasure or Ultracision, paying attention to the surrounding structures. The remnant neck is legated with two endoloops just below the urethral outlet and then it is cut. Staplers are used in older patients with large remnant (with a 10 mm trocar). The remnant is removed through the bigger port site (umbilicus).

The video-assisted technique is performed in babies < 10 Kg. Müllerian remnants are exteriorized through the umbilical port and resected outside the body. A few millimeters of the remnants could be left in case of difficult dissections to reduce the risk of iatrogenic pelvic structure damage.

After surgery the vesical catheter is removed on the 4th post-operative day.

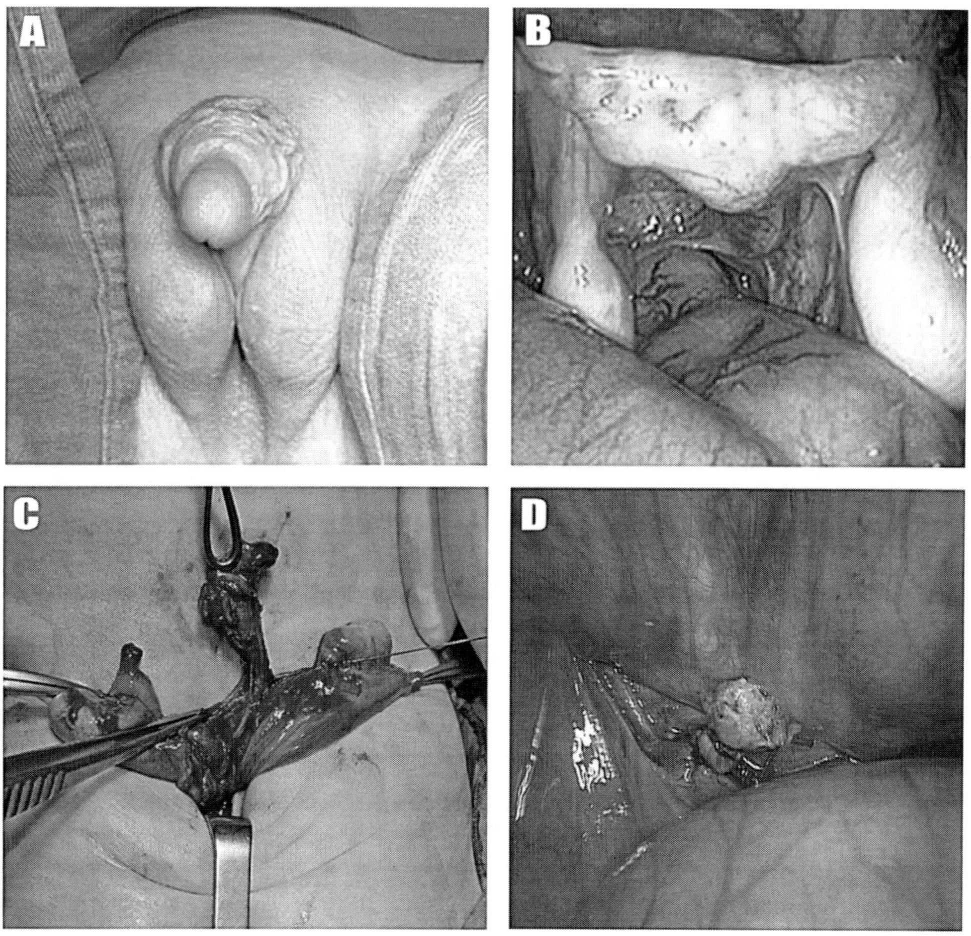

Figure 80. Ambiguous genitalia (A). Video-assisted procedure: the remnant is identified between dysgenetic gonads (A); the remnant is exteriorized through the umbilicus (B) and it is removed after isolation outside the abdomen (C-D).

Complications

Complications are related to the remnant dissection with possible damage of bladder neck, the urethra, the rectum, the uterus, vas, the prostate and the seminal vesicles.

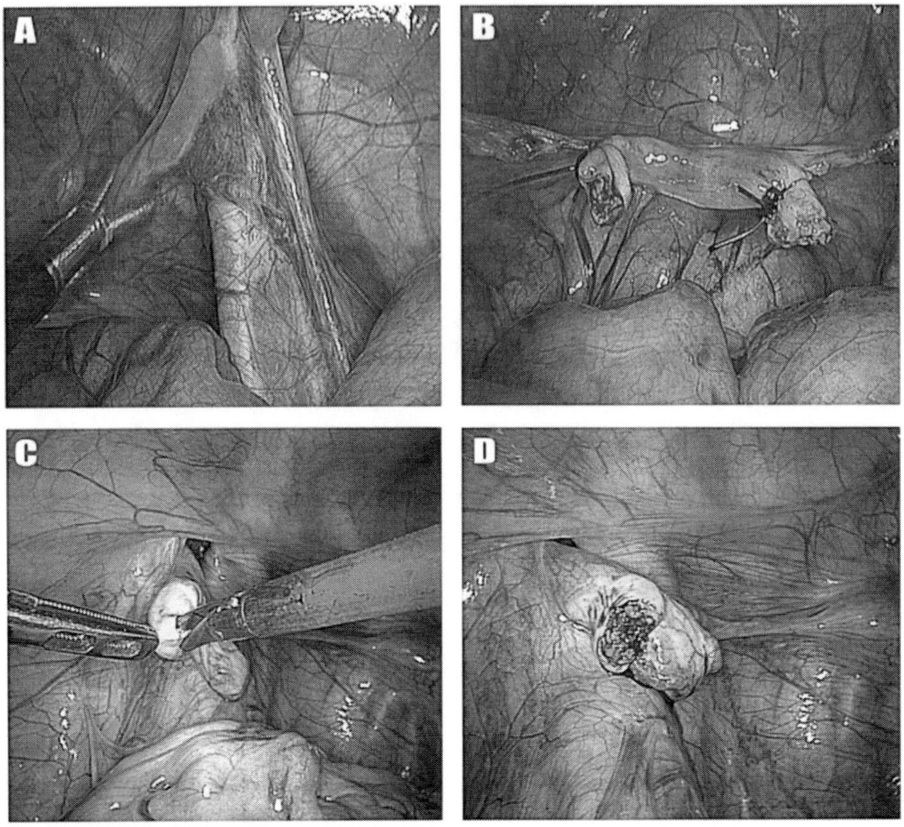

Figure 81. Laparoscopic gonadal biopsy in a case of peripheral androgen insensitivity (A, B). Laparoscopic identification of a gonadal streak (C) and its laparoscopic removal (D). Gonadal streaks are hypoplastic and dysfunctioning gonads with high risk of degeneration.

References

Dénes FT, Mendonça BB, Arap S. Laparoscopic management of intersexual states. *Urol Clin North Am.* 2001 Feb;28(1):31-42.

Holterhus PM. [Intersex and differences of sex development: background, diagnostics, and concepts of care]. *Bundesgesundheitsblatt Gesundheitsforschung Gesundheitsschutz.* 2013 Dec;56(12):1686-94

Jaruratanasirikul S, Engchaun V. Management of children with disorders of sex development: 20-year experience in southern Thailand. *World J Pediatr.* 2013 Jun 17.

Kim KS, Kim J. Disorders of sex development. *Korean J Urol.* 2012 Jan;53(1):1-8.

Öçal G. Current concepts in disorders of sexual development. *J Clin Res Pediatr Endocrinol.* 2011;3(3):105-14.

Ovarian Tissue Cryopreservation

Introduction

Ovarian tissue cryopreservation is an experimental method to restore fertility through surgical tissue collection, cryopreservation and subsequent reimplant in girls who need chemo or radiotherapy and may suffer gonadal toxicity. Tumors are the main indication for a fertility preservation procedure. Indications to perform ovarian tissue cryopreservation are described in Table 14.

Table 15. Indications for ovarian tissue collection for cryopreservation

Neoplasm	Benign pathologies
Rhabdomyosarcoma	*Autoimmune diseases*
Osteosarcoma	Systemic lupus erythematosus
Sarcoblastoma	Nephritic syndromes
Sacral tumors	*Bone marrow transplant*
Wilms tumor	Falciform anemia
Hepatoblastoma	Major thalassemia
Neuroblastoma	*Endocrinal and genetic disorders*
Leukemia	Turner syndrome
Lymphomas	Galactosemia
	Familiarity for premature ovarian failure

The survival rate in patients affected by malignancies has increased thanks to new aggressive chemo and radiotherapy protocols. These protocols, however, may lead to fertility alterations and ovarian function loss. The problem of the loss of ovarian function has addressed research towards techniques that may preserve future fertility. The most widespread is the embryo cryopreservation that requires a stable couple and pubertal patients over 18 years old. Therefore it is not applicable in children or young teenagers.

A recent alternative is the ovarian tissue cryopreservation that offers great promise although still in the experimental stage. Ovarian tissue is preserved until the patient recovers and it is then reimplanted (orthotropic or heterotrophic reimplant). Orthotropic sites of reimplantation are the residual ovary or a peritoneal pocket in the ovarian fossa that permit a spontaneous pregnancy but are not recommended in case of pelvic irradiation. Heterotrophic sites are the subcutaneous forearm or abdominal tissue. Reimplant allows future pregnancies and endocrine function recovery and thus puberty induction. Laparoscopy has given a huge boost to the spread of this technique; surgery moreover does not result in a delay of the oncological treatment. During the surgical procedure it is also possible to move residual gonads in order to reduce effects of local therapy.

The procedure is not applicable in case of ovarian neoplasm, HBV-HCV-HIV-Treponema pallidum infection (for the risk of a new infection after reimplantation);

Prior to surgery all patients undergo the following protocol:

- Hormonal evaluation: FSH, LH, progesterone, estradiol, PRL, testosterone, 17-OH progesterone, estrone, TSH, androstenedione, DHEA-S;

- Virological evaluation: HBs Ag, Ab HCV, HIV, TPHA;
- IL-2, IL-6, IL-8, TNFα;
- Inhibin B, anti-mullerian hormone (ovarian damage indexes);
- Pelvic US: to exclude the presence of pelvic/ovarian masses and to evaluate the ovarian tissue;
- Antibiotic prophylaxis.

Surgery

Undamaged samples should be taken before the beginning of the chemo-radiotherapy. Sometimes it is possible to perform the procedure during the first cycles of therapy.

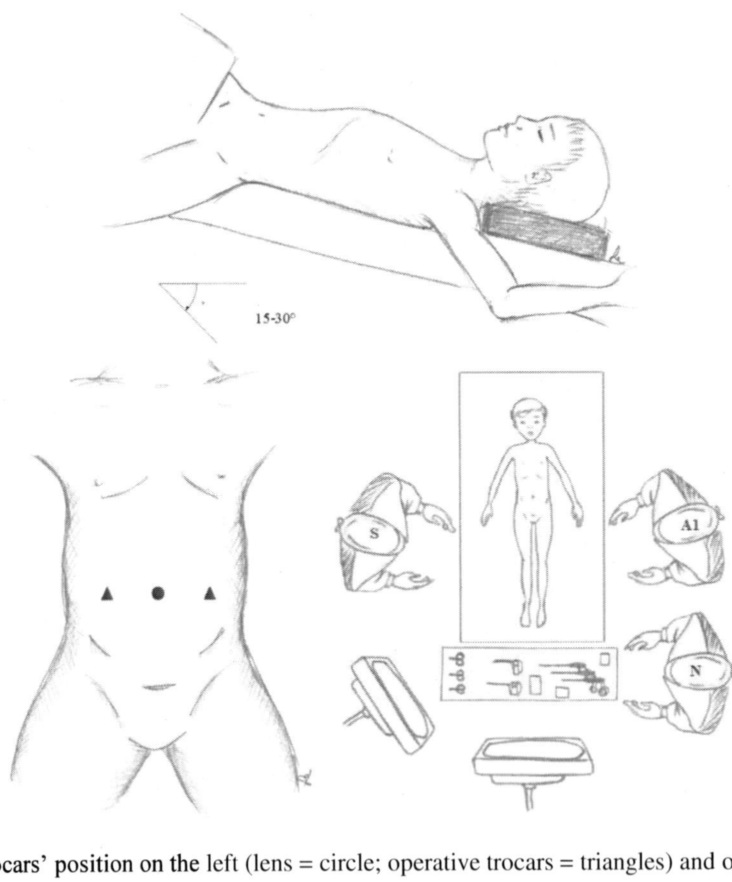

Figure 82. Trocars' position on the left (lens = circle; operative trocars = triangles) and operative set-up on the right.

A 10 mm port for the 0° optic is inserted through the umbilicus with open technique (sub-umbilical semi-circular "smile" incision). Pneumoperitoneum is created with 10 mmHg of pressure and 0.5-1 L/min of flow (depending on patient's size). Two additional operative trocars are inserted under direct vision. The abdominal and pelvic cavities are inspected. Each ovary is grasped with blunt forceps and it is longitudinally cut with cold scissors in order to obtain a sample. Cautery should be avoided during this step because it could damage the tissue. We try to collect almost 2/3 of each ovary with a clean, precise and straight cut.

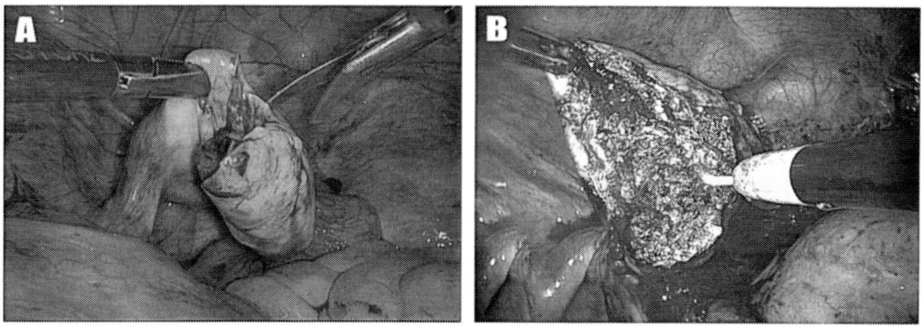

Figure 83. The ovarian tissue is cut with cold scissors (A). Argon gas is used for bleeding control (B).

The specimen is then extracted through the umbilical wound. A finger glove may be useful to avoid the damage of huge samples that are immediately transferred for cryopreservation. Hemostasis is performed at the end of the procedure with bipolar cautery or with Argon plasma coagulator. Accurate washing is useful to remove clots and to exclude the presence of residual bleeding. A pelvic drain is left in all cases. If necessary, gonads can be transposed by fixing them near the anterior-superior iliac spines or the paracolic gutter after ovarian ligament-mesovary section. Alternatively gonads may be fixed to the posterior uterine wall.

The vesical catheter is removed at the end of surgery and the pelvic drain after 24 hours. Antibiotics are administrated for 5 days. Overall hospital stay lasts 1-2 days.

Complications

Although rare, the most feared complication is post-operative bleeding that may lead to hemoperitoneum and can require red blood cell transfusion.

References

Chemaitilly W, Mertens AC, Mitby P, Whitton J, Stovall M, Yasui Y, et al. Acute ovarian failure in the childhood cancer survivor study. *J Clin Endocrinol Metab.* 2006;91:1723–8.

Donnez J, Dolmans MM. Cryopreservation and transplantation of ovarian tissue. *Clin Obstet Gynecol.* 2010;53:787–96.

Donnez J, Jadoul P, Squifflet J, Van Langendonckt A, Donnez O, Van Eyck AS, et al. Ovarian tissue cryopreservation and transplantation in cancer patients. *Best Pract Res Clin Obstet Gynaecol.* 2010;24:87– 100.

Fabbri R, Vicenti R, Macciocca M, Pasquinelli G, Lima M, Parazza I, Magnani V, Venturoli S. Cryopreservation of ovarian tissue in pediatric patients. *Obstet Gynecol Int.* 2012;2012:910698. Epub 2012 Feb 13..

Feigin E, Abir R, Fisch B, Kravarusic D, Steinberg R, Nitke S, Avrahami G, Ben-Haroush A, Freud E. Laparoscopic ovarian tissue preservation in young patients at risk for ovarian failure as a result of chemotherapy/irradiation for primary malignancy. *J Pediatr Surg.* 2007 May;42(5):862-4.

Gracia CR, Chang J, Kondapalli L, Prewitt M, Carlson CA, Mattei P, Jeffers S, Ginsberg JP. Ovarian tissue cryopreservation for fertility preservation in cancer patients: successful establishment and feasibility of a multidisciplinary collaboration. *J Assist Reprod Genet.* 2012 Jun;29(6):495-502.

Green DM, Sklar CA, Boice Jr JD, Mulvihill JJ, Whitton JA, Stovall M, et al. Ovarian failure and reproductive outcomes after childhood cancer treatment: results from the Childhood Cancer Survivor Study. *J Clin Oncol.* 2009;27:2374–81.

Sanchez-Serrano M, Crespo J, Mirabet V, Cobo AC, Escriba MJ, Simon C, et al. Twins born after transplantation of human ovarian cortical tissue and oocyte vitrification. *Fertil Steril.* 2010;93:268.e11–3.

Schmidt KT, Rosendahl M, Ernst E, Loft A, Andersen AN, Dueholm M, et al. Autotransplantation of cryopreserved ovarian tissue in 12 women with chemotherapy-induced premature ovarian failure: the Danish experience. *Fertil Steril.* 2011;95:695–701

W.H. Wallace, A.B. Thomson, T.W. Kelsey. The radiosensitivity of the human oocyte. *Hum Reprod,* 18 (2003), pp. 117–121.

Anesthesiologic Considerations

Pediatric Laparoscopy and Surgical Trauma

Laparoscopic videosurgery is becoming increasingly more important in pediatric surgery for both diagnosis and surgical treatment. Several authors who have compared this technique to traditional surgery for the treatment of some pathologies, have reported reduced surgical trauma, less postoperative pain, reduced perioperative morbidity, a shorter period of postoperative ileus, earlier postoperative mobilization, shorter periods of disability, shorter hospital stays and better cosmetic results in favor of laparoscopic video surgery. Other benefits, compared to traditional "open" operative techniques, include the avoidance of large incisions, less fluid loss, heat and forced retraction of tissues.

Physiopathologic Effects of Pediatric Laparoscopic Surgery

An optimal approach to the planning of anesthesia for laparoscopy entails knowledge of the technical requirements and an understanding of the physiological alterations associated with the procedure.

Physiological changes during laparoscopic surgery are related to the changes resulting from the increased abdominal pressure (IAP) associated with the insufflation of the abdomen, the patient's postural modifications (head-up or head-down), and the CO_2 absorption and its general effects. The magnitude of the physiological perturbations associated with laparoscopy is influenced by the patient's age, the patient's underlying myocardial and respiratory function, and the anesthetic drugs administered.

The airway and cardiovascular systems of children have characteristics that differ from those of adults: the former have less functional residual capacity (FRC), collapse volume is much closer to FRC, and both lung compliance and airway resistance are adversely related to lung size. Infants and young children have fewer alveoli than adults do. The number increases during childhood, from approximately 20 million after birth to 300 million by 8 years of age. Therefore, infants and young children have a relatively small area for gas exchange. The alveolus is small. Alveolar size increases from 150-180 to 250-300 μm during childhood. The infant's systemic vascular resistance is lower. Heart rate plays a more important role in determining cardiac output, and there is a high metabolism and O_2 consumption.

Tension pneumoperitoneum causes an elevation in IAP, which produces important effects on cardiovascular, pulmonary, renal and metabolic function.

Effects on Respiratory System

Pneumoperitoneum and increase in IAP cause cephalic displacement of the diaphragm, resulting in the reduction in lung volumes including vital capacity, total lung volume and FRC. This phenomenon is exacerbated by the cephalic shift of the abdominal contents in the head-down position. Pulmonary compliance is reduced and airway resistance is increased, producing a higher airway pressure for any given tidal volume with an increased risk of hemodynamic changes and barotrauma during intermittent positive pressure ventilation (IPPV). Restriction in diaphragmatic mobility promotes uneven distribution of ventilation to the non-dependent part of the lung, resulting in ventilation-perfusion mismatch with hypercarbia and hypoxaemia. This preferential ventilation is increased further by supine position, inhalational anesthetic agents, and neuromuscular blockade.

Another important respiratory implication is represented by CO_2 insufflation. Insufflated CO_2 is rapidly absorbed across the peritoneum and can lead to an increase in total body CO_2 content. If ventilation is controlled and not changed in response to this increase, then the arterial pCO_2 will rise.

Effects on the Cardiocirculatory System

In recent years, important knowledge has been obtained about the cardiovascular changes induced by pneumoperitoneum in children. Routine clinical measurements, such as heart rate and blood pressure, have been used to assess the hemodynamic changes induced by laparoscopy. Studies so far have shown most effects on blood pressure, which often increases, while there are none or only slight effects on heart rate. Experimental studies on the intraperitoneal insufflation of young animals have also shown an increase in venous return, peripheral arterial resistance with impaired splanchnic circulation, cardiac output and cardiac index. In pigs weighing 3 to 8 kg the presence of hypercarbia during peritoneal insufflation increased heart rate, left ventricular stroke work and cardiac index, without changes in total peripheral resistance or central venous pressure. A study concerning the hemodynamic effects of pneumoperitoneum in healthy infants, by continuous oesophageal aortic blood flow echo-doppler, demonstrated that the abdominal insufflation with a pressure of 10 mmHg resulted in a significant decrease in aortic blood flow and stroke volume, and in a significant increase in systemic vascular resistance.

Another study examined cardiovascular changes associated with intra-abdominal insufflation (10 mmHg) using echocardiography with transthoracic approach. Systolic blood pressure (SBP) and diastolic blood pressure (DBP) increased during intra-abdominal insufflation. Heart rate (HR) remained regular. Pneumoperitoneum was associated with increases in left ventricular end-diastolic volume (EDV), left ventricular end-systolic volume (ESV) and left ventricular end-systolic meridional wall stress (LVESWS). Before, during and after intra-abdominal insufflation, systolic function indexes, left ventricular fractional shortening (LVFS) and ejection fraction (LVEF), underwent slight, insignificant changes. During the surgical procedure LVFS and LVEF remained within a range above 25% and 55%, respectively. Furthermore there are no variations in the LVESWS/LVFS ratio. In this study, pneumoperitoneum induction determined the increase in both EDV and ESV. The EDV is recognized as a good indicator of preload; the increase is mostly due to a drainage effect on the splanchnic circulation, with an increase in venous return to the right heart. The increase in ESV could be partly the result of slightly impaired contractility, probably affected negatively by anaesthetic drugs, and partly of an acute increase in afterload, more correctly expressed as aortic impedance. The myocardial left ventricular performance remains stable in all our patients, as shown by the absence of any modification in the LVFS and LVEF. A parallel increase in ESV explains why LVFS and LVEF did not change significantly. These results could represent the balanced effect of the increase in both preload and afterload induced by elevated intra-abdominal pressure, through a combined action on venous return and aortic impedance.

Pneumoperitoneum in children has a major impact on cardiac volumes and function, mainly through the effect on ventricular load conditions. The acute increase in IAP affects both preload and afterload, while the systolic cardiac performance remains unchanged. The final advice of these studies was to remain prudent before subjecting a child with cardiopathy to laparoscopy. To date, the literature has reported many experiences of laparoscopy in children with cardiac disease, offering reassuring messages about this procedure and its outcome. Today the culture and experience exists to improve or complete the mosaic of pediatric heart diseases, relating the cardiocirculatory changes of laparoscopy to the various pathophysiological and clinical profiles of homogeneous groups of children with similar heart lesions.

Anesthesiological Approach

The studies in the literature consider it very important in pediatric patients to achieve a level of anesthesia, which on the one hand allows a safe execution of the surgical procedure, and on the other does not cause any significant effects on cardiorespiratory function, which is already subject to the pathophysiological changes previously considered.

Modern anesthetic techniques, the wide availability of drugs, and the accuracy of the monitoring of vital signs provide a high level of security in performing anesthesia.

Preoperative Evaluation, Risk Formulation and Informed Consent

Preoperative assessment will, as in all cases, take account of medical and anaesthetic history, allergies and visualization of the venous condition. The physical examination also focuses on the cardiorespiratory system, but begins with the pathology, the global assessment and clinical status of the child. The American Society of Anesthesia developed the classification of Physical Status (ASA) to define a correlation between clinical condition and tolerance to surgery. The evaluation of the risk requires a global view. Correct information about all possible anesthesia techniques (a pamphlet should be given before anesthesiological visit) and in particular about the proposed tailored procedures, must be provided before acquiring the written consent for anesthesia. Specific risks such as difficult airway management, or cardiac, respiratory, neurologic, metabolic conditions are annotated on the anesthesiological chart and on the operatory list.

Premedication and Preoperative Fasting

At the end of the global evaluation a pharmacological medication is considered. Parents are allowed to be present at the induction of anesthesia. Sedative premedication is recommendable: midazolam (500 mcg/kg) by mouth is currently the most frequently used drug. An anticholinergic drug may be given to prevent bradycardia associated with peritoneal insufflation of carbon dioxide. Atropine, however, can be administered during anesthesia induction only after vein placement. A local anesthetic emulsion (lidocaine 25 mg + prilocaine 25 mg) or medicated plaster (lidocaine 70 mg/tetracaine 70 mg, for children over 3 years) is applied on a detectable peripheric vein. Preoperative fasting is indicated for elective surgery, to avoid inhalation syndrome at anesthesia induction. Current indications suggest that fasting must be shorter and has the sole aim of maintaining the stomach empty.

Anaesthetic Management

Anesthesia management can be performed by inhalation or intravenous hypnotics, associated with opioids, neuromuscular blocking agents and adjuvant drugs, if necessary. Sometimes only light general anesthesia is administered combined with regional anesthesia. It is common to avoid the use of nitrous oxide since this may distend the bowel particularly during prolonged procedures where it can be a cause of postoperative nausea and vomiting.

Anesthetic induction techniques include either inhalation techniques with halogenated gases or the use of intravenous anesthetic agents (Tab. 16).

Table 16. Drugs used during anesthesia in pediatric age

Drugs	Induction doses	Maintaining doses
Anesthetic agents		
Sevoflurane *	1-8% (2-3 MAC)	2-3% (1 MAC)
Thiopental	3-6 mg/kg	
Propofol	2.5-3 mg/kg	9-12 mg/kg/h
Opioids		
Fentanyl	1-2 mcg/kg	1-3 mcg/kg/h
Alfentanyl	7-15 mcg/kg	0.5-1,5 mcg/kg/min
Remifentanyl	0.5-1 mcg/kg	0.3-1 mcg/kg/min
Neuromuscular blocking agents		
Atracurium besylate	0.3-0.5 mg/kg	0.2-0.4 mg/kg/h
Cisatracurium besylate	0.15-0.25 mg/kg	0.1-0.3 mg/kg/h
Vecuronium	0.08-0.1 mg/kg	0.06-0.08 mg/kg/h
Rocuronium	0.45-0.6 mg/kg	0.3-0.6 mg/kg/h

* Sevoflurane is a halogenated gas. Its administration is related to MAC (minimum alveolar concentration).

Sevoflurane is the most frequently halogenated inhalational anesthetic drug employed in pediatric anesthesia. The inhalation form, with sevoflurane at an increasing concentration from 1% to 8%, is often adopted in patients younger than 4 years. Inhalation anesthesia allows for a rapid recovery but agitation is at times present and is considered an adverse effect.

The intravenous approach has been more often chosen when a topical anaesthetic cream or plaster has been routinely applied on a visible vein to permit the cannulation without pain. Thiopentone was in the past considered the most commonly used intravenous agent for anesthesia induction. Propofol is now the most frequently used agent for pediatrics.

In many cases tracheal intubation is preceded by a fentanyl or remifentanyl administration and facilitated by atracurium besylate or cisatracurium besylate or vecuronium or rocuronium administration. Depending on the age and the surgical necessity, tracheal intubation was performed both with an oral or nasal tracheal tube (uncuffed in patients younger than 7 yrs., cuffed in patients older than 7 yrs.).

After induction of anesthesia a nasogastric tube should be placed and suctioned. This increases visibility for the surgeon and protects the stomach from injury resulting from instrumentation with the Veress needle, while at the same time lowering the risk of regurgitation during the increase of IAP. This will also usually be required after laparoscopic fundoplication. In operative laparoscopy a vesicle catheter was placed to constantly empty the bladder and to monitor diuresis.

Inhalational or intravenous agents require maintenance of anesthesia. Although brief diagnostic procedures may be performed with laryngeal mask airway and spontaneous ventilation, the majority of laparoscopic surgery procedures require tracheal intubation and controlled ventilation for the duration of the case. Fentanyl or remifentanyl promote adequate anesthesia without interfering with cardiocirculatory stability. The neuromuscular blockade always facilitates the surgical procedure. This enables minute ventilation to be increased to in order to deal with the CO_2 load and to maintain normocarbia. Ventilatory strategies include increasing tidal volume and/or respiratory rate. Peak inspiratory pressures may increase and the pressure limit on pressure-cycled ventilators may need to be adjusted.

The bispectral index is used to observe the anesthesiologic plan and drug consumption but results do not differ from conventional clinical practice.

After starting the pneumoperitoneum the position of the tracheal tube needs to be checked again to exclude an endobronchial position, which can result from the diaphragm and lungs being shifted upwards relative to the tube.

It is important not to exceed an intra-abdominal pressure of 6 mmHg in newborns, 8 mmHg in infants and 12 mmHg in older children so as to minimize the negative effects on cardiocirculatory function and cardiac output. The IAP reading should be clearly visible to the anesthesiologist and documented on the record.

The combination of locoregional with general anesthesia is also practiced during laparoscopic surgery. A variety of locoregional anesthetic techniques have been described starting from neuraxial blocks such as the caudal epidural block and the lumbar epidural block, but currently peripheral nerve blocks, such as the ilioinguinal-iliohypogastric nerve block, the rectus sheath block and the trasversus abdominis plane (TAP) block are widely used. These provide effective pain relief and muscle relaxation for laparoscopy. The pain protection and the use of minimum efficacy doses of drugs are well conjuncted in the combined use of general and locoregional anesthesia techniques in all pediatric ages.

Nevertheless, in contrast to adults, locoregional anesthesia in children is characterized by remarkable hemodynamic stability. In particular, limited cardiovascular modifications are observed along with changes in patient position. This seems to be linked to two factors: the relatively small venous capacity in the lower extremities of children and the relative lack of resting sympathetic peripheral vascular tone. Currently selected local anesthetics for pediatric techniques are left-handed enantiomers (levobupivacaine and ropivacaine) and this makes the technique safer.

Vascular Access, Intraoperative Infusions and Temperature Control

Vascular access is necessary in all types of laparoscopic surgery: the peripheral vein is the first approach at induction of anesthesia; clinical conditions and the severity of surgery will indicate the need for a central venous catheter (CVC) both for the monitoring of central venous pressure (CVP) and for rapid and safe infusions of fluid and blood. Ultrasound guidance during the placement of CVC is currently the best percutaneous procedure.

Fluid replacement is necessary to maintain the hydroelectrolytic homeostasis and acido-basic balance. A correct fluid intraoperative plan should consider the metabolic requirement, pre-operatory fasting, "third space" sequestration, surgery related to fluid/blood loss and particular conditions such as the use of radiant lamps in neonatal age. Intra-surgical crystalloid infusion was 20 ml/kg during the first hour in patients under 3 yrs. and 15 ml/kg for older patients; in the hours that followed, the infusion dosage was 8-10 ml/kg/h for all patients. The infusion used was 1-2% dextrose in polyelectrolite solution or in quarter-strength normal saline solution (0.2% NaCl) and lactated Ringer's solution.

Laparoscopic procedures in pediatric patients are associated with less insensible fluid losses than most equivalent open procedures and reduced heat loss. This is generally beneficial but hypothermia remains a potential risk if the temperature is not measured and steps to prevent it are not taken. A warming mattress, a heat-moisture exchange filter for breathing systems and the use of laparo-insufflator with heated CO_2 are necessary.

Intraoperative Monitoring

The cardiovascular function is monitored by heart rate, systolic blood pressure, and diastolic blood pressure; when clinically necessary the radial arterial catheter and CVC are placed for the invasive monitoring of arterial blood pressure and central venous pressure respectively.

The respiratory function is monitored by peripheral arterial oxygen saturation (SpO_2), end-tidal CO_2 ($EtCO_2$) and measure of respiratory frequency, tidal volume (inspiratory and expiratory), and minute volume, as well as peak inspiratory pressure and mean airway pressure by means of a mechanical ventilator. $EtCO_2$ monitoring is important but it must be appreciated that this may not always accurately reflect arterial carbon dioxide tension ($paCO_2$). Reliance on the use of $EtCO_2$ concentration, as an indicator of $paCO_2$, may occasionally be inaccurate and this is particularly likely in subjects with respiratory diseases, in neonates and small infants or if an excessive IAP increases the dead space during laparoscopy. In some cases, reliance on the $EtCO_2$ may lead to inappropriate ventilation strategies and it may be more appropriate, particularly during prolonged laparoscopic surgical procedures or in neonates and infants, to perform a capillary or arterial blood gas analysis to accurately measure arterial CO_2 tension.

Monitoring also includes body temperature, urine output and inspiratory and expiratory concentration of volatile anesthetics. In pediatric patients the neuromuscular blockade is monitored by stimulating the ulnar nerve using the train-of-four pattern of stimulation.

Postoperative Care and Pain Management

The respiratory and cardiocirculatory effects of the pneumoperitoneum rarely have an adverse effect on postoperative functions; however in some clinical conditions intensive postoperative treatment can be indicated in children after laparoscopic surgery (Tab 17).

Pain following and after laparoscopy results from a variety of maneuvers as well as the surgical trauma, rapid distension of the peritoneum, and excitation of the phrenic nerve with CO_2.

Postoperative pain is best controlled by a multimodal approach consisting of locoregional anesthesia, single-shot infiltration of local anesthetics in laparoscopic working ports, opioids, used especially in intensive care treatments, and non-steroidal anti-inflammatory drugs (NSAIDs) used in the ward (Tab 18). Tramadol is the most common opioid class drug used in the ward. The action of NSAIDs is explained by the inhibition of the activity of both *cyclooxygenase-1*, cyclooxygenase-2 and thereby the synthesis of *prostaglandins* and thromboxanes.

Table 17. Postoperative intensive care in pediatric laparoscopy: admission criteria

Cardiac diseases (Low cardiac output state, congenital heart disease)
Need for vascular expansion
Respiratory diseases (Bronchopulmonary dysplasia, recurrent “ab ingestis” episodes)
Severe neurological, renal, hepatic diseases
Severe diseases with ASA risk class III-IV
Pneumoperitoneum > 180’
Neonate and infant < 3 month with pneumoperitoneum > 60’
High $EtCO_2$ and SpO_2 variations
Major modifications in ventilatory and cardiocirculatory parameters during peritoneal insufflation

Table 18. Doses and method of postoperative administration of tramadol and main non-steroidal anti-inflammatory drugs (NSAIDs) used in children

Drugs	Administration	Dose (kg/day)	N° times (day)	Continuous infusion
Acetylsalicyl acid	oral, intravenous	60-80 mg	4	
Ibuprofen	oral, intravenous	30-40 mg	3-4	
Ketoprofen	oral, intravenous	5-7.5 mg	3	
Ketorolac	oral, intravenous	1-1.5 mg	3	
Naproxen	oral, intravenous	10-20 mg	2	
Paracetamol	oral, rectal	60-90 mg	4-6	
Paracetamol	intravenous	60-90 mg	4-6	
Tramadol	oral, intravenous	2-3 mg	2-3	0.1-0.25 mg/kg/h

References

ASA Committee on Standards and Practice Parameters (2011) Practice Guidelines for Preoperative Fasting and the Use of Pharmacologic Agents to Reduce the Risk of Pulmonary Aspiration: Application to Healthy Patients Undergoing Elective Procedures: An Updated Report by ASA Committee on Standards and Practice Parameters. *Anesthesiology* 114:495-511.

Bozkurt P, Kaya G, Altinas F, Yeker Y, Sarimurat N. Systemic stress response during operations for acute abdominal pain performed via laparoscopy or laparotomy in children. *Anesthesia; 55*:5-9, 2000.

Fahy BG, Barnas GM, Flowers JL, Nagle SE, Njoku MJ: The effects of increased abdominal pressure on lung and chest wall mechanics during laparoscopic surgery. *Anesth Analg* 1995;81:744-50.

Fujimoto T, Segawa O, Lane GJ, Esaki S, Miyano T. Laparoscopic surgery in newborn infants. *Surg Endosc;*13:773-7, 1999.

Gentili A, Iannettone CM, Pigna A, Landuzzi V, Lima M, Baroncini S. Cardiocirculatory changes during videolaparoscopy in children: echocardiographic study. *Paediatr Anaesth* 2000;10:399-406.

Gentili A, Landuzzi V, Pasini L, Lima M. The laparoscopic approach in children with cardiopathy: a mosaic still awaiting completion. *Paediatr Anaesth.* 2014 Mar;24(3):351-2.

Hamza J: Physiologie périnatale. In: Saint-Maurice C (eds): Manuel d'anesthésie pédiatrique. Paris: *Ed Pradel,* 1994:1-16.

Masey SA, Koehler RC, Buck JR. Effect of abdominal distension on central and regional hemodynamics in neonatal lambs. *Pediatr Res* 1985;19:1244-9.

Motoyama EK: Respiratory physiology in infants and children. In: Smith's: Anesthesia for infants and children. St Louis: *Mosby,* 1996:3-67.

Pelosi P, Foti G, Cereda M, Manetti B, Volpe N, Montagna G, Presti A: Respiratory mechanics during laparoscopic cholecystectomy. *Am Rev Respir Dis* 1992;145:A156.

Serafini G, Ingelmo PM, Astuto M, Baroncini S, Borrometi F, Bortone L, Ceschin C, Gentili A, Lampugnani E et al. Preoperative evaluation in infants and children: recommendations of the Italian Society of pediatric and neonatal anesthesia and intensive care (SARNePI) *Min Anest* 2013 Oct 31.

Sfez M, Guérard A, Desruelle P: Cardiorespiratory changes during laparoscopic fundoplication in children. *Paed Anaesth* 1995;5:9-95.

Sfez M. Anesthésie pour coeliochirurgie en pédiatrie. *Ann Fr Anesth Réanim* 1994;13: 221-32.

Strafford MA: Cardiovascular physiology. In: Smith's: Anesthesia for infants and children. St. Louis: *Mosby,* 1996:69-104.

Tobias JD, Holcomb GW, Brock JW, Deshpande JK, Lowe S, Morgan WM. Cardiorespiratory changes in children during laparoscopy. *J Pediatr Surg* 1995;30:33-6.

Tobias JD. Anesthetic management for pediatric laparoscopy and thoracoscopy. In: Lobe TE, Schropp KP, eds. Pediatric laparoscopy and thoracoscopy, 1th edn. Philadelphia: *W B Saunders Company,* 1994:59-66.

In: Laparoscopy
Editor: Christos Iavazzo

ISBN: 978-1-63321-404-0

Chapter 13

Complications of Laparoscopic Surgery

José M. Beleña, M.D., Ph.D.[1,•]
and Mónica Nuñez, M.D.[2,#]
[1]Staff Anesthesiologist, Department of Anesthesiology and Critical Care, Sureste University Hospital, Arganda del Rey, Madrid, Spain
[2]Staff Anesthesiologist, Department of Anesthesiology and Critical Care, Ramón y Cajal University Hospital, Madrid, Spain

Abstract

Laparoscopic surgery is a very common and widely established technique. Benefits include decreased postoperative pain, improved patient satisfaction (including cosmetic results), reduced hospital stay and fewer postoperative complications compared with open techniques. The range of surgical techniques is increasing in complexity and also the kind of patients undergoing these procedures (pluripathological patients, associating co-morbidity). The number of emergency operations performed laparoscopically has been increased as well. Complications of laparoscopic surgery are mainly divided into three groups: complications derived from pneumoperitoneum, complications caused by the surgical procedure and postoperative complications.

The most common alterations caused by the pneumoperitoneum are raised intra-abdominal pressure and physiological effects especially within cardiovascular and respiratory systems, which have significant effects on the patient, especially if they are elderly or have associated morbidity, but also some complications such as severe hypercarbia, cardio-pulmonary compromise, air embolism or gas migration (subcutaneous emphysema, pneumomediastinum and pneumothorax) can occur.

Complications of the operative procedure can be grouped into two categories: complications of access and complications of technique. Complications of access or trocar entry include: hollow or solid viscus perforation, abdominal wall or major vessel injury, incisional hernia and peritoneal tumor cell implantation. In case of complications derived from the surgical technique, we can include: hemorrhage, vascular injury,

• Email: josemariabelena@yahoo.es.
Email: monicamurias@hotmail.com.

retroperitoneal hematoma, bile leak, bile duct injury, bile peritonitis (with or without a bile duct injury).

Postoperative complications include: intestinal perforation, bile leak, retroperitoneal hematoma, pancreatitis, subhepatic abscess and postoperative air embolism.

Complications Derived from Pneumoperitoneum

The most fatal complication in laparoscopy, as in any surgical procedure, is death. The first large series of cases that analyzed this complication goes back to the 70s, specifically from 1975-78. In this series, 25,000 gynecological laparoscopies were analyzed, surgical and diagnostic, founding a mortality rate of 0.008 % [1]. In 1998, on a sample of nearly 30,000 patients undergoing gynecological laparoscopy, also surgical and diagnostic, a mortality of 0.003 % and a morbidity of 0.46 % were obtained [2].

Regarding laparoscopic cholecystectomy series are not that big, but in a meta-analysis published in 1996, mortality can be set between 0.086 and 0.16 %, significantly higher than gynecological laparoscopic procedures, but less than laparotomy cholecystectomies, which reported a mortality rate between 0.66 and 0.74 % [3].

There are other complications, such as those derived from the laparoscopic technique including complications arising from the creation of pneumoperitoneum and insertion of the trocars and those derived from the inlet of the trocars, such as abscesses and hernias or implant tumor cells in the inlet of the trocars. However, in this chapter, we will focus on complications arising from the use of gas for the realization of pneumoperitoneum.

We can distinguish two kinds of complications in this regard, extraperitoneal gas diffusion and gas embolism.

Extraperitoneal Gas Diffusion

Extraperitoneal gas diffusion is one of the most common complications in laparoscopy, its incidence varies between 0.4 and 2% [4]. The most frequent places for pneumoperitoneum gas diffusion are: retroperitoneum, pleural cavity, mediastinum and subcutaneous tissue. In general, the gas flow to these locations comes by a given pressure of pneumoperitoneum.

1. Dissemination to Retroperitoneum

Retroperitoneal space tolerates greater pressures than peritoneum does, so that, the accumulation of CO_2 only involves the disadvantage of the subsequent gas absorption.

2. Diffusion into Pleural Space

Carbon dioxide diffusion into the pleural space will cause a pneumothorax. The mechanism postulated as the cause of pneumothorax is the passage of gas through weak spots or defects in the diaphragm. Usually the pneumothorax will develop subclinical because, as mentioned above, the gas diffusion occurs at low pressure, but it can sometimes manifest by changes in the thoraco-abdominal elastic properties. Intraoperatively, we treat it by increasing PEEP level so we get increased intrathoracic pressures and limit the passage of air from the peritoneal cavity [5].

Pneumothorax is often associated with pneumomediastinum and subcutaneous emphysema [6]. Sometimes there have been described reports involving iatrogenic valve mechanism, either by barotrauma secondary to increased intrapulmonary pressures [7], either by direct surgical trauma such as a pneumothorax after insertion of the trocar and insufflation of CO_2 during a cholecystectomy [8]. In these cases, the use of PEEP aggravates the situation and may need urgent drainage due to the risk of tension pneumothorax.

3. Dissemination to Mediastinum

It usually does not produce symptoms, but sometimes, if severe, it may presents with substernal pain. When it happens, is usually accompanied by subcutaneous emphysema at suprasternal recess.

It is characteristic, though rare, the Hamman's sign, a synchronous snap with the heartbeat which is best heard at the left lateral position. Diagnosis is confirmed by a chest radiograph. It usually does not require treatment, but is eliminated faster when breathing high concentrations of oxygen.

4. Dissemination Subcutaneous Tissue

Subcutaneous emphysema incidence is low and is mainly due to inadvertent extraperitoneal insufflation or insufflation intraperitoneal extension. The causes may be the incorrect position of the trocar or intraoperative mobilization.

The proper use of automatic insufflator CO_2 avoids this complication, since pressure reported at space which is the needle and insufflation stops if it exceeds the preset limit. However, it is not uncommon to produce this type of complication.

Subcutaneous emphysema increases the CO_2 diffusion area and it can result in a significant respiratory acidosis. In any patient undergoing laparoscopic surgery with subcutaneous emphysema, we should auscultate both lungs, verify the ventilator pressures, permanent arterial blood gases and hemodynamic status monitoring.

Monitoring will show increased CO_2 concentrations in the end -tidal ($ETCO_2$) after reaching the plateau. Both of them, emphysema and pneumothorax, an abrupt increase of $ETCO_2$ is detected. When pneumothorax or pneumomediastinum are associated to subcutaneous emphysema, it is more frequent to find blood saturation fall, hypercapnia and respiratory acidosis [9].

In most cases this complication is resolved after abdominal deflation. If emphysema extends to the chest wall and neck, CO_2 can reach the chest or mediastinum and may produce pneumothorax or pneumomediastinum. Whenever we have clinical suspicion, we have to perform a control chest radiography or CT.

It can lead to hypercapnia maintained even after surgery due to gradually reabsortion.

Gas Embolism

Massive gas embolism is the most feared complication in laparoscopic surgery. Its incidence, according to a French study published in 1996 is between 0 - 590 gaseous emboli per 100,000 laparoscopies [10]. Patients who have undergone previous laparotomy are more susceptible to suffer these complications [11].

Passing CO_2 into the bloodstream can result from accidental injection into solid organs or vessels, to the gas inlet through the nozzles open due to vascular tissue dissection, but entry does not occur if the pressure is below 20 mmHg [12]. It is also possible the passage of gas during deflation of peritoneal cavity to the blood by the pressure drop and finally due to the accumulation of gas in the portal system when decompressing the abdomen.

Carbon dioxide has several advantages over other gases for use in laparoscopy, such as not support combustion or being a very soluble gas. Its high solubility prevents the formation of large bubbles and has been shown in animal studies that are tolerated up to 7.5 ml / kg in blood; also prevents nitrous oxide diffuse into CO_2 bubbles and increase their size.

Regarding massive gas embolism clinic, symptoms can be divided into cardiovascular and neurological. With regard to the first, we find right ventricular failure with decreased cardiac output, cape cyanosis, raised jugular venous pressure, tachycardia or bradycardia, severe hypoxemia and pathological heart sounds. As for the neurological manifestations, we can find bilateral mydriasis caused by anoxia, coma, agitation and seizures.

With regard to diagnosis, we would find alterations in the ECG, such as alterations in ventricular axis, arrhythmias or right bundle branch block. $ETCO_2$ value decreases, but it can rise at the beginning. The average pressure in the pulmonary artery rises to 13 mmHg before it is clinically evident. Confirmation of the diagnosis it is showed by the doppler precordial, obtaining more than 2 ml of gas in the right atrium or by esophageal doppler, showing more than 0.05 ml of gas in the right atrium [13].

Treatment consists of removing the peritoneal insufflation, 100% oxygen administration, Durant position (left lateral decubitus and Trendelenburg position, supportive ventricular cardiac massage (internal if possible, because external is less effective), gas suction by central venous catheter and hyperbaric oxygen therapy.

Complications from Laparoscopic Surgical Technique

Laparoscopic surgery is primarily a surgical approach, most of the surgeries, if not all, that are performed by open surgery may be performed laparoscopically, depending on the skills of the surgeon.

Laparoscopic surgery, such any surgery, is capable of having the complications of any surgical procedure regardless of approach.

Specific complications of the laparoscopic approach will be the subject of this section.

Complications from laparoscopic surgical technique are divided into four groups:

- Due to the introduction of the Veress needle, Hasson or different working ports.
- Due to the handling of laparoscopic instruments, more difficult to handle, longer working angle and situations in which the dimension of depth is lost.
- Complications in the gateway of the trocars.
- Complications from the learning curve.

Complications due to the Veress Needle, Hasson Trocar or Introduction of Ports

Important correct use of Hasson and Veress needle , good handling them , check correct placement and if in doubt use the open approach (Figure 1 and 2).

Vascular Injury

Incidence varies from 1% to 6 % depending on the series, most of them are minor vascular lesions of the abdominal wall. Most of the studies refer to epigastric vessel injuries as the most common complication.

In order to avoid it, is important to introduce working ports under direct vision and using transillumination technique. It is also important to control the bleeding immediately in order to avoid a conversion to open surgery due to this cause. Often, the pressure of the trocar is sufficient to cease the bleeding, if points are not applicable to the total thickness of the wall or placing a Foley catheter with inflated balloon which will be removed in the next few hours or the next day [14].

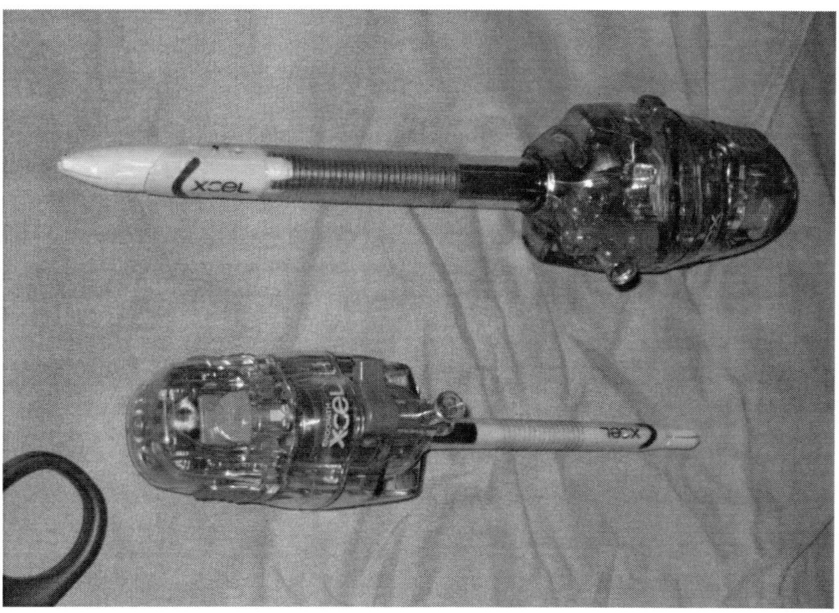

Figure 1. Hasson trocars.

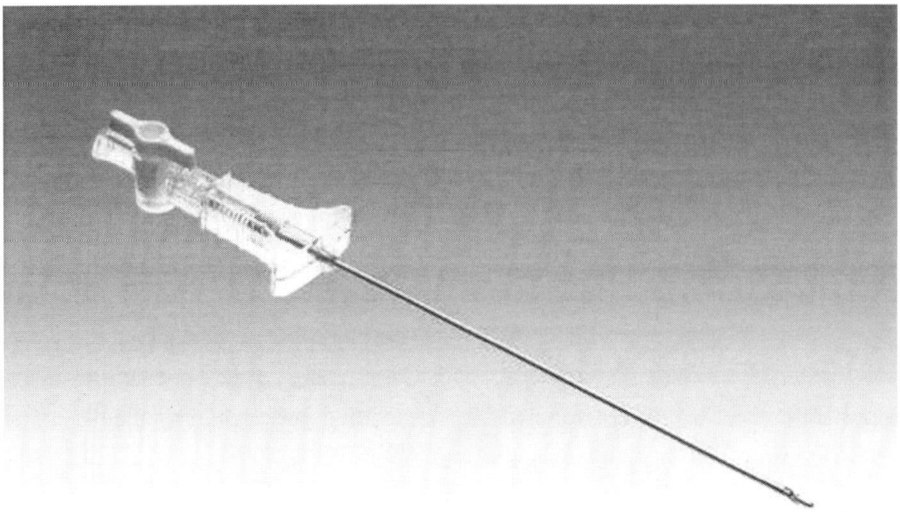

Figure 2. Veress needle.

Major vascular injuries are often the less frequent (0.05%) but its mortality is around 9%. The lesion usually involves retroperitoneal vascular structures and immediate identification is not generally the norm, it usually manifests along the surgery with a hypotensive patient status that should get alert us for an immediate conversion and repair of the vessel. It is important to count on a team of nurses prepared to be able to facilitate the immediate conversion of surgery; conversion of surgery is not a failure of the procedure, but a good clinical judgment.

Intestinal Injury

This is the second most common cause of mortality of laparoscopic surgery. Its incidence varies between 0.1% and 0.3% of cases. Approximately one third of these injuries occur during the access into the abdomen, but it may also occur during removal of instrumental, dissection of structures or electrocautery burns. One of the problems related to this complication is intraoperative difficulty to diagnose it. Most lesions (70%) are diagnosed in the postoperative period and may have already evolved into a severe peritonitis. Depending on the time of occurrence can be classified as [15]:

Early: occur in the first 48 hours after surgery.

Delayed: appear 48 hours after the intervention.

It is produced in many cases by a secondary local inflammatory mechanism after laparoscopic technique.

Perforations are also classified according to the location of the lesion in the gastrointestinal tract or laparoscopic instrument type used. The presence of adhesions or history of previous laparotomies increase risk for perforation. With respect to location, the small bowel injuries are the most common (58%). In laparoscopic cholecystectomy, duodenal injury is the most common lesion. Next in frequency are colon lesions (32%) and finally gastric are rare and account for only 7% of cases. Regarding the material used at the beginning of the intervention, Veress needle and blind trocars puncture used at the beginning of the procedure are those that most frequently cause intestinal perforations.

During the intervention, thermal injury is the most common adverse event. In some cases, these electrical burns are no identified immediately and its symptoms can appear several days after when complete necrosis of the intestinal wall occurs. If it is identified and repaired during surgery, morbidity is low, but if peritonitis is evolved, mortality increases.

Diagnosis of intestinal perforation is often difficult, being masked by factors such as postoperative pain, use of analgesic drugs or use of antibiotics. Persistent abdominal pain, sepsis data or signs of peritoneal irritation, are suggestive of this complication. In many cases the peritoneal irritation is absent. One theory supports the unusual presentation of intestinal perforation in laparoscopic surgery compared to open surgery, based on the lower postoperative immune and metabolic response in the first case. If there is a clinical suspicion, an abdominal CT that allows us to identify intestinal perforation must be performed [16].

Most of the lesions (80%) are treated by conversion to laparotomy for intestinal repair. Conservative management would be based primarily on percutaneous drainage of abscesses and supportive measures such as the use of parenteral nutrition and antibiotics.

Mortality, although it is a rare complication in some published studies it is around 3-6%, especially in those patients progressing to a state of sepsis and multiorgan failure. Moreover, if intestinal injury is associated with vascular injury, mortality increases. Therefore, prevention measures are essential [17].

Bladder Injury

It usually happens if the bladder is full and especially in infraumbilical punctures. If lesion is performed with a Veress needle is usually sufficient a urinary catheter placement. If produced with Hasson trocar, repairing the bladder and a urinary catheter is needed postoperatively.

In some surgical techniques identify ureters is necessary to avoid injury and may even use a previous catheterization is required [18].

Thermal Injury

Because of laparoscopy provides a limited view of the surgical field, it is very easy for even the most experienced surgeon to miss a thermal injury. It is therefore not surprising that intraoperative non-targeted tissue burns are not given higher priority in the differential diagnosis of postoperative complications.

Accidental, unsuspected thermal injuries can result in significant complications during and following surgery, most notably are vessel hemorrhage, organ damage, perforation and peritonitis. Depending on their severity and/or location, these conditions may result in significant morbidity or even death if not detected early enough. Fecal peritonitis following perforation is maybe the most feared complication of thermal damage, with a mortality rate estimated as high as 25% [19].

It is important not to abuse electrocoagulation and remember this action extends beyond the point of application.

Complications Related to Laparoscopic Instruments

Use of laparoscopic instruments (Figure 3) has important weaknesses, the surgeon stops working in 3D, there is no tactile feel and depth, difficulty in handling tissues due to longer and rigid instruments, which exerts leverage.

It is important that the instrument and the structure we are handling not disappear from our visual field, in order to prevent the clamps rotations which involuntarily occur. With this preventive measure we can grasp and release the structure and detect if any injury has occurred and therefore repair it [20].

It is recommended to take a good bite with the laparoscopic forceps, especially when we take small bowel.

In case of small bowel deserosalization is important to repair it at that time, in order to not significantly lengthen operating time [21, 22].

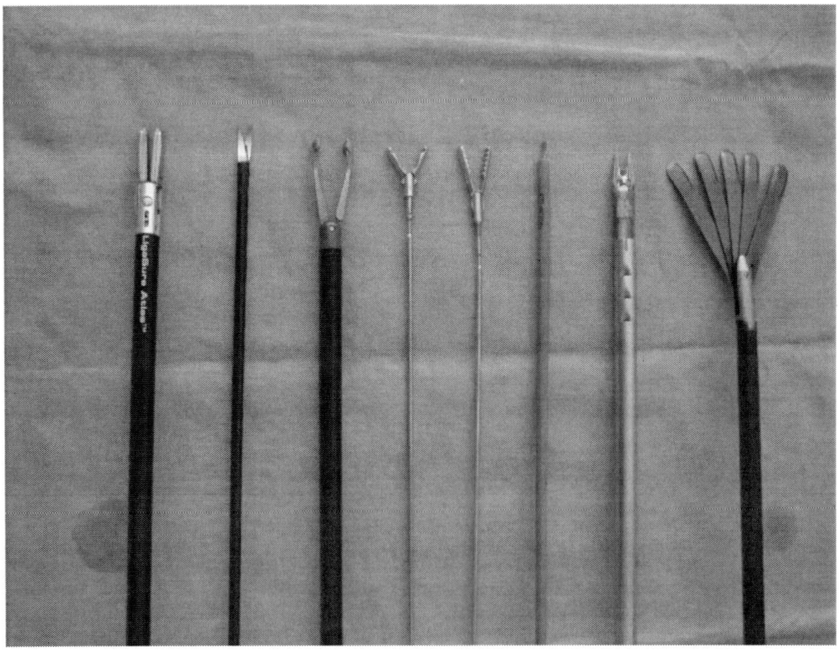

Figure 3. Different laparoscopic instruments.

We can use position change of the patient to take advantage of gravity and mobilize loops to lateralizate them and improve the visual field.

It is therefore important to know the complications that can arise during laparoscopic surgery and know how to fix them, but most important is to avoid them as much as possible.

This is reached by a correct acquisition of theoretical knowledge and proper surgical skills necessary to avoid the learning curve and mistakes in patient. Experimental animals and laparoscopic simulators are the perfect scenario to reach these skills.

Complications Related to Trocars Placement

Trocar insertion through a small 2-3 cm skin incision are necessary to perform a laparoscopy. Despite small incisions, may have the same complications as any surgical incision, but obviously on a small scale. Also common minor complications to any surgical wound, as bruising, hematoma or abscess incision holes, there are other complications, among we would like to highlight the following:

Incisional Hernias

The herniation through the hole of the trocars is found more frequently than expected. Deval et al. [10] first described 40 years ago and since then, its incidence has been underestimated by laparoscopic surgeons. Occurs in 0.2-1% of gynecological laparoscopic procedures [23, 24], but this figure does not reflect the current incidence, because due to the use of increasingly thicker trocars, it is expected that herniation occurs in more cases.

The umbilical hernia is the most frequently type of herniation. Mechanism of production of the hernia may be due to the existence of umbilical hernias preoperatively undiagnosed or the interposition of omentum in the channel of the trocar when removing. In order to avoid this adverse phenomenon, it is advisable to close the fascia of all trocars´ introduction incisions and preexisting umbilical hernia repair if necessary [25].

Implantation of Tumor Cells

Tumor implants in introduction hole of trocars are defined as recurrences in these holes after laparoscopy in cancer patients without peritoneal carcinomatosis [26].

This unfortunate fact was described in 1998 [27] for laparoscopic cholecystectomies with finding malignancy on histopathological examination later. Transumbilical extraction of parts with inapparent tumors, it caused subsequent tumor implants in the parietal canal path.

Extension of the abdominal laparoscopic surgery for cancer has increased the incidence of tumor implants [28]. Implantation of cancer cells have been described following resection of advanced tumors, localized tumors [29] and in biopsies for staging processes. Mechanism responsible for this phenomenon it is not clear. Based on latency period, usually about three months, suggests a massive planting of cells by direct contact with the wound path or trocar [23]. Pneumoperitoneum with CO_2 appears to have an adjunctive role in tumor implantation [30].

Oncological laparoscopic surgery without gas in experimental animal studies, reduces the incidence of cases with tumor implants. The incidence varies widely according to the series consulted and the surgical technique used (0-21%) [23, 27]. Reviewing the cases published in literature, over 65 % occurred in digestive oncology laparoscopy, 17% in gynecological procedures, 14% in thoracoscopy without gas and only 2.5% in urologic surgery. The most common site in all surgical specialties was the extraction port of the surgical specimen [27]. Some measures have been proposed in order to reduce the incidence to 1% (similar to open surgery) [26, 30, 31]:

- Techniques that do not directly manipulate tumor
- Extraction of tumor pieces in protective bags
- Peritoneal washing using nonstick or cytocidal solutions
- Gasless laparoscopy

Complications Related to Learning Curve

Learning curve of laparoscopic surgery, differs slightly from the classical learning process usually related to open surgery. Laparoscopy has been implanted in a relatively short period of time, so that surgeons have virtually all formed simultaneously. Laparoscopic technique has some complications such as injury to common bile duct during cholecystectomy and trocar injuries that have been discussed above. As surgeons have gained experience has seen diminishing injuries attributed to learning curve have diminished as well as the number of laparotomies to resolve complications, increasing cases resolved by laparoscopy [32].

Conversion refers to transforming a laparoscopic technique to conventional open laparotomy. It is precisely the surgeons with little experience, who are often reluctant to convert the technique, persevering and producing unnecessary iatrogenic effects.

Conversion of laparoscopy was studied by Shea et al. [33] in a meta-analysis of more than 25,000 cholecystectomies, which ended in 1,400 conversions (5.5%). The reasons for conversion were:

1. Technical problems: adhesions, significant inflammation, etc., by far the most common cause (55%).
2. Operative findings: choledocholithiasis, advanced cholecystitis, etc. (20%).
3. Perioperative complications: bleeding, bile duct injuries, etc. (14%).
4. Other (9%).

Postoperative Complications

Laparoscopic surgery has revolutionized the field of surgery, using multiple procedures and by different specialties. However, although this technique has many advantages such as less postoperative pain, faster recovery, shorter hospital stay and lower costs, it is not performed without complications.

Knowledge and management of these complications can decrease patients´ morbidity and mortality. This part of the chapter discusses the complications that can occur in the postoperative period.

Intestinal Perforation

Intestinal perforation is the second most common cause of mortality in laparoscopic surgery. Its incidence varies between 0.1% and 0.3% of cases. Approximately one third of these injuries occur during the access into the abdomen, but it may also occur during removal of instrumental, dissection of structures or electrocautery burns.

One of the problems related to this complication is intraoperative difficulty to diagnose it. Most of lesions (70%) are diagnosed in the postoperative period and may have already evolved into a severe peritonitis. Depending on the time of occurrence can be classified as [34]:

Early: occur in the first 48 hours after surgery.
Delayed: appear 48 hours after the intervention.

It is produced in many cases by a secondary local inflammatory mechanism after laparoscopic technique.

Perforations are also classified according to the location of the lesion in the gastrointestinal tract or laparoscopic instrument type used. The presence of adhesions or history of previous laparotomies increase risk for perforation.

With respect to location, the small bowel injuries are the most common (58%). In laparoscopic cholecystectomy, duodenal injury is the most common lesion. Next in frequency are colon lesions (32%) and finally gastric are rare and account for only 7% of cases.

Regarding the material used at the beginning of the intervention, Veress needle and blind trocars puncture used at the beginning of the procedure are those that most frequently cause intestinal perforations.

During the intervention, thermal injury is the most common adverse event. In some cases, these electrical burns are no identified immediately and its symptoms can appear several days after when complete necrosis of the intestinal wall occurs. If it is identified and repaired during surgery, morbidity is low, but if peritonitis is evolved, mortality increases.

Diagnosis of intestinal perforation is often difficult, being masked by factors such as postoperative pain, use of analgesic drugs or use of antibiotics. Persistent abdominal pain, sepsis data or signs of peritoneal irritation scans, are suggestive of this complication. In many cases the peritoneal irritation is absent. One theory supports the unusual presentation of intestinal perforation in laparoscopic surgery compared to open surgery, based on the lower postoperative immune and metabolic response in the first case. When there is a clinical suspicion, an abdominal CT that allows us to identify intestinal perforation must be performed [35].

Most of the lesions (80%) are treated by conversion to laparotomy for intestinal repair. Conservative management would be based primarily on percutaneous drainage of abscesses and supportive measures such as the use of parenteral nutrition and antibiotics.

Mortality, although it is a rare complication in some published studies it is around 3-6%, especially in those patients progressing to a state of sepsis and multiorgan failure. Moreover, if intestinal injury is associated with vascular injury, mortality increases. Therefore, prevention measures are essential [36].

Bile leak

Laparoscopic cholecystectomy is the standard surgical treatment in most patients with gallstones. Its benefits have been clearly demonstrated with respect to the laparotomy and this laparoscopic technique is probably the world´s most widely performed. However, the increase in the number of laparoscopic procedures has also increased the number of complications, with a greater incidence than in the case of open surgery.

The incidence of lesions in the biliary tract in laparoscopic surgery is 0.3%, whereas in open surgery is around 0.2%. In patients with severe chronic cholecystitis or scleroatrophic gallbladder, the risk is higher. There are also studies showing an increased risk of perioperative complications in prolonged procedures. If laparoscopic cholecystectomy lasts more than two hours the risk is four times greater than if the procedure takes 30 to 60 minutes [34].

For this type of injury, Strasberg proposed a classification that can be used in management. According to this, the lesions may be [35] (Figure 4):

- Type A: small bile duct leak in continuity with the common hepatic, cystic or Luschka ducts.
- Type B: partial occlusion of the biliary tree. This unilateral canal is almost always the result of an aberrant right hepatic duct.
- Type C: drain conduit in communication with the common hepatic duct. It is also due to an aberrant right hepatic duct.
- Type D: lateral lesion of extrahepatic ducts due to inadvertedly cannulation of hepatic choledocho during cholangiography.
- Type E (E_1-E_5): circumferential lesion of major bile ducts.

One of the common causes for injury occur when anatomical structures are badly identified, confusing the cystic bile duct with the choledocho, clipping and section the common bile duct. It also may occur with electrocautery burns. These thermal injuries can difficult blood flow to the damaged structure. A burn of bile may manifest as an intraoperative bile leakage or postoperative necrosis and peritonitis or stenosis with ischemia.

With regard to diagnosis, most of the injuries are identified intraoperatively or during immediate postoperative period. In the first case, the injury should be suspected when there is presence of bile in the review of the surgical field. Although intraoperative cholangiography has not been shown to decrease the incidence of bile duct injuries, this should be done to determinate the level and type of injury then proceeding to immediate repair.

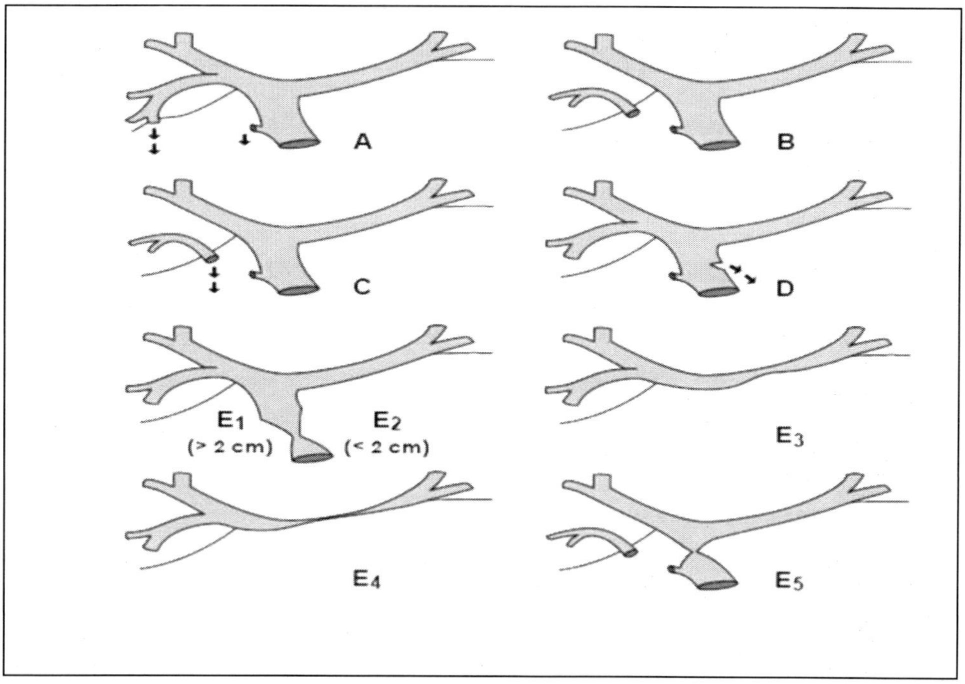

Figure 4. Strasberg Classification: laparoscopic bile duct injuries.

In the postoperative period, often the symptoms are nonspecific but must have a high clinical suspicion when any signs and symptoms such as jaundice, biliary drain output, data sepsis, nausea, vomiting or signs of peritoneal irritation in physical examination. Late clinical presentations usually occur as recurrent cholangitis and secondary biliary cirrhosis.

Regarding diagnostic tests, after initial clinical suspicion, we have to perform analytical tests including liver biochemistry profile. It is possible that in the immediate postoperative period of laparoscopic cholecystectomy GPT increased up to 34% of patients, less frequently bilirubin (9%) or alkaline phosphatase (4%) occurs. However, if liver enzymes increased 24-48 hours after surgery, requires a reassessment of the patient [36]. Abdominal ultrasound is a good diagnostic technique that can demonstrate dilatation of intra and extrahepatic bile duct, finding collections as well. It also can be therapeutic by guiding percutaneous treatments. It is important to note that the absence of sonographic dilatation does not exclude the diagnosis of bile duct injury. Although after cholecystectomy, collections may appear in the gallbladder fossa in 10-14% of patients and the presence of liquid out of this location should not be considered a normal postoperative finding.

Abdominal CT also may show dilated intra and extrahepatic bile duct, collections, parenchyma and liver pedicle. Transhepatic cholangiography (PTC), is an invasive but fast and safe method with a low complication rate, which is able to visualize the entire biliary tree in 98% of patients with dilated bile ducts and up to 75 % of those without dilatation. Since the introduction of endoscopic retrograde cholangiopancreatography (ERCP) and magnetic resonance cholangiopancreatography, indications of PTC have decreased [37].

ERCP is the diagnostic method of choice when the presence of a biliary fistula is suspected, in addition it is a therapeutic option. Magnetic resonance cholangiopancreatography is a method with high sensitivity and specificity. Its advantages include low risks, non-invasive method, requires no contrast and fast realization.

Treatment can be performed intraoperatively or depending on early or late diagnosis. Best treatment option is prevention, which can be achieved with adequate knowledge of the anatomy and the possible variables and conducting a careful surgical technique. Immediate repair will be carried out in the first intervention. We consider an early reoperation when it is carried out in the next few days and late reoperation when it is done from the 6th day on. During the first procedure, conversion to open surgery is in most cases the best treatment option.

In case of biliary fistula diagnosed in the immediate postoperative period, management is conservative in many cases because most close spontaneously. Some studies propose ERCP stent placement or premature papillotomy in order to increase bile flow and accelerate the closure of the fistula [38].

If diagnosis is delayed, treatment will be based on patient resuscitation and treatment of sepsis including drainage of collections. Nutritional support should be maintained until the final repair. Low levels of albumin are associated with a poor prognosis and it is therefore important to correct the nutritional deficit with enteral nutrition. Lack of nutrition can create a dysfunction of intestinal barrier with an increased risk of endotoxemia.

Drainage of collections is usually performed percutaneously, however in the presence of an extensive biliary peritonitis or intraabdominal contamination, surgical scrub and drain placement is necessary. Late diagnosis of the biliary injury may produce systemic inflammatory response syndrome, developing a multiple organ failure secondary to bile peritonitis. The presence of bile peritonitis has proven to be a risk factor for poor prognosis, liver fibrosis can appear after 6-12 months of injury if the management is not adequate [38].

With regard to the use of endoscopic techniques for repairing minor injuries in the bile duct, it is important to consider etiology and location of the damaged structure, the experience of endoscopy team, the cost of the procedure and the possibility of short and long term monitoring. In many cases it can be an adjuvant treatment to surgery. A prerequisite for an injury to be treated by percutaneous and/or endoscopic is the continuity condition of biliary tree.

Retroperitoneal Hematoma

Injury of a large retroperitoneal vessel is a serious complication in laparoscopic approach. Its incidence is around 0.1%. Up to 75%, it usually occurs after insertion of the Veress needle or trocar [39].

Early diagnosis of vascular injury is essential, considering that delay is an important factor to increase postoperative morbidity and mortality. However, there is often a delay in diagnosis because the retroperitoneal bleeding vascular lesion is not visible in the field. If a bulge of retroperitoneum is produced, elevating intestine and producing that pneumoperitoneum is insufficient despite being correct [40].

During the immediate postoperative period patients show tendency to hypotension and severe anemia. Clinical and analytical alterations should make us think about the diagnosis. If retroperitoneal hematoma diagnosed intraoperatively, in most cases needs conversion to laparotomy. In case of postoperative diagnosis, patients require urgent surgical reoperation [41].

Subhepatic Abscess

Incidence of postoperative infectious complications in laparoscopic surgery is low, unless it occur secondary to other complications (intestinal perforation, bile leak, etc). Hollow viscus injuries are more frequent in patients with adhesions and previous interventions or inflammatory processes. Routine use of nasogastric tube during surgery and urinary catheterization decrease the risk of this type of injury and facilitate viewing of the surgical field.

Repair can be performed laparoscopically in case of intraoperative diagnosis, but in most cases required conversion to open surgery. If intraoperative diagnosis of the injury does not occur, it leads to immediate postoperative peritonitis.

During laparoscopic cholecystectomy may occur accidental perforation of the gallbladder (15-40 % of cases), bile and gallbladder stones output during the procedure. Output of gallbladder stones to the peritoneal cavity occurs in up to two thirds of patients. It is important to make an effort to recover laparoscopically gallstones dropped into the peritoneal cavity, which can form subhepatic adhesions and abscesses by lefting them in the abdominal cavity (0.1-2.9% of laparoscopic cholecystectomies). Formation of subhepatic abscess is more common in cholecystectomy for acute cholecystitis, in case of bile infection or calcium bilirubinate gallstones. Symptoms usually appear in the early postoperative period, being unusual late manifestation [42].

Conducting a successful laparoscopic technique, recovery gallstones and extensive washing in case of gallbladder drilling, added to the experience of the surgeon are essential to avoid a laparotomy and possible complications caused by gallstones left.

Intra-abdominal abscess or wound infection may also occur during dissection or surgical removal of surgical specimen by extending bacteria inside the abdomen or in the access area.

Diagnosis of septic complications following abdominal surgery can be difficult; in this sense postoperative pain, presence of paralytic ileus and hemodynamic or ventilatory support may mask the signs of an acute abdomen. In addition, most of the data of infection such as hyperthermia and leukocytosis, are also part of the normal response to postoperative stress, being masked clinical profile.

Postoperatively, the presence of persistent sinus tachycardia (> 120 bpm), respiratory dysfunction with inability to extubate the patient, fever maintained, tendency to hypotension, hyperglycemia or the appearance of a paralytic ileus after the 7th postoperative day should make us suspect source of intra-abdominal sepsis. Early diagnosis and treatment are essential because the patient can progress to multiorgan failure with high mortality [43]. Suspecting infection it is important to culture specimens (blood, fluid drains, etc). Empiric broad-spectrum antibiotic therapy has to be initiated. In most cultures is isolated *E.Coli, Enterococcus* and *Klebsiella pneumoniae*. In addition to appropriate antibiotic therapy is essential in these patients to identify the location of the septic focus and proceed to drain it. In terms of imaging test, CT is the most sensitive test, although ultrasound is more specific for detecting abandoned gallstones. The ultrasound image of the abscess is usually visualized as a hyperechoic lesion with acoustic shadowing. The CT is usually seen as a hypodense mass with peripheral ring of contrast enhancement.

A single subhepatic or subphrenic abscess can be drained through an extraperitoneal or under the height of the 11th rib subcostal approach, enabling open the peritoneal cavity without exposing the contents of the abscess drainage. Sometimes the definitive treatment is surgical approach.

Postoperative Air Embolism

Gas embolism (GE) is a rare complication (15 interventions/100,000/year) but with a high mortality (70-90%). It is produced by the passage of CO_2 to the venous system and then through the right ventricle to the pulmonary circulation. The gas can also pass to arterial blood circulation in any organ causing ischemia. There are two conditions that are required in order to produce GE: the first one is a direct communication between the gas source and the vascular system, the second one is a favorable pressure gradient of gas inlet to circulation. These conditions occur during laparoscopic surgery at different times during the procedure. Considering the time of onset of symptoms the GE is classified as early (initial), during the procedure and after deflating. The first two are intraoperative complications and were treated in another part of the chapter. GE after deflation is less frequent and difficult to explain. Experimental studies suggest that CO_2 could be "trapped" in the splanchnic vessels in a high concentration, favored by the gradient of CO_2 during the procedure. When abruptly release the neumoperitoneum, CO_2 may form small bubbles in the circulation in the same way that occurs with the nitrogen in the sudden decompression of divers. In this case the symptoms may appear in the immediate postoperative period or deferred in general in relation to active and passive mobilization of the patient [44]. Clinical is related to the amount of gas that enters the circulation and with the organ affected by the ischemia. Most GE are subclinical, however, if it is clinical, differential diagnosis with symptomatic pulmonary thromboembolism, ACVA or myocardial infarction is difficult. Crepitus in the neck vessels is uncommon but diagnostic.

Diagnosis is usually suspected in patients with acute onset of clinical support during the more risky moments of the procedure. Hemodynamic and respiratory monitoring usually helps us for diagnosis. Control of expiratory pCO_2 ($ETCO_2$) by capnography is useful since the passage of CO_2 into the bloodstream, producing an initial increase in pCO_2 followed by a sharp drop from pulmonary embolism. It is followed by hypoxia and fall in O_2 saturation with hypotension sharp decrease in cardiac output. The absorption of CO_2 produced mixed, respiratory and metabolic acidosis. Other diagnostic procedures such as echocardiography, CT scan or pulmonary arteriogram is made on the basis of clinical status.

Most effective treatment is prevention: careful puncture gas, repeated aspiration, initial injection of gas at low flow and work with the least intra-abdominal pressure. Use of other less soluble gases like Argon also increases the risk of GE [45]. After initial treatment begins, supportive measures with vasopressors and mechanical ventilation with high oxygen concentration are necessary. In patients with a large gas bubble obstructing the right ventricular outflow, Trendelenburg position and left lateral position can reposition the air at the tip of the right ventricle allowing the pulmonary circulation (Durant maneuver). Gas extraction is also recommended by a central venous catheter in the event that the patient already had channeled. The channeling of central venous access for resuscitation is often difficult. Closed cardiac massage is an option and that chest compression could break a big bubble in other small to pass the pulmonary circulation. Hyperbaric oxygen urgent therapy is usually inaccessible in most hospitals, but is the only one that has shown a reduction in mortality.

References

[1] Healy M., Strunin L. Anaesthesia and laparoscopic cholecistectomy. *Baillere´s Clin. Anaesth.*, 1992; 4: 819-45.

[2] Chapron C., Querleu D., Bruhat M. A. et al. Surgical complications of diagnostic and operative gynaecological laparoscopy: a series of 29,966 cases. *Hum. Reprod.,* 1998; 13: 867-72.

[3] Shea J. A., Healy M. J., Berlin J. A. et al. Mortality and complications associated with laparoscopic cholecystectomy. A meta-analysis. *Ann. Surg*., 1996; 224: 609-20.

[4] Kallam S. B., Reamy J. A., Collins R. L. Pneumomediastinum and subcutaneous emphysema during laparoscopy. *Cleve. Clin. J. Med*., 1992; 57: 639-42.

[5] Joris J. L., Chiche J. D., Lamy M. L. Pneumothorax during laparoscopic funduplication: diagnosis and treatment with positive end-expiratory pressure. *Anesth. Analg*., 1995; 81: 993-1000.

[6] Pascual J. B., Baranda M. M., Tarrero M. T. Subcutaneous enphysema, pneumomediastinum, bilateral pneumotorax and pneumopericardium alter laparoscopy. *Endoscopy,* 1990; 22: 59.

[7] Perez J. E., Alberts W. M., Mamel J. J. Delayed tension pneumothorax alter laparoscopy. *Surg. Laparosc. Endosc*., 1997; 7: 70-2.

[8] Whiston R. J., Eggels K. A., Morris R. W. et al. Tension pneumothorax during laparoscopic cholecystectomy. *Br. J. Surg*., 1991; 78: 1325.

[9] Wahba R. W., Tessler M. J., Kleiman S. J. Acute ventilatory complications during laparoscopic upper abdominal surgery. *Can. J. Anaesth*., 1996; 43: 77-83.

[10] Bazin J. E., Schoeffer P. Anesthésie pour chirugie par voie laparoscopique. *Encycl. Méd. Chir. (Elserier, Paris) Anesthesie-Reanimation,* 1996; 6p: 36-569-A-10.

[11] Cottin V., Delafose B., Viale J. P. Gas embolism during laparoscopy: a report of seven cases in patients with previous abdominal surgical history. *Surg. Endosc*., 1996; 10: 166-9.

[12] Bazin Je., Gillart T., Rasson P. et al. Haemodynamic conditions enhacing gas embolism after venous injury during laparoscopy: a study in pigs. *Br. J. Anaesth*., 1997; 78: 570-5.

[13] Mann C., Boccara G., Fabre J. M. et al. The detection of carbon dioxide embolism during laparoscopy in pigs: a comparison of transesophageal doppler and end-tidal carbon dioxide monitoring. *Acta Anaesthesiol. Scand*., 1997; 41: 281-6.

[14] Dubois F., Icard P., Berthelot G. et al. Coelioscopic cholecystectomy; *Ann. Surg.,* 1990; 211:60-62.

[15] Van der Voort M., Heijnsdijk E. A. M., Gouma D. J. Bowel injury as a complication of laparoscopy. *Br. J. Surg*., 2004; 91: 1253-8.

[16] Gerges F. J., Kanazi G. E., Jabbour-khoury S. I., et al. Anesthesia for laparoscopy: a review. *J. Clin. Anesth.*, 2006; 18: 67-78.

[17] Bishoff J. T., Allaf M. E., Kirkels W., et al. Laparoscopic bowel injury: incidence and clinical presentation. *J. Urol.,* 1999; 161: 887-90.

[18] Blanco-Engert R., Díaz R., Gascón M., et al. [Postoperative complications in bowel laparoscopic surgery]. *Cir. Esp.*, 2002; 72 (2).

[19] Brill A. I., Feste J. R., Hamilton T. L. et al. Patient Safety During Laparoscopic Monopolar Electrosurgery - Principles and Guidelines. *JSLS*, 1998; 2(3): 221–225.

[20] Lacy A. M., Garcia Valdecasa J. C., Delgado S.; Castells A., Taura P., Pique Jm., et al. Laparoscopy-assisted colectomy for treatment of non-metastatic colon cancer : a randomised trial. *Lancet,* 2002¸359 2224-9.

[21] Townsend C., Beauchamp R., Evers B.; Mattox K. Sabiston Treatise of Surgey. 17th ed. Madrid: Elsevier Saunders, 2005.

[22] Law W. L., Lee Y. M., Choi Hk., Seto C. l., Ho Jw. Impact of Laparoscopic Resection for Colorrectal Cancer on Operatives Outcomes and survival. *Annals of Surgery*, 2007; 246 (2): 339-40.

[23] Deval B., Mekouar O., Fritel X. et al. Incisional hernia after surgical laparoscopy: a case of hepatic ligament incarceration and review of the literature. *Contracept. Fertil Sex.,* 1997;25(1): 66-8.

[24] Lajer H., Widecrantz S., Heisterberg L. Hernias in trocar ports following abdominal laparoscopy. A review. *Acta Obstet. Gynecol. Scand.*, 1997; 76(5): 389-93.

[25] Áñez C., Saludes J., Pelegrí D. et al. [Anesthesia for abdominal surgery. Laparoscopic techniques]. In: Torres Treatise of Anesthesia and Resuscitation. *Arán Editors. Madrid,* 2001: 2243-84.

[26] Cotlar A. M., Mueller C. R., Pettit J. W. et al. Trocar site seeding of inapparent gallbladder carcinoma during laparoscopic cholecystectomy. *J. Laparoendosc. Surg.,* 1996; 6(1): 35-45.

[27] Reymond M. A., Schneider C., Hohenberger W. et al. The pneumoperitoneum and its role in tumor seeding. *Dig. Surg.*, 1998; 15(2): 105-9.

[28] Martinez J., Targarona E. M., Balagué C. et al. Port site metastasis. An unresolved problem in laparoscopic surgery. *A review. Int. Surg.*, 1995; 80(4): 315-21.

[29] Schaeff B., Paolucci V., Thomopoulos J. Port site recurrences after laparoscopic surgery. *A review. Dig. Surg.* 1998; 15(2): 124-34.

[30] Reymond M. A., Schneider C., Kastl S. et al. The pathogenesis of port-site recurrences. *J. Gastrointest. Surg.*, 1998; 2(5): 406-14.

[31] Neuhaus S. J., Texler M., Hewett P. J. et al. Port-site metastases following laparoscopic surgery. *Br. J. Surg.*, 1998; 85(6): 735-41.

[32] Chapron C., Querleu D., Bruhat M. A. et al. Surgical complications of diagnostic and operative gynaecological laparoscopy: a series of 29,966 cases. *Hum. Reprod.,* 1998; 13(4): 867-72.

[33] Shea J. A., Healey M. J., Berlin J. A. et al. Mortality and complications associated with laparoscopic cholecystectomy. A meta-analysis. *Ann. Surg.*, 1996; 224(5): 609-20.

[34] Csendes A., Navarrete C., Burdiles P., et al. Treatment of common bile duct injuries during laparoscopic cholecystectomy: endoscopic and surgical management. *World J. Surg.,* 2001; 25: 1346-51.

[35] Krähenbühl L., Sclabas G., Wente M. N., et al. Incidence, risk factors, and prevention of biliary tract injuries during laparoscopic cholecystectomy in Switzerland. *World J. Surg.,* 2001; 25: 1325-30.

[36] Strasberg, S. M., Hertl M., Soper N. J., et al. An analysis of the problem of biliary injury during laparoscopic cholecystectomy. *J. Am. Coll. Surg.,* 1995; 180: 101-25.

[37] Gazzaniga G. M., Filauro M., Mori L. Surgical treatment of iatrogenic lesions of the proximal common bile duct. *World J. Surg*., 2001; 25:1254-9.

[38] Connor S., Garden O. J. Bile duct injury in the era of laparoscopic cholecystectomy. *Br. J. Surg*., 2006; 93: 158-68.

[39] Saville L. E., Woods M. S. Laparoscopy and major retroperitoneal vascular injuries. *Surg. Endosc*., 1995; 9: 1096-100.

[40] Guloglu R., Dilege S., Aksoy M., et al. Major retroperitoneal vascular injuries during laparoscopic cholecystectomy and appendectomy. *J. Laparoendosc. Adv. Surg. Tech. A*., 2004; 14: 73-6.

[41] Alcázar M. T., Ornaque I., Delgado M. A., et al. [Abdominal aortic injury as a complication of laparoscopic cholecystectomy]. *Rev. Esp. Anestesiol. Reanim*., 2004; 51: 452-5.

[42] Joshi G. P. Complications of laparocopy. *Anesthesiol. Clin. North America*, 2001; 19: 89-105.

[43] Kirshtein B., Domchik S., Mizrahi S., et al. Laparoscopic diagnosis and treatment of postoperative complications. *Am. J. Surg*., 2009; 197: 19-23.

[44] Cunningham A. J. Anesthetic implications of laparoscopic surgery. *Yale J. Biol. Med.,* 1998; 71: 551-78.

[45] Kirchhoff P., Dincler S., Buchmann P. A multivariate analysis of potential risk factors for intra- and postoperative complications in 1316 elective laparoscopic colorectal procedures. *Ann. Surg*., 2008; 248: 259-65.

In: Laparoscopy
Editor: Christos Iavazzo
ISBN: 978-1-63321-404-0

Chapter 14

Intestinal Complications in Laparoscopic Surgery

Ignacio Brunel, Elisa Moreno Palacios, Javier De Santiago and Ignacio Zapardiel
Gynecology Oncology Department. La Paz University Hospital, Madrid, Spain

Abstract

Laparoscopic surgery potentially involves intestinal complications that surgeons should understand, identify and treat properly. Intestinal complications, which represent between 0.08% and 0.3% of all laparoscopic complications, present a mortality rate of 20% according to various studies. Intestinal injuries, such as thermal or mechanical injuries, hernations, or acute intestinal obstruction resulting from severe adhesions, may occur during the abdominal access or during the surgical procedure.

Literature has described several risk factors present in intestinal lesions. The presence of previous abdominal surgeries or processes that involve adherence syndromes such as endometriosis or pelvic inflammatory disease are particularly important. Furthermore, several studies have analyzed different laparoscopic entry techniques, but have not found conclusive evidence as to which may be the safer one.

Since the timing of diagnosis and adequate treatment of these injuries determine their prognosis, when the intestinal injury is not diagnosed during surgery it is essential to recognize the symptoms and apply correct treatment as soon as possible.

Introduction

Laparoscopy is the art of examining the abdominal cavity and its contents through small incisions. It requires insertion of canulas through the abdominal wall, distension of the abdominal cavity with gas (pneumoperitoneum) and an illuminated telescope.

It is considered as minimally invasive surgery, although it is not exempted from complications. Intestinal and vascular lesions are specific complications of this type of surgery. In some cases laparotomy conversion is required to solve them.

Abdominal structures can be injured during abdominal access or during the surgical procedure itself [1]. To diminish the morbid-mortality of these lesions it is indispensable to identify and repair them during the same laparoscopic procedure. Late diagnosis may have devastating consequences for the patient.

Risk factors for laparoscopic complications have been described in the literature. Laparoscopic surgeons should identify these factors and carry out different strategies to prevent these complications from happening. When any risk factor is present, it is mandatory to perform an exhaustive examination of the abdominal cavity before closure. Up to half of the intestinal lesions are diagnosed 24hours after surgery [2].

The rate of entry-related complications is less than 1% [3], 75% of which are intestinal injuries. Abdominal structures most frequently damaged are the small intestine 25%, the iliac artery 19%, the colon 12%, and the liver 2% [2].

We should not forget that intestinal lesions are associated with a 3.6% mortality rate [4].

On the other hand, there are long-term complications related with the closure of the abdominal wall, which can be avoided with correct surgical closure techniques.

Anatomical Considerations

The abdominal cavity extends from the diaphragm to the pelvis. The transverse mesocolon divides it in two regions, the supramesocolic and the inframesocolic regions.

- The supramesocolic region is composed of the left and right hypochondriums and epigastrium region in the center.
- The inframesocolic region is composed superiorly of the left and right lumbar regions and the umbilical region in the center, and inferiorly of the left and right iliac regions and the hypogastric region in the middle.

The gastrointestinal tract is composed of the stomach, the small intestine, the colon, and the rectum.

The stomach is located in the supramesocolic region of the abdomen. Its size depends on its repletion grade. It is vascularized by branches of the celiac trunk. Two branches irrigate the minor curvature, thc right and left gastric arteries. Two branches irrigate major curvature, the right and left gastroepiploic arteries. Short gastric arteries from the splenic artery irrigate the fundus.

The small intestine is divided in duodenum, jejunum and ileum. The duodenum is located retroperitoneally, and presents an intimate relationship with the head of the pancreas. The vascularization is provided by the gastroduodenal and superior mesenteric artery.

The jejunum and ileum are attached to the retroperitoneum by the mesenterium. They are vascularized by the superior mesenteric artery.

The colon is divided in four portions: ascending, transverse, descending, and sigmoid colon. The ascending and descending colon are retroperitoneal structures and are vasculirazed by the superior mesenteric artery. The transverse and sigmoid colon are intraperitoneal organs, and are vascularized by the inferior mesenteric artery.

The colon's blood flow is protected by multiple anastomosis between branches of the superior and inferior mesenteric arteries, as well as by the marginal colon artery, also called arc of Riolan, that runs in the meso of the transverse colon.

The greater omentum or epiplon covers the gastrointestinal tract. This is a large peritoneal fold composed by the fusion of four peritoneum layers. This structure can be injured during abdominal access in laparoscopy.

The liver is situated in the right hypochondrium. Its inferior border crosses obliquely the abdominal wall from the 10º right rib to the 7º left intercostal space, which is located in the epigastric region. The right lobe of the liver is located subcostally in its totality, with a length of 5-6cm. The bottom of the gallbladder protrudes through the inferior edge of the liver.

The stomach is located in the left hypochondrium, less elevated than the right hypocondrium. The stomachs corpus and fundus are occult behind the condrocostal articulations from the 5º to the 9º cartilage. Although depending on its repletion status it can adopt different sizes and forms.

The spleen is positioned in the upper part of the left hypochondrium from the 8º to the 10º intercostal space, hidden by the stomach.

The small intestine is covered by the omentum and occupies the mesocolic region. It is connected to the retroperitoneo by the mesentery, which provides the blood flow to the bowel. The superior mesenteric artery arises from the aorta at the level of L1 (supramesocolic), although it emerges in the inframesecolic region after crossing the uncinate process of the pancreas and the horizontal portion of the duodenum. The inferior mesenteric artery arises from the aorta at the level of L3, behind the horizontal portion of the duodenum, above to the aorta's bifurcation that takes place at the level of L4.

Risk Factors

Laparoscopic surgery has a theoretical risk of bowel injury. Several risk factors can increase this risk. For example:

- Previous abdominal or pelvic surgeries.
- Peritonitis of any etiology: pelvic inflammatory disease, perforated appendicitis, etc.
- The presence of other abdominal or pelvic disorders related to abdominal adhesions as endometriosis, cancer, inflammatory bowel or pelvic disease.
- The stomach's repletion status during surgery.

There are other risk factors not patient-dependent that should be considered, such as the surgeon's experience and the complexity of the surgery [5].

Just about every patient that undergoes surgery will develop abdominal adhesion. These adhesions can be established between different abdominal structures or with the abdominal wall, particularly at the cicatrix points. The most frequent site of adhesions is between the epiplon and the abdominal wall at the cicatrix point. The cicatrix point is of major significance, due to the fact that up to 68.9% of the intestinal lesions are produced in patients with previous surgeries or adhesion-related disorders.

However, the risk of developing abdominal adhesions is not the same for every patient. There are several factors that can influence in the development of adhesions and their extension:

- The type of surgical incisions. Transverse incisions, as Pfannenstiel incisions, are associated with lower rate of adhesions than longitudinal ones [6].
- Number of laparotomies. The risk of developing adhesions increases with each laparotomy [6, 7, 8].
- Visceral or parietal peritoneum damage. In animal studies, adhesions seem to be more intense when the visceral peritoneum is injured [9]
- Complications during surgery. Hemorrhage and infections increase the risk of developing adhesions [10, 11, 12].
- Surgery type. Some surgeries, such as cholecystectomy and Nissen fundoplication [13], are related with higher rate of adhesions.

Access to the abdominal cavity is the one challenge of laparoscopy that is particular to the insertion of surgical instruments through small incisions. Access is therefore associated with intestinal and vascular complications. At least 50% of the complications occur prior to the commencement of the intended surgery. The majority of the complications occur during the insertion of the primary umbilical trocar. Several entry techniques intended to diminish entry related complications have been described: The closed or classical technique, with the introduction of the Veress pneumoperitoneum-needle directly; or the open (Hasson) technique, direct trocar insertion without prior pneumoperitoneum. It would seem that the open technique should reduce the risk of lesions, but this has not been demonstrated in the literature.

In 2008 a Cochrane revision concluded that there was no difference in the complication rate between the open and closed entry-techniques. However, the small sample size analyzed and the low incidence of intestinal lesions [14] limits the implications of this study with regard to the detection rate of these lesions.

On the other hand there are retrospective studies that suggest that the open technique reduces the risk of severe complications [3,15,16]. Therefore there is no clear evidence in favor of any technique. However special attention should be considered in patients with risk factors for intestinal lesions.

Trocars positioning in the abdomen is specific of the surgical procedure to be performed. If the patient presents scars, abdominal wall meshes or umbilical hernias, trocars should be located avoiding these areas because of the risk of intestinal adhesions at these levels. Auxiliary access points for Veress needle insertion may be used.

Several auxiliary access points have been described. An example can be the Palmer Point, located 3cm below the left subcostal border in the midclavicular line. Access points can be located also in the ninth or tenth intercostal spaces, where the Veress needle is inserted directly through the intercostal space at the anterior axillary line, along the superior surface of the lower rib, in order to avoid injury of the neurovascular bundle [16].

Gastrointestinal Injuries during Abdominal Access

Intestinal injuries in laparoscopy have been classically attributed to the use of electrosurgical elements. By now we know that 30-50% are entry-related complications, either with the closed or open access techniques [1,18-21].

According to the study performed by Chapron in 56 patients, 18 of them presented intestinal injuries during abdominal access (36%). In 6 patients (10.7%) the intestinal lesion occurred during the introduction of the Veress needle, in 9 patients (16.1%) during the placement of the umbilical trocar, and in 3 patients (5.3%) during the placement of the hypogastric trocar [22] (Figure 1,2).

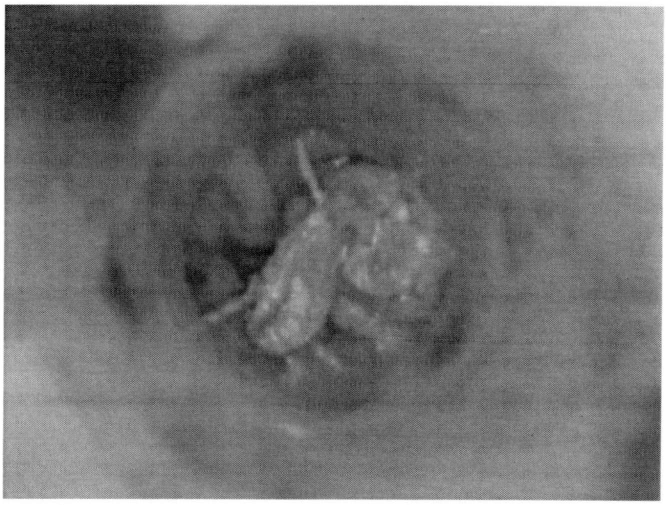

Figure 1. Direct view of trocar injury.

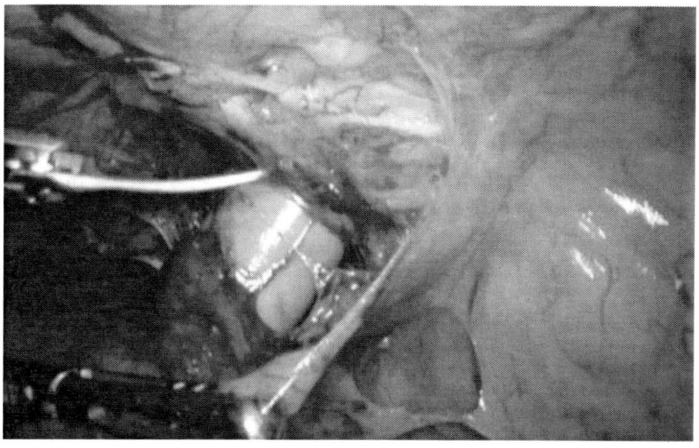

Figure 2. Trocar injury.

Intestinal injuries caused by the introduction of the Veress needle are of minor severity. This can explain the small frequency with which they are reported. Nevertheless, once the Veress needle is in the abdominal cavity its movements ought to be cautious, due to the fact that if the bowel has been injured, the size of the lesion can augment with the movements, aggravating the situation [5].

The small intestine is the organ most frequently injured, although the stomach, liver, and colon can be injured when auxiliary access points are used [23, 24].

Stomach

Stomach lesions are rare in laparoscopy, representing only 1.6% of all gastrointestinal injuries during primary entrance [2, 22], and 10% during secondary trocar placement (2).

There are several strategies that can help us prevent gastric injuries: Introducing a nasogastric tube after the anesthetic induction to empty the stomach; performing an adequate neumoperitoneum before introducing the primary trocar [25]; positioning the patient in a trendelemburg position before introducing the Veress needle (only when the access point are the Palmer or the subcostal points).

Finally, it is important to consider that complicated anesthetic inductions can provoke stomach spasms, favoring incidental stomach injuries [26].

Small Intestine and Colon

The small intestine, which occupies the majority of the abdominal cavity, is the organ most frequently injured. It accounts for up to 25% of the entry-related intestinal lesions, and 10% of the injuries caused by the introduction of secondary trocars [2].

Colon lesions represent only 12.2% of the gastrointestinal injuries occurring during primary abdominal access [2].

When the surgical procedure is concluded, it is essential to perform a meticulous inspection of the abdominal cavity in order to detect intestinal lesions. Injuries are detected by observing output of feces through the needle or the trocar, by visualizing feces in the abdominal cavity, or by detecting hematomas in the intestinal serosa or the muscularis propria. When abdominal adhesions or umbilical hernias are suspected, it is recommended primary abdominal access through Palmer point with a mini laparoscope to visualize the abdominal cavity. This mini laparoscope allows the introduction of the primary trocar under direct vision avoiding adhesions [27].

Another element that has been considered to prevent intestinal injuries is the use of disposable trocars, which present a security resort system. However, evidence is inconclusive, and does support recommending its use [28, 29].

Gastrointestinal Injuries during Surgical Procedures

Intestinal lesions can occur during the surgical procedure itself. They may be caused by the use of electrosurgical elements, dissection or direct manipulation of the bowel, which are responsible of two-thirds of the intestinal lesions [22].

Electrosurgical elements use high frequency energy to coagulate, cut and desiccate structures. These instruments can have different electrode configuration, monopolar or bipolar.

Monopolar energy may produce damage either by direct contact or by stray currents that produce distant injuries. This occurs if the electrodes are not properly isolated, or the return electrode is harmed. Bipolar energy uses lower voltage and a closed energy circuit. These characteristics practically eliminate the risk of distant injuries. When the device is activated for a long period, it reaches high temperatures, may cause damage to adjacent, or even distant structures, by direct contact [30].

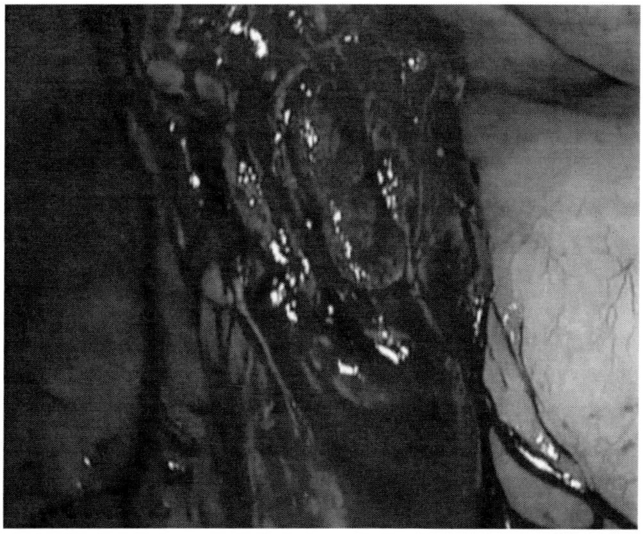

Figure 3. Bowel injury.

The risk of electrical injuries during laparoscopy is estimated in 18.8%, although this frequency varies in different studies. Monopolar energy is associated with a higher rate of visceral injuries than bipolar energy, which is explained by their characteristics [22]. Electrical energy may cause burns to the intestine, producing a necrotic area that leads to perforation in a variable period of time. This causes a latent clinical course, delaying the diagnosis and aggravating the prognosis [20] (Figure 3).

Visceral damage can be produced also during tissue dissection, especially in patients with intense adherence syndrome. The risk of injuries depends on the type of surgery. Complex surgeries present higher risk of structure damage [19].

In summary, the frequency of intestinal injuries during laparoscopy depends on the type of surgery, the patient's characteristics, and the correct use of the electrosurgical elements.

Diagnosis

The most important prognostic factor of intestinal lesions is the time to diagnosis. The best prognosis is when lesions are detected and repaired during the same surgical procedure in which they are produced. However, in most cases lesions are not detected during surgery. Thus, it is very important to recognize the symptoms caused by these lesions.

Usually after any type of surgical procedure there is a progressive recovery. If recovery is delayed, structure damage should be suspected. Symptoms can appear from 12 hours up to 5 days after laparoscopy. Commonly intestinal lesions appear with fiber, absence of bowel sounds, peritoneal irritation, abdominal distention, ileus, nausea and vomiting. If the treatment is delayed, sepsis symptoms can appear [31]. However, in some occasions intestinal injuries have an insidious presentation, manifesting nonspecific symptoms such as tachycardia, malaise or general pain [21]. Also atypical symptoms can appear, such as anorexia, diarrhea, low fiber and normal bowel sounds without leukocytosis. Intestinal injuries have also been related with intense and persistent pain in the trocar insertion point [32].

If an intestinal injury is suspected, imaging tests and blood recount should be carried out to help confirm the diagnosis. Leukocytosis with neutrophilia can be found in the blood count often accompanied with the elevation of acute phase reactants. Although acute phase reactants are not useful for diagnosis because of their low specificity, they help monitor treatment response. In severe cases, leucopenia can be found.

Abdominal x-rays is a cheap and simple test, which in many cases may allow to confirm the diagnosis. It is important to keep in mind that close to 40% of patients present neumoperitoneum during the first 24 hours after laparoscopic surgery. In these cases a computerized tomography (CT) is needed [33, 34].

The presence of any of these symptoms is usually enough to suspect and treat intestinal injuries without recurring to multiple test, which can delay its diagnosis and treatment.

Treatment

Intestinal injuries are treated differently depending on their characteristics, such as their number, localization, size, viability of the intestinal portion injured (blood flow), and whether or not they are associated with peritonitis.

When an intestinal perforation is suspected, broad-spectrum antibiotics should be administered immediately. The most adequate antibiotic depends on the bacteria present in each portion of the gastrointestinal tract. Gram-negative bacilli and gram-positive cocci predominate in the small intestine. Gram-negative bacilli, anaerobes and enterococci predominate in the colorectal tract.

If the lesions occur in the gastroduodenal or the small intestinal, the antibiotic recommended is Cefazolin (2gr IV). If there is a colorectal lesion either Cefazolin (2gr), Cefotetan (2gr IV) or Cefoxitin (2gr IV), always associated with Metronidazole (500mgr IV), are appropriate. If the patient is allergic to beta-lactams, other options are available as Clindamycin (900 mgr IV) or Vancomycin (15mgr/Kgr IV), associated with Levofloxacin (500mgr IV) or Aztreonam (2gr IV) [35].

In general small lesions produced by the Veress needle can be treated conservatively with broad-spectrum antibiotics. When larger lesions are diagnosed surgical reparation is needed. The surgical procedure required depends on the size of the injury and the conditions of the intestinal segment affected. Small lesions, with conserved blood flow and no peritonitis can be repaired with a two-layer loose points suture, using a 3-0 dissolvable thread. On the other hand, if the lesion affects a larger area, has a decreased vascularization, or peritonitis is present, intestinal resections are required. Posterior anastomosis can be performed in the same procedure. Otherwise a temporal colostomy is needed [36] (figure 4,5).

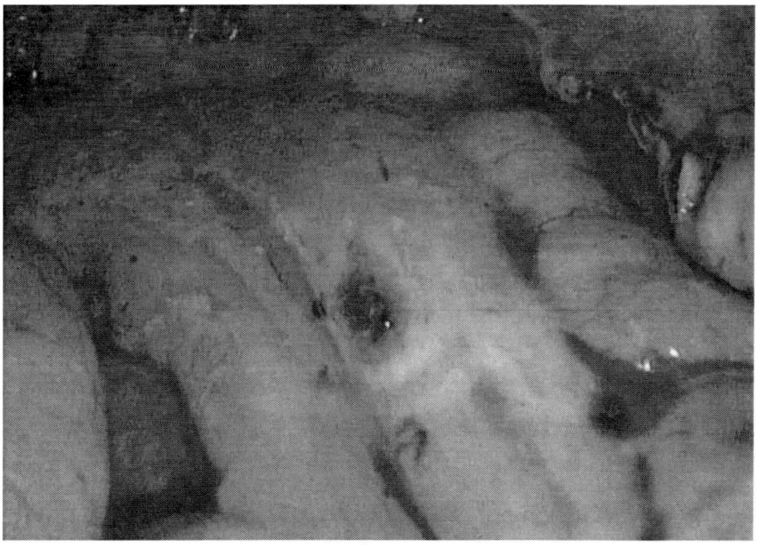

Figure 4.Thermal injury.

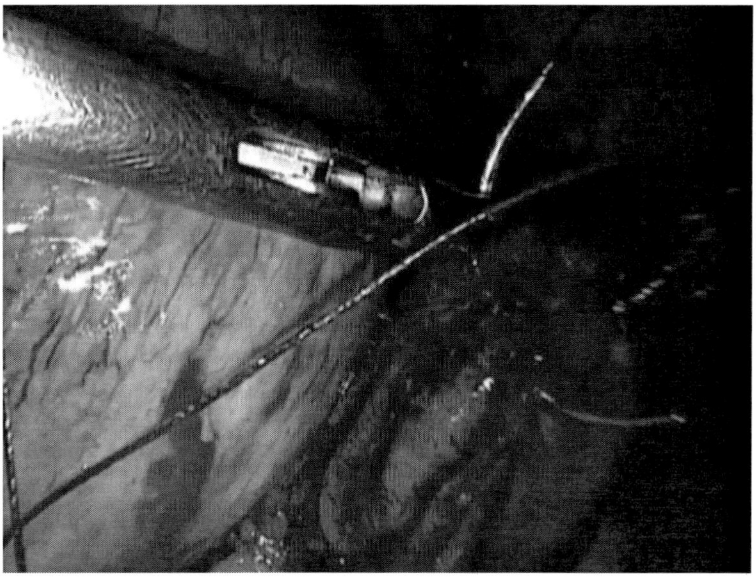

Figure 5. Suture of bowel.

If during surgery a thermal intestinal injury is detected, it ought to be repaired with an adequate technique before closure [39]. Two techniques have been described. One consists of reverting and superposing healthy intestine margins. The second one consists of resecting the damaged tissue with healthy margins of 1-2 cm, and performing a posterior anastomosis [37].

Rectovaginal Fistula

Obstetrical traumas are responsible for approximately 88% of rectovaginal fistulas, being a rare complication of laparoscopy. Their frequency rises when low intestinal resections are performed. They can also appear as a consequence of non-diagnosed or erroneously treated intestinal injuries [38]. 10% of rectovaginal fistulas are associated with low colorectal resections.

This percentage has increased in the last decade with the use of endostapleres (39). Rectovaginal fistulas have also been reported after laparoscopic sacrocolpopexy performed to repair genital prolapse, although with low frequency [40].

Its diagnosis is clinical. Patients refer output of gas or stool through the vagina. Sometimes it is not observed in the physical examination. In these cases complementary test such as a CT, magnetic resonance, endoanal ultrasound or colonoscopy are needed [41].

Rectovaginal fistulas can be treated only with surgical repair. Different surgical approaches (vagina, anus or perine) can be used depending on the location of the fistula and the ability of the surgeon. Sometimes intestinal resections with posterior anastomosis are required to treat them [42]. Surgical repair of rectovaginal fistulas achieve rates of success of about 44% to 100% [44].

Prognosis

Intestinal injuries are the third most frequent cause of death by laparoscopy, after anesthetic complications and vascular lesions [43]. Their prognosis is intimately related to the timing of diagnosis and treatment. Global mortality is estimated in 3.6% of patients with intestinal lesions.

Some studies claim that if the lesion is diagnosed and treated during the same surgical procedure, no mortality is associated [31]. Mortality increases by 20% if they are not diagnosed during surgery [20, 21]. Intestinal injuries are not detected during surgery in two-thirds of the cases [22]. Mechanical injuries are diagnosed on average 1.3 days (with a range of 0 to 4 days) after the surgical procedure, while electrosurgical injuries are diagnosed on average 10.4 days (with a range of 0 to 38 days) after the surgical procedure.

Conclusion

In the last decade there has been an increase in the number of intestinal lesions diagnosed during laparoscopy. Laparoscopic surgeons are becoming increasingly aware of this risk, reducing the morbidity and mortality of intestinal injuries [44]. It is essential to be aware of the risk of intestinal lesions in laparoscopy as well as the importance of a timely diagnosis to improve the prognosis of these lesions.

References

[1] Magrina JF. Complications of laparoscopic surgery. *Clin. Obstet Gynecol*, 2002 45, 469-80.

[2] Chandler JG, Corson SL, Way LW. Three spectra of laparoscopic entry access injuries. *J. Am. Coll Surg*, 2001 192, 478-90.

[3] Molloy D, Kaloo PD, Cooper M, Nguyen TV. Laparoscopic entry: a literature review and analysis of techniques and complications of primary port entry. *Aust N J Z Obstet Gynaecol*, 2002 42, 246-54.

[4] Bhoyrul S, Vierra MA, Nezhat CR, et al. Trocar injuries in laparoscopic surgery. *J. Am. Coll Surg,* 2001 192, 677–83.

[5] Brosens I, Gordon A. Bowel injuries during gynaecological laparoscopy: A multinational survey. *Gynaecol Endosc*, 2001 10, 141–5.

[6] Brill AI, Nezhat F, Nezhat CH, Nezhat C. The incidence of adhesion after prior laparotomy: a laparoscopic appraisal. *Obstet Gynecol*, 1995 85, 269–72.

[7] De Cherney AH, di Zerega GS. Clinical problem of intraperitoneal postsurgical adhesion formation following general surgery and the use of adhesion prevention barriers. *Surg. Clin. North Am*, 1997 77, 671–88.

[8] van der Krabben AA, Dijkstra FR, Nieuwenhuijzen M et al. Morbidity and mortality of inadvertent enterotomy during adhesiolysis. *Br. J. Surg*, 2000, 87, 467–71.

[9] Wallwiener D, Meyer A, Bastert D. Adhesion formation of the parietal and visceral peritoneum: an explanation for the controversy on the use of autologous and alloplastic barriers? *Fertil Steril*, 1998 69, 132–7.

[10] Gamal EM, Metzger P, Szabo G et al. The influence of intraoperative complications on adhesion formation during laparoscopic and conventional cholecystectomy in an animal model. *Surg Endosc* 2001 15, 873–7.

[11] Gadallah MF, Torres-Rivera C, Ramdeen G, Myrick S, Habashi S, Andrews G. Relationship between intraperitoneal bleeding, adhesions, and peritoneal dialysis catheter failure: a method of prevention. *Adv. Perit Dial*, 2001 17, 127–9.

[12] Szabo G, Miko I, Peto K, Brath E, Nagy P, Gamal EM. Laparoscopic versus open cholecystectomy: reaction in the liverbed. *Magy Seb*, 2005 58, 106–10.

[13] Al-Took S, Platt R, Tulandi T. Adhesion-related small-bowel obstruction after gynecologic operations. *Am. J .Obstet Gynecol*, 1999 180, 313-5.

[14] Ahmad G, O´Flynn H, Duffy JM, et al. Laparoscopic entry techniques. Cochrane *Database Syst Rev* 2012; 2:CD006583.

[15] Fuller J, Ashar BS,Carey-Conrado J. Trocar-asociated injuries and fatalities: an analysis of 1399 reports to the FDA. *J. Minim Invasive Gynecol*, 2005 12, 302-7.

[16] Azebedo JL, Azebedo OC, Miyahira SA, et al. Injuries caused by Veress needle insertion for creation of pneumoperitoneum: a systematic literature review. *Surg Endosc,* 2009 23, 1428-32.

[17] Palmer R. Safety in laparoscopy. *J. Reprod Med,* 1974 13, 1-5.

[18] Härkki-Sirén P, Kurki T. A nationwide analysis of laparoscopic complications. *Obstet Gynecol,* 1997 89, 108-12.

[19] Härkki-Siren P, Sjöberg J, Kurki T. Major complications of laparoscopy: a follow-up Finnish study. *Obstet Gynecol*, 1999 94, 94-8.

[20] Jansen FW, Kapiteyn K, Trimbos-Kemper T, Hermans J, Trimbos JB. Complications of laparoscopy: a prospective multicentre observational study. *Br. J. Obstet Gynaecol*, 1997 104, 595-600.

[21] Brosens I, Gordon A, Campo R, Gordt S. Bowel injury in gynecologic laparoscopy. *J. Am. Assoc Gynecol Laparosc,* 2003 10, 9-13.

[22] Chapron C, Pierre F, Harchaoui Y, Lacroix S, Béguin S, Querleu D, Lansac J, Dubuisson JB. Gastrointestinal injuries during gynaecological laparoscopy. *Hum. Reprod,* 1999 14, 333-7.

[23] Sigman HH, Fried GM, Garzon J, Hinchey EJ, Wexler MJ, Meakins JL, Barkun JS. Risks of blind versus open approach to celiotomy for laparoscopic surgery. *Surg. Laparosc Endosc.* 1993 3, 296-9.

[24] Philosophe R. Avoiding complications of laparoscopic surgery. *Fertil Steril*, 2003 4, 30-9.

[25] Chapron C, Querleu D, Bruhat MA, et al. Surgical complications of diagnostic and operative gynaecological laparoscopy: A prospective multicenter observational study. *Br. J. Obst Gynaecol*, 1997 89, 108-112.

[26] Loffer FD, Pent D. Indications, contraindications and complications of laparoscopy. *Obstet Gynecol Surg*, 1975 30, 407-27.

[27] Golan A, Sagiv R, Debby A, Glezerman M. The minilaparoscope as a tool for localization and preparation for cannula insertion in patients with multiple previous abdominal incisions or umbilical hernia. *J. Am. Assoc Gynecol Laparosc*, 2003 10, 14-6.

[28] Oshinsky GS, Smith AD. Laparoscopic needles and trocars: an overview of designs and complications. *J. Lapaoendosc Surg*, 1992 2, 117-25.

[29] Leibi BJ, Kraft K, Schmedt CG, Bittner R. Access techniques for endoscopic surgery types f trocars, ports and cannulae an overview. *Minim Invasive Ther Allied Technol*, 2001 10,5-10.

[30] Vilos GA, Rajakumar C. Electrosurgical generators and monopolar and bipolar electrosurgery. *J. Minim Invasive Gynecol*, 2013 20, 279-87.

[31] Binenbaum SJ, Goldfarb MA. Inadvertent enterotomy in minimally invasive abdominal surgery. *JSLS*, 2006 10, 336-40.

[32] Bishoff JT, Allaf ME, Kirkels W, Moore RG, Kavoussi LR, Schroder F. Laparoscopic bowel injury: incidence and clinical presentation. *J. Urol,* 1999 161, 887-90.

[33] Farooqui MO, Bazzoli JM. Significance of radiologic evidence of free air fllowing laparoscopy. *J. Reprod Med.* 1976;16:119.

[34] Chichom Mefire A, Weledji PE, Verla VS, Lidwine NM. Diagnostic and therapeutic challenges of isolated small bowel perforations after blunt abdominal injury in low income settings: analysis of twenty three new cases. *Injury.* 2014 45, 141-5.

[35] Bratzler DW, et al. Clinical practice guidelines for antimicrobial prophylaxis in surgery. *Surg. Infect.* 2013 14, 73-156.

[36] Jo EJ, Lee YY, Kim TJ, Choi CH, Lee JW, Bae DS, Kim BG. Management and outcome of rectal injury during gynecologic laparoscopic surgery. *J. Minim Invasive Gynecol,* 2013 20, 166-71.

[37] Thompson BH, Wheeless CR Jr. Gastrointestinal complications of laparoscopy sterilization. *Obstet Gynecol*, 1973 41, 669-76.

[38] Senatore PJ., Jr Anovaginal fistulae. *Surg. Clin. North Am.* 1994 74, 1361–1375.

[39] Kosugi C, Saito N, Kimata Y, Ono M, Sugito M, Ito M, et al. Rectovaginal fistulas after rectal cancer surgery: Incidence and operative repair by gluteal-fold flap repair. *Surgery,* 2005 137, 329–336.

[40] Chan CM, Liang HH, Go WW, To WW, Mok KM. Laparoscopic sacrocolpopexy for uterine and post-hysterectomy prolapse: anatomical and functional outcomes. *Hong Kong Med. J,* 2011 17, 301-5.

[41] Champagne BJ, McGee MF. Rectovaginal fistula. *Surg. Clin. North Am.*, 2010 90, 69-82.

[42] van der Hagen SJ, Soeters PB, Baeten CG, van Gemert WG. Laparoscopic fistula excision and omentoplasty for high rectovaginal fistulas: a prospective study of 40 patients. *Int. J. Colorectal Dis,* 2011 26, 1463–1467.

[43] Nordestgaard AG, Bodily KC, Osborne RW Jr, Buttorff JD. Major vascular injuries during laparoscopic procedures. *Am. J. Surg*, 1995 169, 543-5.

[44] Swartz MJ, Faiena I, Cinman N, et al. Laparoscopic bowel injury in retroperitoneal surgery: current incidence and outcomes. *J. Urol,* 2010 184, 589-594.

Index

#

A

B

C

D

E

F

I

N

O

P

Q

R

S

T

U